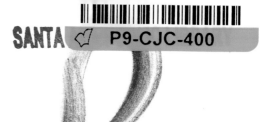

1001
NATURAL
REMEDIES

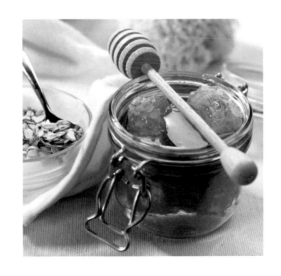

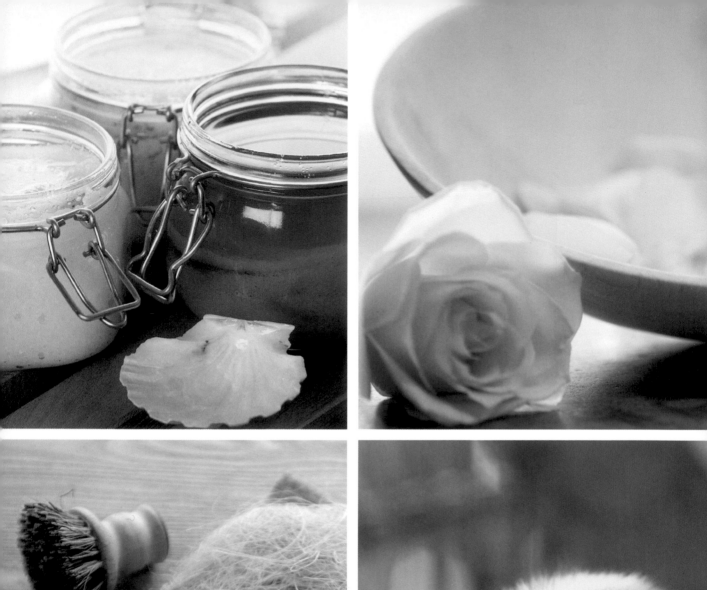
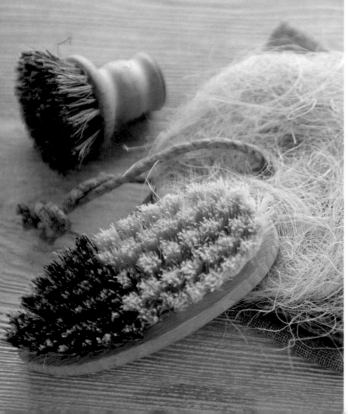
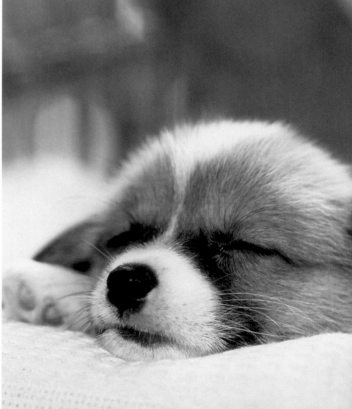

1001
NATURAL
REMEDIES

Produced by

The Philip Lief Group, Inc.

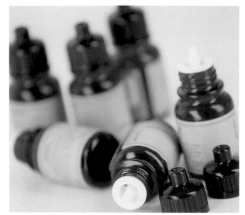
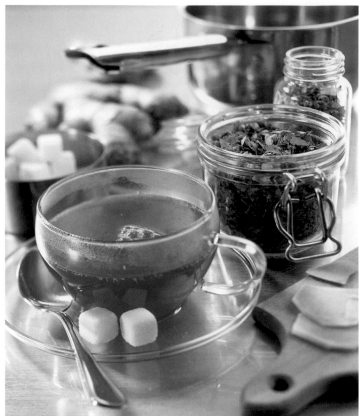
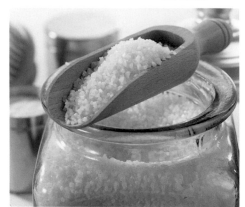
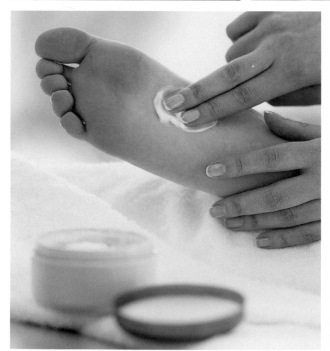
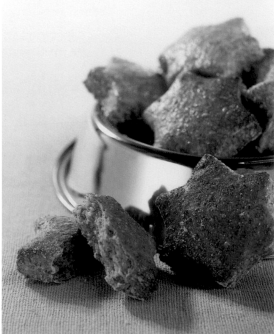

Contents

NATURAL HEALTH REMEDIES 6

How to make and use herbal teas, creams, compresses, and other treatments for a wide range of ailments, including headaches, indigestion, backache, diaper rash, and nausea. Also featured throughout are quick tips on staying healthy and improving well-being.

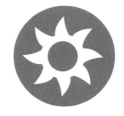

NATURAL BEAUTY 60

Discover how to make luxurious creams, masks, shampoos, massage oils, cleansers, exfoliants, bath salts, aftershaves, lip balms, and many other beautifying potions based on essential oils, witch hazel, rose petals, lemon juice, and other natural products.

NATURAL HOUSE & GARDEN 118

A collection of sweet-smelling air fresheners, furniture polishes, kitchen and bathroom cleaners, stain removers, garden sprays, and more, all made with gentle, environmentally friendly products such as essential oils, baking soda, vinegar, and herbs.

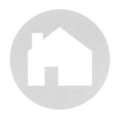

NATURAL PET CARE 160

Tips, hints, and remedies involving safe, natural ingredients such as herbs, garlic, and natural supplements to keep your cat and dog healthy and happy and to treat common ailments such as parasites, muscle strains and sprains, and digestive upsets.

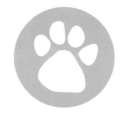

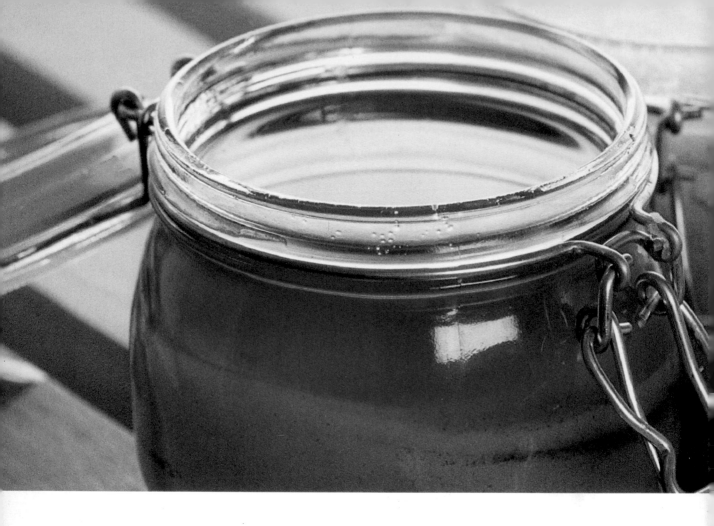

NATURAL
HEALTH
REMEDIES

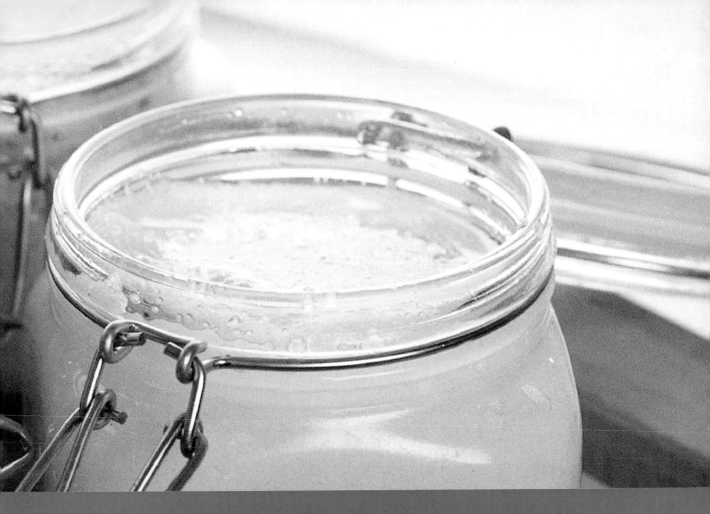

"Our bodies know how to heal themselves," my father was fond of saying as I was growing up. This idea fascinated me and started me on a lifelong journey of learning how to use nature's medicines. For the past 25 years, I have relied solely on natural remedies for treating all kinds of illnesses, from simple colds and stomach upsets to cystitis and bronchial infections.

I recently spent three days caring for a close friend who had come down with a bad case of the flu. He was achy, feverish, and miserable, so I did all the things my mother used to do for me when I was sick—plus a few extras that I have learned along the way. On the morning of the fourth day, he was in tip-top shape, ready to return to his normal life.

Considering how sick he had been, I was surprised at how quickly he recovered. He told me it was because he had been given such wonderful care, and I realized once again how important love is to healing. Home remedies give us the opportunity to nurture, and to bring the intangible yet essential ingredient of love into healing.

In this chapter on natural health remedies you will find all kinds of suggestions for treating the most common health problems that you are likely to encounter, from headaches and diarrhea to coughs and varicose veins. You will also find various recommendations for buying, storing, and preparing natural remedies.

Natural Medicines

Natural medicines include herbs, essential oils, homeopathic remedies, nutritional supplements, and common items such as ice, sea salt, and garlic. All of the ingredients for the remedies in this chapter can be found at natural food stores. With the increasing popularity of natural medicines, you can probably find most of them at many pharmacies and large supermarkets as well. Although medicine cabinets are generally located in the bathroom, heat and humidity are damaging to herbs, essential oils, and supplements. Find a cool, dark, dry cabinet or closet in which to store your natural medicines.

Essential oils

When you are buying essential oils, always look for the best quality. The oils are distilled from particular plants and are at their most potent when pure, undiluted, and unadulterated. They evaporate easily, so store them in tightly capped, dark glass bottles, and they will retain their potency for about three years. **Caution:** Unless indicated, do not apply essential oils directly to the skin (some oils can burn). Never take an essential oil internally unless a trained professional directs you to do so.

Dried herbs

Many of the recipes in this chapter require you to make your own herbal remedies, so always select the finest quality herbs. Your herbal medicines will only be as potent as the herbs you make them with. Look for herbs that are brightly colored and fragrant. Store each herb individually in its own tightly lidded glass container. Properly stored, herbs will retain their medicinal properties for one year. Herbal salves and oils will stay fresh for approximately six months if stored in the refrigerator.

Taking herbal remedies

Herbal medicines come in three forms: teas (infusions), capsules, and extracts (tinctures). You will gain the most benefit from herbal remedies if you know the best ways of preparing and taking them. **Caution:** Pregnant women, nursing mothers, and women trying to conceive should consult a healthcare practitioner before taking any herbal medicine.

Herbal teas

Herbal teas are the traditional and time-proven way to use herbs and are inexpensive. Teas are excellent for treating digestive upsets because the herbs quickly come into contact with the gastrointestinal tract. They are also useful for treating urinary tract infections because the fluids help flush the bladder. On the other hand, making a herbal tea is more time-consuming than taking a capsule or extract. Teas do not extract all of the medicinal properties of certain herbs, such as goldenseal and kava, and some herbs taste unpleasant.

WHEN YOU SHOULD SEE YOUR DOCTOR

Natural remedies are effective for most of the common conditions that you would ordinarily self-treat. The following health problems and injuries require immediate medical attention:

- bones that are fractured, broken, or dislocated
- bites from animals or humans

- a high fever (equivalent to 105°F (40.5°C) in adults; 103°F (39.4°C) in children; 100°F (37.7°C) in infants under six months old), or any fever that persists for more than three days
- injury to the head, neck, or spinal cord
- unexplained lumps

- puncture wounds and other severe wounds
- third-degree burns or extensive second-degree burns
- unconsciousness or recurrent dizziness
- vomiting blood, vomiting that persists for more than two days, or vomiting and diarrhea in infants

Capsules

Capsules are convenient and familiar. They provide exact doses and are an easy way to take herbs with less-than-pleasant tastes. On the other hand, capsules contain dried herbs which are finely ground—a process that exposes more of the surface area of the herb to damage from heat, light, and oxygen, and speeds up loss of potency. Always buy capsules from a reputable manufacturer and use them within three months.

Liquid extracts

Liquid herbal extracts, also known as tinctures, contain a broader spectrum of the healing properties of a plant than teas. This is because certain compounds will dissolve in alcohol but not in water. Liquid extracts have a shelf life of between three and five years. Convenient to take, they are highly concentrated—a quarter to half a teaspoon of extract is roughly equivalent to a cup (250ml) of herbal tea—and are absorbed quickly by the blood. On the other hand, extracts contain alcohol, which you may wish to avoid. Alcohol-free extracts are made with vegetable glycerin, which is less effective at dissolving some compounds. Most of the alcohol in an extract will evaporate if you measure the dosage into a cup and add a quarter of a cup (60ml) of boiling water. Allow to cool before drinking.

Standardized extracts

Standardized extracts are capsules or liquid extracts that are processed to contain a specific amount of what experts believe is the herb's primary

---

YOUR NATURAL MEDICINE CHEST

The following herbs, essential oils, and other items are those that I consider indispensable for a basic natural medicine chest for the home:

- Arnica—as a gel or cream for muscle strains and bruises
- Calendula—as a gel, cream, or salve for burns, cuts, scrapes, and insect bites
- Chamomile—as dried flowers for stress and stomach upsets
- Echinacea—as an extract or capsules for colds, flu, cuts, infections, and scrapes
- Elderberry—as an extract for colds and flu
- Epsom salts—for muscle soreness, relaxing, and relieving tension
- Eucalyptus—as an essential oil for respiratory congestion and muscle soreness
- Ginger—as fresh root for colds, respiratory congestion, nausea, and stomach upsets
- Lavender—as an essential oil for stress, insomnia, and headaches
- Sea salt—for sore throat gargles and for bath salts
- Tea tree—as an essential oil for skin infections and insect bites
- Valerian—as an extract for mild pain relief and insomnia

---

active ingredient. But there may be other ingredients in the herb that are just as important. If you're treating a serious condition, such as high blood pressure (hypertension), it's a good idea to use a standardized extract. For general use, try a whole-herb extract first. If you don't get the results you want after a month, switch to a standardized extract and see if there is a noticeable difference. When in doubt, always consult a medical herbalist for guidance.

When to take herbs

Take liquid extracts in a small amount of warm water about 15 minutes before meals—the herbs are quickly absorbed into the bloodstream on an empty stomach. Capsules are best taken after meals to reduce the possibility of stomach upset. Herbal teas can be taken either before or after meals.

Determining dosages for children

To tailor a dose of a natural medicine to a child, follow this guideline: all the adult doses recommended in this chapter are for a 150lb (68kg) person; a child's dose should be adjusted in proportion to the child's weight. For example, if the adult dose of a remedy is one teaspoon, the dose for a 50lb (23kg) child would be one-third of a teaspoon. In general, teenagers can take adult doses. But always adjust the doses of medicines for children under 12 years of age. When in doubt, check with a qualified medical herbalist.

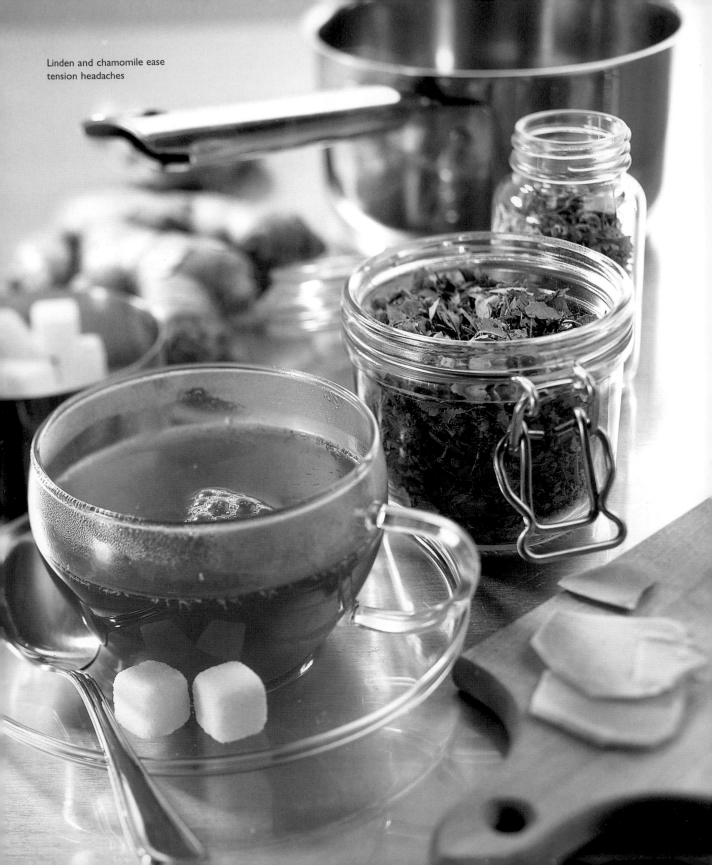

Linden and chamomile ease
tension headaches

Headaches

Tension headaches are caused by anxiety, nervous tension, eyestrain, poor posture, or tight muscles in the shoulders or neck. Migraine headaches are caused by an expansion of blood vessels in the head. Headaches can also be caused by colds and the flu, allergies, PMS, and digestive problems.

1 Herbal tea for tension headaches

Ginger decreases the production of pain-causing chemicals in the body. Chamomile and linden are mild relaxants that help ease emotional and physical tension.

1 teaspoon fresh chopped ginger root
1 cup (250ml) water
1 teaspoon dried chamomile
1 teaspoon dried linden

Simmer the ginger in the water in a covered pot for five minutes. Remove from the heat. Add the chamomile and linden and steep for 10 minutes. Strain, sweeten the tea if desired, and drink it hot.

2 Ease headaches with an aromatherapy compress

Lavender eases physical and mental stress and marjoram has deeply relaxing properties. Add five drops each of lavender and marjoram essential oils to a basin of cool water. Soak two washcloths in the water and lightly wring out. Lie down and apply one cloth to your forehead and one to the back of your neck. Rest for 30 minutes.

3 Lavender massage

To ease a tension headache, massage your temples with a couple of drops of lavender essential oil.

4 Take valerian for pain

Valerian helps relieve the pain of tension or migraine headaches. Take half a teaspoon of valerian extract diluted in warm water every 30 minutes until the pain has abated (up to three teaspoons a day).

5 Footbath for headache relief

To help relieve a headache, try immersing your feet in a bucket of water—as hot as you can stand it—for 15 minutes. At the same time, wring out a cloth in ice water and place the cold compress on your forehead, temples, back of the neck, or wherever the pain is concentrated. Hot water dilates blood vessels and increases blood flow to the feet, while the cold compress constricts blood vessels in the head, reducing the volume of blood flow and thereby reducing pain.

6 Loosen mucus

Spicy foods, such as horseradish and hot peppers, increase the flow of blood and loosen the secretions of mucus in the sinuses. This has the effect of relieving the congestion that causes sinus headaches.

7 Massage away tension headaches

A simple acupressure massage can help relieve a tension headache. Place your fingers at the top of your spinal column, where your neck meets your skull. Move your fingers out 1–2in (5cm) along the base of your skull until you find a small indentation on either side. These points will feel slightly tender as you apply pressure. Apply firm pressure with the pads of your fingers, making a small rotating motion with your fingers. The more deeply you massage the points, the better. Breathe deeply, and imagine that you are releasing tension with each exhalation. Continue for one to three minutes, and repeat as often as you desire.

8 Ginger for migraines

At the first sign of a migraine headache, mix a heaping one-fourth of a teaspoon of powdered ginger into a glass of water and drink it. Ginger contains anti-inflammatory and pain-relieving compounds that may be able to halt a migraine attack.

Anxiety & Stress

Chronic stress impairs adrenal gland function, which can lead to a weakened immune system and degenerative diseases. Although herbs are wonderful allies during times of stress, it is important to identify the underlying cause of anxiety rather than rely on the power of sedative herbs.

9
Chamomile and catnip herbal tea

Herbs are wonderful allies during times of stress. Chamomile and catnip are relaxing and mildly sedative.

1 cup (250ml) boiling water
1 teaspoon dried chamomile
1 teaspoon dried catnip

Pour the boiling water over the herbs. Cover, steep for 10 minutes, and strain. Sweeten with honey if you desire. Drink three cups daily.

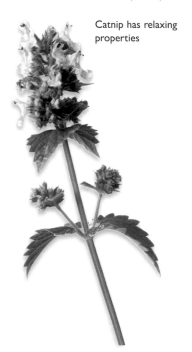

Catnip has relaxing properties

10
Eat well for stress protection

The adrenal glands are an integral part of the endocrine system of hormones. They play a key role in regulating the body's response to stress. Avoid foods that tax your adrenal glands, particularly caffeine, sugar, and alcohol. Nutrients that are important for supporting adrenal health are vitamin C, pantothenic acid (vitamin B5), vitamin B6, magnesium, and zinc. Vitamin C is found in many fruits and vegetables, including cantaloupe, broccoli, red peppers, oranges, and strawberries. Rich sources of pantothenic acid include avocados, eggs, chicken, mushrooms, salmon, and yogurt. Lentils, tempeh, trout, tuna, and bananas are good sources of vitamin B6. Zinc is found in pumpkin and sesame seeds, black beans, oysters, and mussels. Foods rich in magnesium include almonds, corn, halibut, tofu, and peas.

11
Supplements for combating stress

Various supplements will fortify the body against emotional stress. These include vitamin B complex (take 50mg twice a day), which supports the adrenal glands; and magnesium (take 500mg once a day) and calcium (take 1,000mg once a day), which both have natural tranquilizing effects.

12
Take time out for yourself

Think you cannot possibly take time to relax? That's a clear signal that you really need to. Schedule a minimum of two 15-minute breaks every day to calm and center yourself. Meditate, soak in an aromatherapy bath, listen to calming music, or just do nothing. In addition, schedule an appointment with yourself once a week for tea, a massage, a walk with a friend, or something else that makes you feel good. Record these times on your calendar just as you would any other important appointment.

13
Lavender inhaler

To relieve stress and anxiety, place a drop of lavender essential oil onto a handkerchief or tissue, and inhale as often as desired.

14
Improve stress resistance with ginseng

Siberian ginseng is excellent for strengthening the adrenal glands and helping the body adapt more easily to physical and emotional stress. Buy an extract that has been standardized for eleutheroside (regarded as the primary active compound in ginseng),

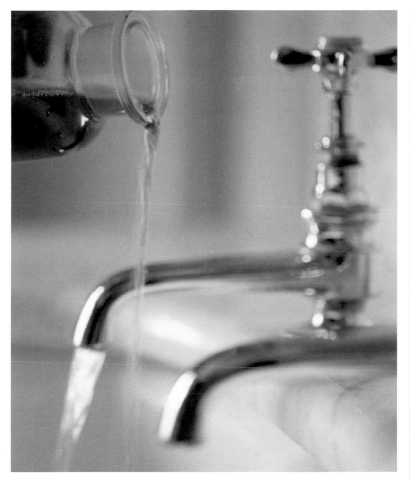

Take time out for yourself and relax in an aromatherapy bath

16
Stress-relieving bath

Lavender, sandalwood, and ylang ylang essential oils make a soothing bath. Epsom salts are rich in magnesium, which helps ease physical and emotional tension.

2 cups (250g) Epsom salts
5 drops lavender essential oil
5 drops sandalwood essential oil
2 drops ylang ylang essential oil

Add the Epsom salts as you fill the bathtub with warm water. Add the essential oils to the bath, stirring the oils into the water just before you enter the tub. Relax deeply in the bath for at least 20 minutes and make the experience more luxurious with candlelight, a bath pillow, and a thick robe to wrap up in afterward.

17
Breathe to relax

Consciously slowing down your breathing into a rhythmic pattern gives your body and mind the message to relax. Sit or lie in a comfortable position. Take a deep breath. Exhale completely through your slightly open mouth. Close your mouth and inhale slowly through your nose to a mental count of five. Hold your breath for a count of five. Then exhale completely through your mouth to a count of 10. Take your time but make your exhalation take twice as long as your inhalation. Inhale again and repeat the cycle for a total of five breaths. Practice this at least twice daily, and whenever you feel tense or anxious.

and take approximately 250mg twice a day. It is safe to take for up to six weeks. **Caution:** If you have high blood pressure, consult your doctor before taking any type of ginseng.

15
Valerian sedative tea

Valerian is a powerful but safe herbal sedative and is helpful in cases of extreme stress and anxiety.

I cup (250ml) boiling water
I teaspoon dried valerian root

To prepare valerian tea, pour the boiling water over the dried root and cover to prevent the evaporation of the herb's therapeutic essential oils. Steep for 10 minutes, and strain. Try to drink up to three cups a day. Because valerian has a very strong flavor, you may prefer taking the herb in a capsule or as an extract. Take one or two 300–500mg capsules, or a half to one teaspoon of extract, up to three times a day. **Caution:** Valerian may cause headaches and muscle spasms. Do not exceed the quantities or take it for long periods.

Depression

Many people turn to herbal or prescription antidepressants at the first sign of feeling low. But feelings are important messages from your body and mind. It is far better to pay heed to the message and to take appropriate steps to restore balance to your life before resorting to drugs, herbal or otherwise.

18
Herbal help for depression

If your depression is not transitory, St. John's wort may help. The capsule form is widely available. Take 300mg, three times daily, of a standardized extract that contains 0.3 percent hypericin and 5 percent hyperforin—the primary active compounds. Allow six weeks for the herb to begin working. **Caution:** Do not take St. John's wort during pregnancy or with other medicines without first consulting your doctor.

19
Nurture yourself with aromatherapy

Self-nurturing is always called for when you're feeling low and in need of a lift. An aromatherapy bath with lavender and bergamot relaxes your body and mind and has mood-elevating properties. Run yourself a warm bath, and add 10 drops of lavender essential oil and five drops of bergamot essential oil. Soak for a good 20 minutes.

20
Walk to lift depression

A brisk 45-minute walk stimulates your body to produce endorphins, natural mood-elevating chemicals. Try it the next time you feel down, and practice preventive mental healthcare by taking a walk every day.

21
Keep a journal

Keeping a journal can help you gain an insight into your emotions. Sit down and write for 20 minutes each day; don't think about the grammar, punctuation, or whether what you are saying is interesting. Just write whatever comes to mind and don't censor yourself. You'll find that putting your thoughts on paper will help you sort through painful emotions, clarify decisions, and keep your life on track.

Dried lavender is soothing and relaxing

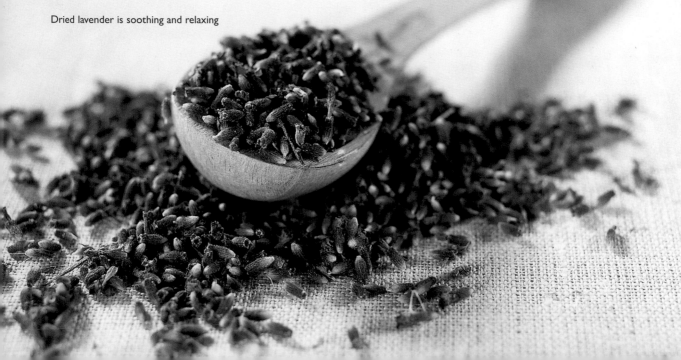

Insomnia

Many cases of insomnia are caused by tension, anxiety, or stimulants such as caffeine. Eliminate all stimulants from your diet and try these natural sleep inducers.

22
Tips for restful sleep

In the couple of hours before bed, read a relaxing book, take a warm bath, or listen to soothing music. Go to bed at a regular time, and try to stick to it—even on weekends—to accustom your body to sleeping at a specific time. Ensure your bedroom is as quiet as possible and completely dark. Invest in room-darkening blinds, curtains, or drapes.

23
Fresh air

You'll sleep more restfully with plenty of fresh air, so keep your windows open a little, even in winter.

24
Relax in an Epsom salts bath

If you're having trouble sleeping, try soaking in an Epsom salts bath just before bed. Epsom salts are rich in magnesium, which is an excellent muscle relaxant and sedative for the nervous system. Add two cups (250g) of Epsom salts to a bathtub and fill the tub with water that is as close as possible to body temperature. To enhance the relaxing effects, add 10 drops of lavender essential oil. Soak in the bath for 20 minutes, and go to bed immediately after toweling dry to avoid stimulating your body and mind.

25
Herbal sedative

Valerian and hops calm the nervous system and relieve insomnia. Mix 1fl oz (30ml) of valerian extract and half a fluid ounce (15ml) of hops extract in a dark glass bottle. Take a teaspoon of the mixture in a small amount of warm water 30 minutes before bed. Repeat the dose if necessary. **Caution:** Valerian may cause headaches and muscle spasms. Do not exceed the quantities or take valerian for long periods. Do not use hops if you have depression.

26
Sip passionflower tea

Passionflower and chamomile make a gentle tea for restful sleep.

1 cup (250ml) boiling water
1 teaspoon dried passionflower
1 teaspoon dried chamomile

Pour the water over the herbs, cover, and steep for 10 minutes. Strain and drink 30 minutes before bed.

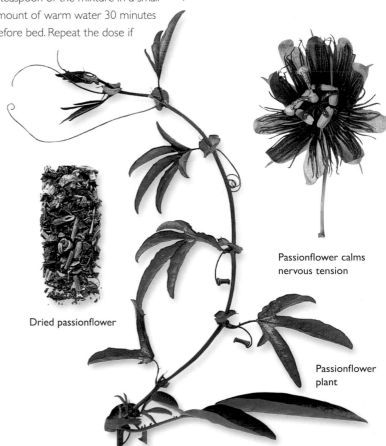

Dried passionflower

Passionflower calms nervous tension

Passionflower plant

Jet Lag

Disorientation, irritability, and sleep disturbances are symptoms of jet lag and are caused by the body trying to reset its internal biological clock to a different time schedule. Flying across time zones requires adjustments in the regulation of heart rate, body temperature, hormone levels, and sleep patterns.

27
Reset your inner clock

To overcome jet lag, get out into the sun as early in the day as possible when traveling. Sunlight helps reset your biological clock.

28
Minimize jet lag

To minimize jet lag, fly during the day if possible. This enables you to arrive at your destination, take a walk, have dinner and go to bed on the local schedule, all of which will help you adjust more quickly. Avoid the impulse to nap as soon as you arrive—it will only make it more difficult for you to get accustomed to the local time.

29
Exercise to overcome jet lag

Exercise as soon as possible after you arrive at your destination. A brisk 30-minute walk aids relaxation and sleep. Try to continue exercising every day when you travel. Regular exercise makes your body more resilient and helps you adapt to stressors (such as flying) more quickly.

30
Get help with melatonin

Melatonin, a hormone produced by your body that sends the signal that it's time to sleep, can be extremely effective in combating jet lag. Take a 1mg tablet of melatonin one hour before you want to go to sleep. Try taking it for several days, until you feel acclimated to the local time.

31
Ease travel stress with essential oils

Essential oils can ease the emotional stress of traveling and help your body come into balance more quickly. To help you relax your body and mind before going to bed, soak in a warm bath with six drops each of lavender and sandalwood essential oils.

Fatigue

Many factors can contribute to fatigue, including mental and physical tension, a nutrient-poor diet, lack of sleep or exercise, and improper breathing habits. Fatigue can also be a symptom of blood-sugar disturbances, low thyroid function, or a chronic illness, so consult your doctor if it persists.

32
Get enough sleep

How much sleep you need depends on many things, including your age and levels of stress and activity. As a general rule, most people need about eight hours a night. If you need an alarm clock to wake up, you probably aren't getting enough sleep.

33
Clean up your diet

Eliminate caffeine, alcohol, and all concentrated sugars from your diet as they stress your adrenal glands and drain your vitality. To rebuild adrenal health and energy, eat a balanced whole-food diet that includes two to three servings daily of lean protein foods (chicken, fish, eggs, or legumes) and a high-potency multivitamin and mineral supplement.

34
Exercise daily

Even if you feel tired, walking will relieve tension, oxygenate your cells, and build endurance. Try to get at least 30 minutes of moderate aerobic exercise every day. Meditative, flowing types of exercise, such as yoga and tai chi, enhance organ and gland function as well as build energy.

Eye Conditions

Common eye conditions include black eyes, conjunctivitis, and eye strain. In a black eye, tiny capillaries close to the surface of the skin around the eye leak blood into the surrounding tissue. Symptoms of conjunctivitis, or pinkeye, include redness of the eye and sensitivity to light, a "gritty" feeling when blinking, and a watery discharge from the eye. Symptoms of eyestrain include fatigue, headache, and eye soreness.

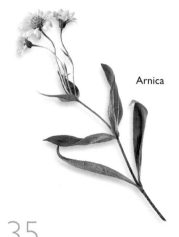

Arnica

35
Heal a black eye with arnica

Arnica fosters the healing process by stimulating the circulation, relieving pain, and easing swelling. Apply arnica gel to the injured area twice a day until the skin has returned to normal. **Caution:** Keep arnica out of the eyes. Do not apply arnica to cut or broken skin.

36
Apply ice to ease the pain of a black eye

As soon as possible, apply an ice pack to the injury. Ice provides immediate pain relief, reduces swelling, and arrests bleeding by constricting the damaged blood vessels. Use a cold gel pack or an ice pack wrapped in a thin cotton towel to prevent burning the skin. Apply the cold pack to the eye for 10 minutes, take a five-minute break, and reapply for 10 minutes. Repeat the cycle until the swelling and pain are relieved.

37
Apply compresses to a black eye

After the first day or two, when the swelling begins to go down, apply alternating hot and cold compresses to the affected area to increase circulation and speed healing. Apply a very warm washcloth for five minutes, followed by an ice-cold washcloth for one minute. Repeat the cycle three times, twice a day.

38
Soothe conjunctivitis with goldenseal

A lukewarm eyewash prepared from goldenseal can soothe irritation and fight infection.

1 cup (250ml) boiling water
1 teaspoon powdered goldenseal root

Pour the boiling water over the goldenseal root. Cover, and steep for 15 minutes. Strain the liquid through a paper coffee filter to remove all the herb particles. Rinse the affected eye with approximately a third of a cup (80ml) of the lukewarm solution three times a day. Note that goldenseal may stain clothing and towels, so try not to splash yourself.

39
Calendula compress for conjunctivitis

A warm compress made with calendula tea can relieve the itching and discomfort of conjunctivitis. Calendula has antiviral and antibacterial properties and encourages healing.

1 cup (250ml) boiling water
2 tablespoons dried calendula

To prepare the tea, pour the boiling water over the calendula. Steep in a covered container for 15 minutes and strain. Dip a clean, thin cotton washcloth into the liquid and wring it out slightly. Apply the warm calendula compress to the affected eye. Continue to reapply a compress every few minutes for 15 minutes or more at a time (reheating the tea if necessary). Repeat this several times each day.

40
Preventing eyestrain

Many people spend a great deal of time engaged in focusing on close-up activities, such as reading, computer work, or watching television. But to maintain healthy and relaxed vision, your eyes need the practice of focusing on distant objects. If you work on a close-up activity, prevent yourself from developing eyestrain by trying something as simple as looking out of the window for a few minutes every half hour.

41
Eye exercises for eyestrain

Several exercises will help you to relieve your eyestrain. Focus on the tip of your nose, and then shift your focus to an object across the room. Repeat this several times. Now slowly roll your eyes in a circle, looking upward as far as you can, to the left, down, and to the right. Repeat in the opposite direction. Close your eyes, gently cup your hands over your eyes to create complete darkness, and relax for a minute. Remember to breathe and relax (see No. 17) while you are doing these exercises.

42
Compresses for eyestrain

Applying hot then cold compresses to your strained eyes will increase the circulation of blood and promote relaxation. Prepare two bowls of water—one comfortably hot and the other ice cold. Dip a washcloth into the bowl of hot water, wring it out, and apply it to your closed eyes after a minute, replace the hot cloth with a cold cloth. Repeat several times, ending with a cold compress.

Ear Infections

Middle ear infections are most common in childhood. They often follow a cold, when congestion prevents the middle ear from draining normally and causes fluids to stagnate, creating a breeding ground for bacteria and viruses. The resultant swelling exerts pressure on sensitive nerve endings, causing excruciating pain. If the infection does not begin to subside with home treatment within 24 hours, consult your doctor.

43
Prevent ear infections

Allergies, especially food allergies, are often a factor in chronic middle-ear infections. Avoid common food allergens such as dairy products, wheat, corn, oranges, eggs, and peanut butter. **Caution:** Consult a dietitian before restricting a child's diet.

44
Boost immunity with echinacea

Give echinacea extract to boost immune function. Children over six can be given half a teaspoon three times a day, while children under six should be given a quarter of a teaspoon three times a day.

45
Use garlic oil to fight infection

Garlic oil ear drops are excellent for fighting ear infections. Mince one large bulb of fresh garlic and place it in a heavy pot with enough olive oil to cover it by one inch (25mm). Cover the pot, and warm gently over low heat for one hour. Cool, strain the oil

through several layers of cheesecloth, and refrigerate in a covered glass jar. To use the oil, warm a small amount in a metal spoon over a candle flame to a comfortable temperature (test the warmth of the oil on the back of your hand.) Suction the oil in an ear dropper, place two drops into the ear canal, and plug with a cotton ball. Repeat the treatment every hour as needed, until symptoms subside. **Caution:** Do not use garlic oil to treat swimmer's ear (an inflammation of the external ear canal), or if you suspect a punctured eardrum.

46
Avoid pollutants

Airborne pollutants from cigarette smoke and wood-burning stoves are associated with a higher incidence of middle-ear infections. Avoid these irritants when possible.

47
Ease the earache

Wrap a warm hot-water bottle in a soft cloth and place it over the ear to help ease the pain of an earache. Make sure the water in the bottle is not too hot.

Mouth & Gum Disorders

Canker sores on the tongue, insides of the cheeks, or gums last from one to two weeks. Red, soft, and bleeding gums are a sign of gingivitis, caused by bacteria that feed on plaque. Bad breath is generally caused by poor dental hygiene or by gastrointestinal disorders. If it persists, consult your doctor.

48
Sea salt rinse for canker sores

To help heal canker sores, rinse your mouth several times a day with a mixture of half a teaspoon of sea salt dissolved in half a cup (125ml) of warm water.

49
Dab on myrrh for healing sores

The resin from the myrrh tree has been used for centuries in Ayurvedic medicine for healing mouth ulcers. It has antiseptic and antimicrobial properties and is also rich in tannins, which help heal irritated mucous membranes. Open a capsule of powdered myrrh and apply it directly to the sores several times a day.

50
Licorice for long-term relief from sores

Deglycyrrhizinated licorice (DGL) stimulates your body to produce protective mucus, encourages healing of the mucous membranes, and fights the microorganisms that may cause canker sores. Buy chewable DGL tablets that have had the compound glycyrrhizic acid removed (as this acid can cause water retention and high blood pressure). Take one or two 380mg tablets (letting them dissolve completely in your mouth) three times a day. You can use this remedy as often as necessary and may want to consider taking DGL long-term (for at least three months) if you suffer from chronic canker sores.

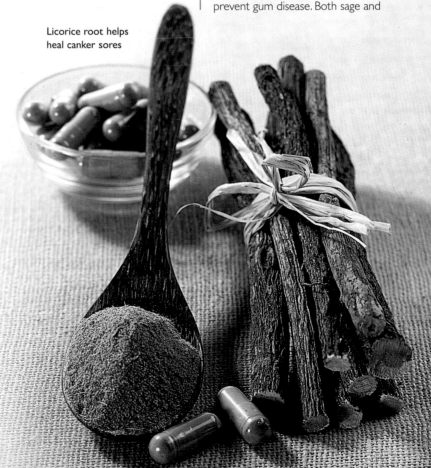

Licorice root helps heal canker sores

51
Preventing canker sores

If you are prone to canker sore outbreaks, specific foods may be contributing factors. The most common culprits are highly acidic foods, such as citrus fruits, tomatoes, pineapple, and vinegar, but other foods can be problematic. Note what you ate the day or two prior to an outbreak to identify potential triggers.

52
Sage mouth rinse for healthy gums

Rinsing your mouth daily with a solution of sage tea and sea salt helps prevent gum disease. Both sage and sea salt are mildly antiseptic, relieve inflammation, and promote healing. Because they are astringent, they also help tighten gum tissue.

1 cup (250ml) boiling water
2 teaspoons dried sage
1/2 teaspoon sea salt

Pour the boiling water over the sage, cover, and steep for 15 minutes. Strain, add the sea salt, and cool to lukewarm. Using approximately a quarter of a cup (60ml), swish the mixture around your mouth after brushing your teeth. Use the rest of the mouthwash within two days.

53
Sea salt for healthy gums

Rinse your mouth and gums with a solution of an eighth of a teaspoon sea salt dissolved in a quarter of a cup (60ml) warm water after flossing and brushing your teeth. Sea salt is a mild antiseptic that helps tighten the gums and keep them healthy.

54
Myrrh mouth rinse for healthy gums

Myrrh's powerful antimicrobial and astringent properties help kill bacteria and protect gum tissue.

1/2 cup (125ml) warm water
1/4 teaspoon sea salt
1/4 teaspoon myrrh extract

Mix the ingredients together. Using a quarter of a cup (60ml), rinse your mouth thoroughly twice daily after brushing and flossing teeth.

55
Goldenseal poultice for sore gums

A poultice made from goldenseal and myrrh provides intensive healing for sore gums. Mix a few drops of myrrh extract and goldenseal powder to make a thick paste. Wrap it in sterile gauze. Place it next to the affected area for one hour; repeat twice a day.

56
Dietary solutions for bad breath

Sluggish intestines are often a factor in generating bad breath. To keep your gastrointestinal tract in top form, eat a high-fiber diet with plenty of fresh fruits and vegetables and whole grains. In addition, take a daily supplement of *Lactobacillus acidophilus*—available in capsule form at health food and nutrition stores— to maintain a healthy population of beneficial intestinal flora. Dehydration can also cause stale or sour breath; drink at least six glasses of water daily to stay well hydrated.

57
Preventing bad breath

Cleaning your teeth daily removes odor-causing food particles that accumulate between your teeth. Be sure to brush your tongue, too. Floss your teeth once a day and brush them at least twice daily—preferably after every meal. If you cannot brush after a meal or snack, at least rinse your mouth with water.

58
Neutralize mouth odors

Baking soda is an excellent tooth cleanser and neutralizes mouth odors. Scoop up a teaspoon in your hand, coat a damp toothbrush with it, and use as you would any toothpaste.

59
Breath freshener

To freshen your breath, try chewing on a small handful of either fennel or anise seeds.

60
Mouth-freshening rinse

Conventional mouthwashes can actually cause bad breath because the alcohol they contain dries out the mucous membranes in your mouth. Instead, use a mouth rinse made with peppermint and witch hazel to freshen breath.

1 teaspoon witch hazel extract
1/2 teaspoon vegetable glycerin
3 drops peppermint essential oil
1/2 cup (125ml) water

Mix the ingredients together and shake well. Rinse your mouth with the mouthwash after brushing your teeth, or anytime you want to freshen your breath.

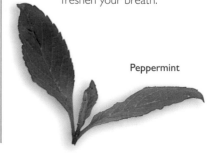

Peppermint

Psoriasis

Psoriasis is a skin disorder characterized by red, thick, and scaly patches that occur most often on the torso, elbows, knees, and scalp. It tends to come and go sporadically, and is thought to be an autoimmune condition.

61
Healing sunshine

Judicious sunbathing several times each week (while being very careful not to burn your skin) can often help heal the scaly patches characteristic of psoriasis.

62
Reduce inflammation

Omega-3 essential fatty acids help reduce the inflammatory compounds involved in psoriasis. Eat cold-water fish, such as salmon, sardines, and mackerel, at least three times a week, and take one tablespoon of flaxseed oil daily.

63
Improve your protein digestion

Poor protein digestion creates toxins that may contribute to psoriasis.

$^{1}/_{2}$ teaspoon herbal bitters tonic
$^{1}/_{4}$ cup (60ml) warm water

Mix the herbal bitters digestive tonic in the warm water. Take the mixture approximately 15 minutes before each meal to stimulate the flow of your digestive fluids and improve your digestion.

64
Heal skin with chamomile

Chamomile has both cleansing and cooling properties and acts like an antihistamine. To help calm the inflammation of psoriasis patches and to stimulate healing of the skin, apply a cream containing chamomile to your skin three times a day.

65
Detoxify with sarsaparilla

Sarsaparilla helps detoxify the body and, as a tea, has a long history of use for treating skin conditions such as psoriasis.

2 teaspoons dried sarsaparilla root
1 cup (250ml) water

Prepare the sarsaparilla tea by simmering the dried root in water in a covered pot for 10 minutes and strain. Drink up to three cups (750ml) a day. Alternatively, take half a teaspoon of liquid sarsaparilla extract diluted in a small amount of warm water, three times a day.

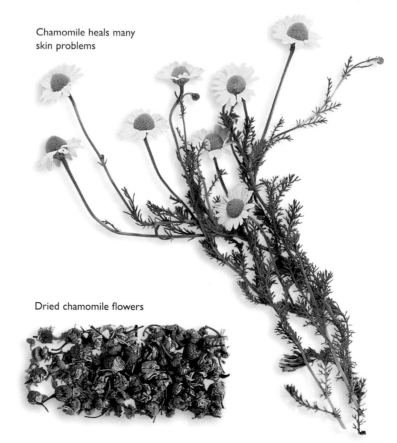

Chamomile heals many skin problems

Dried chamomile flowers

Bites, Stings, & Rashes

Bites, stings, and rashes can cause painful reactions and feelings of discomfort. Occasionally, an insect bite or sting can cause a severe allergic reaction, which requires emergency medical attention. By applying the following remedies to bites and stings, you can greatly speed healing and alleviate itching.

66
First aid for bites and stings

If you have been stung by an insect such as a bee, remove the stinger by carefully scraping a credit card or a fingernail across the skin. Apply ice immediately to any bite or sting to relieve the pain and to stop the toxin from spreading through your body. Wash the area with an antiseptic solution composed of equal amounts of tea tree essential oil and witch hazel extract.

67
Stop itching

Mix one teaspoon of cosmetic clay with enough water to make a paste. Add three drops of peppermint essential oil. Apply to a bite or sting.

68
Draw out toxins with charcoal

Apply a paste of activated charcoal to insect bites and stings to draw out the toxins that cause inflammation, swelling, and itching. Activated charcoal is also available in capsules. Open a couple of capsules, mix the charcoal with a few drops of water, and apply to a bite or sting. After half an hour, wash off the charcoal paste.

69
Herbal lotion to relieve itching

Witch hazel is a mild astringent and helps calm inflammation, while peppermint cools irritated skin and relieves itching. Lavender is both anti-inflammatory and antimicrobial.

1fl oz (30ml) witch hazel extract
20 drops peppermint essential oil
20 drops lavender essential oil

Combine the ingredients in a small bottle. Shake well, and apply with a cotton ball as often as desired.

70
Heal a skin rash with clay

Apply a poultice of cosmetic clay, aloe vera gel, and peppermint essential oil to treat a rash caused by a plant. Cosmetic clay is drying and aloe vera encourages healing. Peppermint oil cools and temporarily relieves itching.

2 tablespoons cosmetic clay
Aloe vera gel to mix
2 drops peppermint essential oil

Mix the clay with enough aloe vera gel to make a thin, spreadable paste. Add the peppermint essential oil, spread onto the rash, and let it dry. Reapply the poultice mixture as often as you wish.

Honeybees can cause painful stings

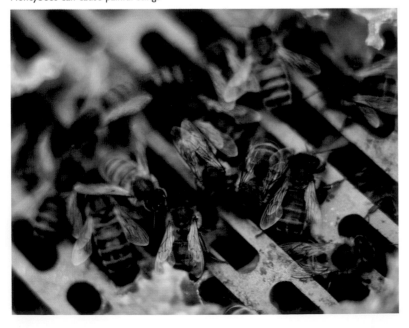

71
Relieve a plant rash

If you've been exposed to poison ivy, wash the affected area thoroughly with lukewarm water and a concentrated shampoo or dish soap to remove the irritating oils. Lather twice, and rinse thoroughly.

72
Ease an itchy rash with an oatmeal bath

A soothing bath with oatmeal and lavender essential oil soothes the itchy, irritated skin of a rash.

2 cups (200g) rolled oats
10 drops lavender essential oil

Grind the oats in a blender into a fine powder. Add to a tub of warm water along with the lavender oil. Soak for 20 minutes, and pat your skin dry without rinsing.

73
Fight rash infection with goldenseal

Rashes caused by plants, including poison ivy, may sometimes become infected. A mixture of raw, unfiltered honey and goldenseal applied to the rash fights infection and encourages healing. Goldenseal has antimicrobial properties and helps dry and heal the weeping rash. Raw honey is also antiseptic and soothes irritation. Mix equal parts of honey and powdered goldenseal, and spread onto the rash. Cover with a gauze bandage. Change the dressing twice daily until the rash has healed.

Head Lice

Head lice are easily spread from one person to another through hats, combs, towels, and contact with an infested person's hair. Lice feed on blood from the scalp, and cause intense itching and sores. Herbal and essential oil remedies offer a safe and effective alternative to chemical products. Use the following natural remedies to kill and remove lice, and repeat treatments after one week to kill any new lice that may have hatched.

74
Essential oil treatment

Rosemary and lavender essential oils help kill lice.

1fl oz (30ml) olive oil
10 drops rosemary essential oil
10 drops lavender essential oil

Mix the ingredients, dampen the hair, and massage the oil thoroughly into the hair and scalp. Cover with a shower cap and leave for an hour. Follow with Lice-removing shampoo and Anti lice hair rinse (see Nos. 75, 76).

75
Lice-removing shampoo

Follow the essential oil treatment by shampooing with neem, an herb used in Ayurvedic medicine to remove parasites, and thyme. Mix one tablespoon of a shampoo containing neem with three drops of thyme essential oil. Lather up, and wait five minutes before thoroughly rinsing with warm water. Follow with Anti lice hair rinse (see No. 76). **Caution:** Thyme is a potent natural insecticide and is irritating to the skin and scalp. Do not exceed the recommended amount and never apply it undiluted.

76
Anti lice hair rinse

Follow the Lice-removing shampoo (see No. 75) with a hair rinse that helps soften the glue that attaches the nits (lice eggs) to the hair. The rosemary and lavender essential oils help eradicate any remaining lice.

2 cups (500ml) warm water
2 cups (500ml) apple cider vinegar
6 drops rosemary essential oil
6 drops lavender essential oil

Mix the ingredients together and rinse the hair and scalp thoroughly with the mixture after shampooing. Cover the hair with a shower cap for 15 minutes, and then comb it with a lice comb (a special fine-toothed comb available at pharmacies). Rinse the hair and scalp again thoroughly with warm water.

77
Prevent reinfestation

To prevent lice from finding new homes, be sure to wash all combs, brushes, clothing, bedding, and towels in hot water. Thoroughly vacuum carpets and upholstered furniture, including car seats and headrests.

Bacterial Skin Infections

Boils are red, swollen, and tender eruptions. Impetigo causes tiny blisters, usually around the nose and mouth. Body odor is often caused when bacteria on the skin react with perspiration. You can treat all these with natural remedies but if they don't respond, or if they are severe or persistent, consult your doctor.

78
Treating a boil

Never squeeze a boil because you might force the bacteria into the bloodstream and spread the infection through the body. Hot compresses help draw the boil to a head, so it can safely rupture, drain, and then heal. Soak a washcloth in hot water and place it on the boil. Cover the washcloth with a dry towel to retain heat. When it cools, resoak the cloth in hot water and reapply. Repeat for 15 minutes, three times a day.

79
Tea tree for boils

Tea tree essential oil has powerful antimicrobial properties and helps to fight infection. Apply a drop of undiluted tea tree oil to the boil several times a day until the eruption has healed.

80
Fight infection with echinacea

Echinacea boosts the function of your immune system and helps fight the bacteria that cause infections. Take half a teaspoon of echinacea extract three times a day for up to 10 days.

81
Tea tree for impetigo

Tea tree is antibacterial and helps dry impetigo blisters. Lavender essential oil helps alleviate inflammation.

1 tablespoon almond oil
$^1/_2$ teaspoon tea tree essential oil
$^1/_2$ teaspoon lavender essential oil

Combine the ingredients in a tightly capped bottle. Apply with a cotton ball to the blisters three times a day.

82
Calendula for impetigo

Calendula is a powerful antimicrobial but is gentle enough for infants. Make a strong tea by pouring one cup (250ml) of boiling water over two tablespoons of dried calendula. Cover, steep for 20 minutes, and strain. Soak a washcloth in the warm tea and apply to the impetigo blisters for 10 minutes, three times a day.

83
Detoxify to prevent body odor

A simple detox program may help reduce toxins expelled through your skin. For two days, eat only vegetables and vegetable broth, and drink at least six glasses of water. Take one tablespoon of psyllium husks in the morning with a glass of water, followed by another glass of water.

84
Reduce odor by avoiding certain foods

Avoid eating fried foods or baked goods, which may contain rancid fats or oils that contribute to offensive body odor. Also avoid otherwise healthful foods, such as onions, garlic, and curry spices, which all contain potent essential oils that may be released through your skin.

85
Chlorophyll foods to combat odor

To improve liver function and so combat body odor, eat foods high in chlorophyll, such as kale, collards, watercress, and other dark leafy greens. Or take a teaspoon mixed in liquid twice a day of chlorophyll-rich supplements such as spirulina, chlorella, and barley grass.

86
Oils to neutralize odor

Spray the following mixture under your arms when needed to help stop the growth of odor-causing bacteria.

2fl oz (60ml) distilled witch hazel extract
10 drops grapefruit-seed extract
10 drops cypress essential oil
10 drops lavender essential oil

Mix the ingredients in a small spray bottle and shake well before using.

Fungal Skin Conditions

Ringworm may appear anywhere on the skin or scalp, and the ring-shaped rash can be tough to eradicate. Athlete's foot is a red, itchy, cracked, and scaly rash that usually begins between the toes and sometimes spreads to other parts of the feet. Antifungal herbs and essential oils will eradicate the tenacious fungus, but you also have to take steps to prevent reinfection.

87
Boost your immunity

Fungi are opportunistic so the stronger your immune system, the less likely they are to hang around. Take half a teaspoon of echinacea extract twice daily for 10 days, take a break for three days, and repeat the dosage for an additional 10 days.

88
Prevent ringworm spreading

Ringworm is highly contagious so change clothing, towels, and bedding daily. Wash items in hot water and dry in a hot dryer to kill the fungi.

89
Antifungal spray

Apple cider vinegar restores the healthy acidity of the skin to help it become more resistant to fungal growth. Lavender is antimicrobial and soothes itching and inflammation.

$^{1}/_{2}$ cup (125ml) apple cider vinegar
$^{1}/_{2}$ teaspoon lavender essential oil

Combine the ingredients in a spray bottle and shake. Spray onto your skin once a day after showering.

90
Fight ringworm with essential oils

Tea tree oil is a powerful antifungal and one of the best remedies for fungal skin infections. Lavender oil relieves itching and irritation, and also helps subdue the intense medicinal smell of tea tree oil. Mix together equal parts of tea tree essential oil and lavender essential oil and apply to the rash twice daily.

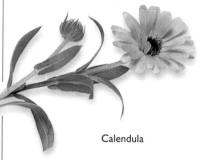

Calendula

91
Calendula antifungal foot soak

Calendula fights the athlete's foot fungus and encourages skin healing.

2 cups (500ml) boiling water
4 tablespoons dried calendula flowers
$^{1}/_{4}$ cup (60ml) apple cider vinegar

Pour the water over the flowers, cover, and steep until lukewarm. Strain, and pour into a basin large enough to hold your feet. Cover your feet with warm water and add the vinegar, which increases skin acidity and discourages fungal growth. Soak your feet twice daily for 20 minutes.

92
Healing foot spray

Tea tree combats the athlete's foot fungus, while aloe soothes irritated, itchy skin.

4fl oz (125ml) aloe vera juice
$^{1}/_{2}$ teaspoon tea tree essential oil

Combine the ingredients in a spray bottle. Shake well before using, and apply twice daily. Let your feet air-dry before putting on socks or shoes. Continue using this spray for at least one month, even after symptoms have disappeared, to ensure that the fungus has been eliminated.

93
Prevent reinfection of your feet

Dry your feet well after bathing, especially between your toes, where the athlete's foot fungus usually takes hold. A hairdryer can be helpful for thorough drying. Change your socks every day (more often if you exercise and your feet get sweaty), and choose cotton socks over synthetic fibers. Alternate shoes so that you aren't wearing the same pair every day. Wear rubber flip flops in public showers or locker rooms—the fungus that causes athlete's foot thrives in such environments and is easily spread.

Viral Skin Infections

The virus that causes warts enters through a crack in the skin. Although warts generally disappear on their own, you can hasten their demise with natural remedies. Because warts are contagious and can spread, avoid picking, scratching, or otherwise irritating them. The herpes simplex virus, which causes cold sores and genital herpes, lives in nerve endings. An outbreak is often precipitated by emotional tension or by physical stressors such as menstruation or too much sun.

94
Eliminate warts with tea tree oil

Tea tree essential oil has powerful antiviral properties and can help eliminate warts. Apply undiluted tea tree oil with a cotton swab directly to the wart several times a day.

95
Boost immune function with echinacea

Opportunistic organisms such as warts are a sign that your immune system is not functioning up to par. Take a course of echinacea to stimulate your immune system to overcome the virus. Take half a teaspoon of echinacea extract twice a day for 10 days. After a break of three days, repeat the dosage for an additional 10 days.

96
Fight warts with garlic

A poultice of crushed raw garlic has powerful antiviral properties and can get rid of a wart in a few days. Because the essential oils in raw garlic can burn your skin, it's important to protect the skin around the wart with a layer of vitamin E oil; prick a vitamin E capsule with a pin and spread the oil onto your skin. Mash a clove of garlic, apply to the wart, and cover with an adhesive bandage. Remove the bandage after 24 hours. A blister usually forms, and the wart should fall off within one week.

97
Resisting herpes

To increase resistance to the herpes virus during times of susceptibility, take half a teaspoon of echinacea extract three times daily for up to 10 days. Garlic is a potent antiviral; to keep the virus in check, eat one or two cloves of raw garlic daily.

98
Ice cube rescue

If you feel the tingling sensation of an impending herpes outbreak, rub an ice cube on the area. This sometimes stops a cold sore from erupting.

99
Helping to heal herpes with calendula

Calendula has antiviral properties and encourages the healing of herpes outbreaks. Prepare a strong tea by pouring one cup (250ml) of boiling water over two tablespoons of dried calendula. Cover, steep for 20 minutes, and strain. Apply with a cotton ball to the blisters several times daily.

100
Dry herpes blisters with tea tree oil

Tea tree essential oil is a powerful antiviral and helps dry the herpes blisters. Dilute with an equal amount of vegetable oil to prevent irritation of the skin and sensitive mucous membranes. Dab a small amount onto the blisters four times a day.

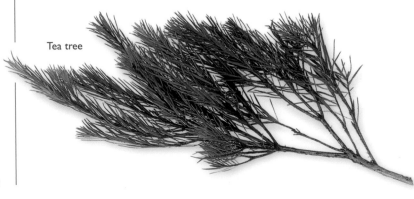

Tea tree

Skin Damage

When the skin is damaged—by a cut, burn, blister, or bruise—keep it clean and use herbs to help prevent infection and to speed healing. Treat a burn at once to prevent further damage. A blister creates a natural cushioned bandage that protects damaged skin and promotes healing. Treat a bruise promptly to minimize bleeding, reduce soreness, and speed recovery time.

101
Soap and water

Clean cuts and wounds thoroughly with a mild natural soap and lukewarm water to remove dirt and bacteria and to reduce the risk of infection.

102
Honey for wounds

Raw, unprocessed honey contains a natural antibiotic that has been proven to be effective against infectious organisms. Clean the wound, smooth on a thin layer of honey, and apply a bandage. Reapply the honey and change the bandage twice daily.

103
Stop bleeding with yarrow

The flowering tops of yarrow contain a number of natural wound-healing ingredients that encourage blood coagulation, ease pain, and relieve inflammation. Open a capsule of powdered yarrow and sprinkle it onto the cut. Apply gentle pressure to the cut with a clean cloth until the bleeding stops.

104
Yarrow compress

You can use liquid yarrow extract to make a compress to stop the bleeding from a cut. Dilute one teaspoon of yarrow extract in half a cup (125ml) of warm water. Soak a clean cloth in the solution, and apply with firm pressure to the wound.

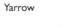

Yarrow

Yarrow flowers

Dried yarrow

Yarrow leaves

105
Heal cuts with comfrey

Comfrey is rich in allantoin, which has been proven to speed up the regeneration of cells. After a scab has formed, apply a salve containing comfrey to a cut or wound to encourage healthy skin renewal.
Caution: Because comfrey is so effective, it should not be applied to an open cut or wound as it might encourage the skin at the surface to heal prematurely, which could cause an abscess.

106
First aid for burns

Immediately immerse the affected area in ice-cold water until the burning sensation subsides (at least five minutes). This eases pain and inflammation and will often prevent a blister from forming. If a blister does form, don't puncture it. When the blister ruptures naturally, leave the protective skin intact and wash it thoroughly with an antiseptic skin wash made by mixing equal parts echinacea extract and water.

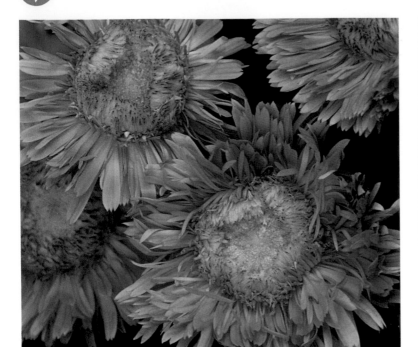

Calendula fights infection and promotes healing

107
Aloe vera burn remedy

Freshly prepared aloe vera gel can speed up the healing of burns and fight the bacteria that cause infection. Vitamin C, vitamin E, and lavender essential oil can also promote skin healing and help preserve the fresh aloe.

½ cup (60g) peeled, sliced aloe leaf
1,000mg powdered vitamin C
800 IU vitamin E oil
1 teaspoon lavender essential oil

Place all the ingredients into a clean blender and blend thoroughly. Store the mixture in a clean glass jar in the refrigerator, and apply it several times a day to a burn. This mixture will stay fresh for approximately two months in the refrigerator.

108
Heal burns with calendula

Calendula fights infection, soothes inflammation, and promotes healing. After cooling a burn (see No. 106), apply calendula gel and bandage the affected area lightly. Clean the burn and reapply the gel and a fresh bandage every day until the burn has healed.

109
Quick aloe burn relief

Grow a small potted aloe vera plant in a sunny kitchen window. For quick burn relief, slice off a small piece of the leaf, slit it open, and apply the inner gel to the burn as needed.

110
Treating a blister

If you must break a blister (such as when your shoe rubs against one on your foot), puncture it gently with a sterilized needle. Don't peel off the remaining skin. To prevent infection, wash the area with a solution of equal parts echinacea extract and water twice daily until the skin begins to heal. Cover with an adhesive bandage during the day but remove it at night to allow the blister to dry.

111
Heal a blister with witch hazel

Soak a cotton ball in witch hazel extract, place on the blister, and cover with an adhesive bandage. Change the cotton every six hours.

112
Aloe vera blister bandage

Aloe vera has astringent and tissue-healing properties and makes a simple herbal bandage for blisters. Peel a thin slice from a fresh aloe vera leaf and place it directly onto the blister. Cover with an adhesive bandage. Change the bandage twice daily until the blister has healed.

Aloe vera

113
Comfrey salve for broken blisters

After a blister breaks, clean it and apply comfrey salve twice daily to help regenerate new skin.

114
Cool a bruise

Apply an ice pack or a cold gel pack to a bruise at once. Cold helps stop the bleeding and relieves swelling and pain. Hold the pack on the bruised area for 15 minutes, and then reapply 10 minutes later. Depending on the severity of the bruise, repeat this two or more times for the first day.

115
Arnica for bruises

Arnica has anti-inflammatory and pain-relieving properties and will significantly lessen soreness. Apply a liberal amount of arnica gel or oil to the bruised area three or four times a day. **Caution:** Do not use arnica on broken skin.

116
Apply heat to ease a sore bruise

After the first 24 hours, apply heat to the bruised area. Heat improves circulation—which helps the blood to be reabsorbed—and alleviates stiffness and soreness. Use a hot-water bottle or soak in a hot bath. Add seven drops of rosemary essential oil to a bath to further improve circulation.

Snoring

Snoring is caused by a partial obstruction of the throat passage that restricts the flow of air during inhalation. Allergies, upper respiratory infections, obesity, and anatomical abnormalities can all cause snoring. No remedies are guaranteed to stop snoring but here are a few tricks to try, including foods to avoid, and tips on keeping your bedroom free from allergens.

117
Use a golf ball to stop snoring

Most people who snore do so when they are sleeping on their backs. To discourage this kind of snoring, make a special sleep shirt by sewing a golf ball into the pocket of a T-shirt and wear the shirt backward to bed. The ball is just uncomfortable enough to prevent the snorer from sleeping on his or her back.

118
Elevate the bed to relieve snoring

You can sometimes relieve snoring by slightly elevating the head of your bed. You only need to raise it by approximately 2in (5cm) and this can be done simply by placing a block of wood under each of the legs at the head end of the bed.

119
Dietary relief from snoring

Dairy products are common food allergens that create excess mucus and exacerbate congestion in the respiratory system. Try eliminating all dairy foods for two weeks to see if it relieves snoring. In addition, try to avoid alcohol and other sedatives for several hours before going to bed because they have a relaxing effect on the throat muscles and can make snoring worse.

120
Allergy-proof the bedroom

Allergies can be a contributing factor in chronic snoring. Try to make your bedroom as allergy-proof as possible by installing an air filter, keeping pets out, and getting rid of feather pillows and comforters. Keep dust and other particles at a minimum by vacuuming and dusting the room thoroughly at least once a week.

121
Clear congestion to relieve snoring

A sudden or unusual bout of snoring in a nonsnorer may be caused by congestion associated with an upper respiratory infection. To clear this congestion, take a hot shower or bath just before bed and apply a mentholated balm to the throat and chest.

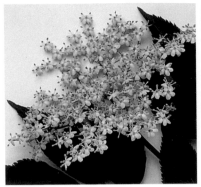 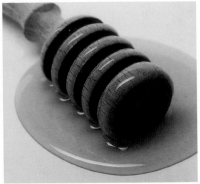 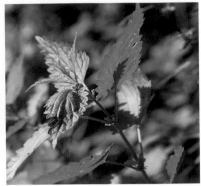

Elderflower, honey, and nettle all provide relief from hay fever

Sensitivities & Intolerances

Some people have an immediate and life-threatening allergic reaction to foods such as peanuts, which requires emergency medical attention. Here, however, we offer remedies that can help relieve some of the common symptoms of sensitivities and intolerances. These include sneezing, itchy and watery eyes, nasal congestion, inflammation, fatigue, and headaches.

122
Herbal eyewash

Calendula is soothing and healing, elderberry is anti-inflammatory, and eyebright is astringent and relieves irritation of the eyes.

1 cup (250ml) boiling water
1 teaspoon dried calendula
1 teaspoon dried elderflower
1 teaspoon dried eyebright

Pour the boiling water over the dried herbs. Cover, and steep for about 15 minutes. Strain through a coffee filter to remove all herb particles. Use as an eyewash, or soak cotton balls in the herbal tea and apply to your eyes at least three times a day for 10 minutes. Apply eyewash more often if you need it.

123
Eat local honey

Look for honey that is made by bees in your locality. Eat it regularly because it can help desensitize you to pollens in your environment.

124
Hay fever relief

Bioflavonoids in citrus peel can help to ease allergy symptoms via a mild antihistamine effect. Chop up the peels and white inner rinds of oranges and lemons (preferably organic). Place in a pot and barely cover with water; simmer, covered, for 10 minutes. Sweeten the mixture to taste with honey and eat one teaspoon three times a day.

125
Nettle tea

Steep a teaspoon of dried nettle in one cup (250ml) of boiling water for 10 minutes. To help relieve a respiratory allergy, drink up to four cups (1 liter) of the tea daily. Or take two capsules of freeze-dried nettle or half a teaspoon of nettle extract four times a day until symptoms abate.

126
Prevent allergies with quercetin

Quercetin is an antioxidant that inhibits the release of histamine, the inflammatory compound primarily responsible for the uncomfortable symptoms of respiratory allergies. Foods that are naturally rich in quercetin include citrus fruits, purple and yellow onions, and buckwheat. Concentrated quercetin is also available in capsules; take 500mg twice daily between meals. Quercetin acts to prevent allergies and so works best when started a month prior to the start of allergy season. Continue taking it throughout the season.

127
Peppermint inhalation

To relieve the sinus dryness and headaches caused by allergies, try this steam inhalation. Bring a large pot of water to a boil, remove from heat, and add two teaspoons of dried peppermint. Cover, and steep for five minutes. Remove the lid, and make a towel tent over your head and the pot, taking care to not burn yourself with the steam. Breathe in the warm steam for 10 minutes. Peppermint's healing properties are in its fragrant essential oils, so the more minty your peppermint smells, the better. Peppermint acts as a decongestant and, combined with warm steam, it opens up the sinuses. In addition, the herb has relaxing properties that help ease headache pain.

128
Eliminate food allergens from your diet

A rotation diet requires increasing the variety of foods eaten and not eating any specific food more than once every four days. Such a diet helps remove allergens and alleviate food sensitivities. You can choose from a wide range of additive-free whole foods. Base your diet on fresh vegetables and fruits, low-fat animal and vegetable proteins (avoiding dairy products), seeds and nuts, whole grains, and extra-virgin olive oil. Choose brown rice, quinoa, millet, and amaranth over gluten-containing grains (wheat, rye, barley, and oats) if gluten sensitivity is a particular problem.

Sinusitis

Colds, flu, allergies, and air pollution can cause sinus infections or chronic sinus inflammation. Symptoms of sinusitis include nasal congestion, pressure or pain in the sinuses, headache, and a yellowish-green mucus discharge. To get rid of a sinus infection, you need to relieve the congestion and eliminate the invading microorganisms.

129
Eucalyptus to relieve sinus congestion

Inhaling hot steam loosens and thins the mucus in your sinuses so that it can be expelled. Eucalyptus essential oil has powerful antimicrobial properties, and peppermint essential oil has a strong penetrating fragrance that helps open sinus passages.

1½ quarts (2 liters) boiling water
5 drops eucalyptus essential oil
2 drops peppermint essential oil

Carefully pour the boiling water into a heatproof bowl and then add the essential oils. Make a towel tent over your head and the bowl, and breathe in the steam for 10 minutes. Take care to not burn yourself with the steam. Repeat twice daily.

130
Relieve pain with compresses

To ease pain and encourage drainage of mucus, apply hot compresses to your sinuses. Eucalyptus oil helps decongest stuffy nasal passages and the heat eases pain. Add three drops of eucalyptus essential oil to a small basin of hot water. Soak a thick

cotton washcloth in the water and place it over your sinuses, being careful not to burn yourself. Rewet the cloth when it cools and reapply for a total of 10 minutes. Repeat the compress treatment several times a day as desired.

131
Strengthen immunity

To help your body overcome a sinus infection, take echinacea and garlic. Echinacea boosts immune function and garlic has powerful antimicrobial properties. Take half a teaspoon of echinacea extract three times a day for 10 days. You can repeat the dosage after a three-day break if necessary. Eat one to two cloves of raw garlic each day to strengthen your immune response.

132
Drink hot liquids

To relieve sinusitis, drink plenty of fluids to thin mucus secretions. Hot liquids are especially helpful—try peppermint tea for its decongesting properties, and vegetable or chicken soup with a clove of chopped raw garlic to fight infection.

Bronchitis

Bronchitis is an inflammation of the lungs and often follows an upper respiratory infection. It can also be a chronic condition that is intensified by air pollution, smoking, or colds. Symptoms include fever, coughing that produces yellow mucus, and sometimes chest pains and difficulty breathing.

133
Infection fighters

Herbal antibiotics such as echinacea, goldenseal, and garlic fight infection and boost your immune response. Take half a teaspoon of echinacea extract and a quarter of a teaspoon of goldenseal extract three times a day for up to 10 days. In addition, eat a clove of raw garlic twice daily until the infection has cleared. **Caution:** Do not take goldenseal if you have high blood pressure or are pregnant.

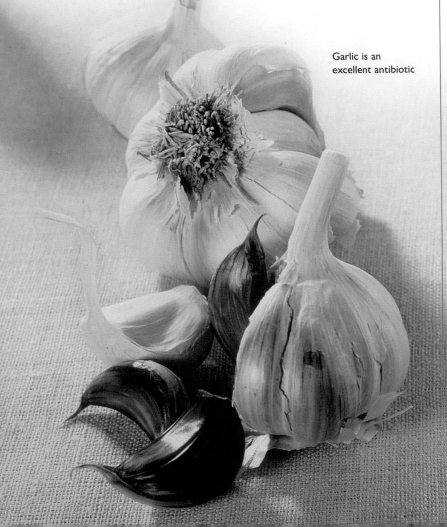

Garlic is an excellent antibiotic

134
Soothing mullein tea

Mullein leaves are rich in mucilage, a gelatinous substance that soothes irritated mucus membranes and bronchial passages. Marshmallow root also contains mucilage and has a slightly sweet taste, which tempers the flavor of the slightly bitter and astringent mullein.

1 cup (250ml) boiling water
1 teaspoon dried mullein leaf
1 teaspoon dried marshmallow root

Pour the water over the herbs, cover, and steep for 15 minutes. Strain, sweeten if desired, and drink three to four cups daily.

135
Loosen congestion in the chest

Eucalyptus loosens chest congestion and fights respiratory infection.

1½ quarts (2 liters) boiling water
3 drops eucalyptus essential oil

Carefully pour the boiling water into a heatproof bowl. Add eucalyptus essential oil, and cover your head and the bowl with a large towel. Inhale the steam for 15 minutes, taking care to not burn yourself. Repeat as often as desired.

Coughs

Colds, flu, allergies, or irritation of the bronchial tubes are the primary causes of coughs. Coughs that bring up mucus should not be suppressed because the body is trying to expel mucus and bacteria from the lungs. Dry coughs, however, are generally nonproductive and only further irritate the bronchi.

136
Quick cough reliever

Scoop up half a teaspoon of honey and add a squeeze of lemon. Let it dissolve slowly in your mouth before swallowing. Repeat when needed. **Caution:** Don't give unpasteurized honey to children under two.

137
Onion and honey syrup

The resins in onions are expectorant and antimicrobial. Honey helps loosen congestion. Finely chop a large onion, cover with honey, and warm in a covered pot over a low heat for 40 minutes. Store in a glass bottle in the refrigerator. Take half to one teaspoon every 15 to 30 minutes until the cough is relieved. **Caution:** Don't give unpasteurized honey to children under two.

138
Herbal cough syrup

Thyme, licorice root, and aniseed loosen mucus congestion and relax the respiratory tract. Honey thins mucus secretions, preserves the syrup, and soothes a raw, irritated throat. For a more potent syrup that can ease spasmodic coughs, try adding wild black cherry bark, which acts as a powerful sedative.

- 1 tablespoon aniseed
- 1 tablespoon dried licorice root
- 1 tablespoon dried wild black cherry bark (optional)
- 2 cups (500ml) water
- 1 tablespoon dried thyme
- 1 cup (250ml) honey
- **(To make and use, see below)**

139
Ease a cough with peppermint oil

Peppermint's strong menthol scent breaks up congestion and helps ease spasmodic coughing. Dab a drop of peppermint oil under your nose. If your skin is sensitive, dilute the oil with an equal amount of vegetable oil. For young children, place a drop or two of the oil on a pajama collar or pillow instead of the skin.

MAKING AND USING HERBAL COUGH SYRUP

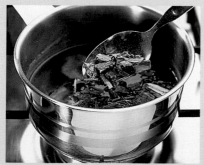

1 Simmer the aniseed, licorice root, and wild black cherry bark (if you have chosen to include it) in the water in a covered pot for 15 minutes.

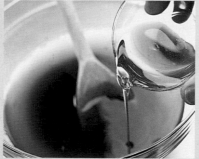

2 Remove from the heat, add the thyme, cover, and steep until room temperature. Strain, and add honey, warming the tea gently, if necessary, to dissolve the honey.

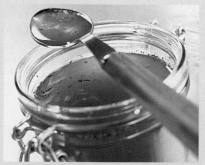

3 Store in a covered glass jar in the refrigerator, where it will keep for three months. Take one teaspoon as often as needed to relieve a cough.

Sore Throats

Sore throats are upper respiratory tract infections that are usually caused by viruses but occasionally by bacteria. A sore throat often accompanies a cold or the flu, lasts for about three days, and may cause a mild fever. Natural remedies treat the infection and soothe the inflammation.

140
Gargle with cayenne

Cayenne will temporarily relieve the pain of a sore throat. Make a gargle of half a cup (125ml) of warm water, one tablespoon of lemon juice, one teaspoon of salt, and a dash of powdered cayenne. Gargle several times a day.

141
Fight viruses with garlic

Garlic is a powerful ally for your immune system and is excellent for fighting the viruses that cause most sore throats. Eat two cloves of raw garlic daily at the first inkling of a sore throat. Chop finely and add to hot miso or chicken soup just before serving. The heat of the soup will also temporarily soothe your throat.

142
Boost immunity

Echinacea stimulates your immune system to overcome the infection. Elderberry prevents the virus from replicating. Take half a teaspoon of echinacea extract and one teaspoon of elderberry extract three times a day in a quarter of a cup (60ml) of warm water.

143
Soothe pain with marshmallow tea

Marshmallow contains a water-soluble fiber that soothes irritated tissues. Ginger and peppermint both help relieve inflammation.

1 teaspoon marshmallow root
1 cup (250ml) water
1 teaspoon chopped fresh ginger root
1 teaspoon dried peppermint

Simmer the marshmallow root and ginger root for five minutes in water in a covered pot. Remove from the heat, add peppermint, cover, and steep for an additional 10 minutes. Strain, sweeten if desired, and drink as often as needed.

144
Gargle to encourage healing

A warm gargle made from sage tea and sea salt eases sore throat pain and promotes healing. Sage contains astringent compounds that relieve pain temporarily, and sea salt has mildly antiseptic properties.

1 cup (250ml) boiling water
2 teaspoons dried sage
½ teaspoon sea salt

Pour the water over the sage, cover, and steep for 10 minutes. Strain, add sea salt, and gargle with the warm solution several times a day.

Echinacea helps boost immune function

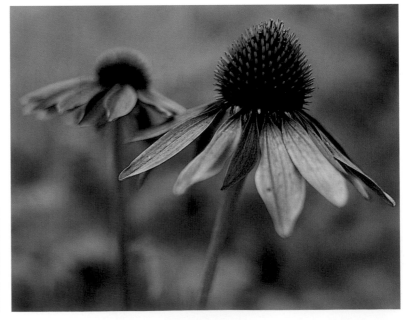

Colds, Flu, & Fever

Many cold and flu symptoms are similar—sore throat, cough, congestion, runny nose, and general achiness—but the flu is a more severe ailment. Sometimes there is a fever. If body temperature reaches over 103°F (39.4°C), or if a fever persists for more than three days, consult a doctor. Both colds and the flu are caused by viruses. The symptoms of a cold or flu are created by the body's attempt to rid itself of the virus; natural remedies support rather than suppress the body's efforts.

145
Prevent colds and flu

Astragalus is a Chinese herb that strengthens immunity. Take it in the early fall for at least a month. Simmer a teaspoon of dried, shredded astragalus in one and a quarter cups (300ml) of water for 15 minutes in a covered pot. Strain, and drink two cups (500ml) daily. Or take a quarter of a teaspoon of astragalus extract in a little warm water twice daily.

146
Boost immune function

During a cold or a bout of the flu, take half a teaspoon of echinacea extract three times a day for up to 10 days to boost your immunity.

147
Hot teas and broths

When you are battling a cold or a bout of the flu, drink plenty of hot herbal teas, vegetable broths, and chicken soup. Hot liquids make good decongestants, and as they heat the throat, they slow the reproduction cycle of the virus.

148
Eat garlic

Eat one clove of finely chopped raw garlic twice a day. To avoid stomach upset, eat garlic with meals.

149
Fight the flu with elderberry

In Europe, elderberry is traditionally used to treat the flu; compounds in elderberries disarm the flu virus and prevent it from replicating. Take one tablespoonful of elderberry syrup three times a day to help fight the flu.

150
Chase chills with ginger

Ginger tea loosens nasal congestion, eases a sore throat, and relieves chills.

3 teaspoons fresh grated ginger root
2 cups (500ml) water
2 tablespoons lemon juice
1 tablespoon honey

Simmer the ginger and water in a covered pot for 10 minutes. Remove from the heat, strain, and add lemon juice and honey. Drink as desired.

151
Stop a virus with zinc

To shorten the duration of a cold, suck on zinc gluconate lozenges. Cold viruses reproduce in the throat, and zinc kills them on contact. Take 15 to 25mg of zinc gluconate in lozenge form every two hours (up to 10 lozenges a day) for up to one week.

152
Relieve congestion with essential oils

Try an herbal steam inhalation using tea tree and eucalyptus essential oils. Tea tree has antiviral and antibacterial properties, and eucalyptus helps drain mucous congestion.

1½ quarts (2 liters) boiling water
2 drops tea tree essential oil
2 drops eucalyptus essential oil

Pour boiling water into a heatproof bowl and add the oils. Cover your head and the bowl with a large towel. Inhale the steam for 10 minutes, without burning yourself.

153
Relief from muscle aches and chills

Epsom salts are rich in magnesium, a natural muscle relaxant. Eucalyptus oil eases muscle aches and its steam will temporarily relieve sinus congestion.

2 cups (250g) Epsom salts
10 drops eucalyptus essential oil

Mix the ingredients and add to a hot bath. Soak for 20 minutes to relieve your aches and chills.

154
Fight the flu with herbal tea

Elderflowers and peppermint help lower the fever associated with the flu and to decongest the airways.

2 cups (500ml) boiling water
1 teaspoon dried peppermint
1 teaspoon dried elderflowers

Pour the boiling water over the herbs in a teapot, cover and steep for 15 minutes. Strain, add honey if desired, and drink four cups a day.

155
Ease sore throat pain

To ease the pain of a sore throat, gargle several times daily with warm saltwater, which has mild astringent and antiseptic properties. Dissolve three-quarters of a teaspoon of sea salt in one cup (250ml) of warm water. For more suggestions, see Sore Throats on page 34.

156
Soothe cold symptoms with massage

A chest and back massage with a blend of eucalyptus, lavender, and peppermint essential oils helps relieve chest congestion, opens the sinuses, and eases the achy feeling that often accompanies a cold or the flu.

4fl oz (125ml) almond oil
20 drops eucalyptus essential oil
20 drops lavender essential oil
5 drops peppermint essential oil

Mix the ingredients in a tightly capped bottle and shake well. Apply one teaspoon or more to the chest and back and massage into the skin.

157
Menthol cough drops

To ease the nagging cough that accompanies a cold or the flu, suck on cough drops made with menthol, which has an antispasmodic action.

158
Cough relief

To alleviate a cough associated with a cold or the flu, take a thyme syrup.

1 cup (250ml) boiling water
2 tablespoons dried thyme
½ cup (125ml) honey

Pour the boiling water over the thyme, cover, and steep for about 20 minutes. Strain, and add honey. If necessary, warm the tea over a gentle heat to completely dissolve the honey. Store in a dark glass bottle. Take one teaspoon as often as you need. For more suggestions, see Coughs on page 33.

Thyme soothes nagging coughs

159
Cool down with yarrow

Yarrow reduces inflammation and increases circulation to the surface of the skin. This promotes sweating and helps reduce a fever without suppressing the immune system.

2 cups (500ml) boiling water

3 tablespoons dried yarrow

Pour the water over the yarrow, cover, and steep for 20 minutes. Strain, and add the tea to a tubful of lukewarm water. For a sponge bath, dilute the tea with an extra 16fl oz (500ml) of lukewarm water before using.

160
Herbal tea for lowering a fever

Ginger, peppermint, and elderflower stimulate circulation and encourage perspiration, helping lower a fever naturally and safely.

1 cup (250ml) boiling water

2 teaspoons chopped fresh ginger root

1 teaspoon dried peppermint

1 teaspoon dried elderflower

Pour the water over the herbs. Cover, and steep for 10 minutes. Strain, sweeten if desired, and drink hot, up to four cups (1 liter) a day.

161
Drink fluids

Drink plenty of fluids during a fever. At least two quarts (2.5 liters) or more daily of pure water, mild herbal teas, and diluted fruit juices will keep your body well hydrated.

162
Relieve chills with hot baths

Epsom salts ease muscle aches, and ginger essential oil is warming.

2 cups (250g) Epsom salts

5 drops ginger essential oil

Mix the ingredients and add to a hot bath. Soak for 15 minutes.

163
Lavender relief

Lavender has anti-inflammatory and cooling properties. Add three drops of lavender essential oil to a basin of lukewarm water. Soak a sponge in the water basin and wipe the forehead, the back of the neck, the insides of the elbows, the backs of the knees, and the soles of the feet.

Irritable Bowel Syndrome

Irritable bowel syndrome (IBS) is characterized by diarrhea, constipation, gas, abdominal pain, and bloating. Although there is no structural problem with the colon, the normal rhythmic, wavelike contractions that move waste through the intestinal tract become irregular and spastic.

164
Replenish intestinal flora

Improve the general health of your intestinal tract by making sure it has a flourishing population of friendly intestinal flora. Eat a cup (250ml) daily of yogurt that contains live *Lactobacillus acidophilus* organisms. Or buy a good-quality supplement and follow the directions on the label.

165
Eat a high-fiber diet

Eating sufficient fiber keeps waste moving smoothly through your intestines. Avoid wheat bran, which can be too irritating for a sensitive colon. Increase your intake of fruits and vegetables. Eat a bowl of oatmeal daily as it contains fiber and a slippery substance called mucilage which soothes the lining of irritated intestines. You might also try a fiber supplement such as psyllium: start with half a teaspoon stirred into a glass of water and work up to one to two tablespoons a day. It's important to gradually increase the amount of fiber in your diet—too much too soon can cause gas and bloating.

166
Avoid allergenic foods

Certain foods may trigger symptoms of IBS. To find out which ones may affect you, keep a food and symptom diary for two weeks. Common culprits include caffeine, artificial sweeteners (especially sorbitol), citrus fruits, dairy products, fatty foods, as well as gas-producing foods such as beans and cabbage.

167
Relieve IBS symptoms with herbs

An herbal mixture of chamomile, hops, and fennel seed can relieve intestinal cramping and gas pains, and promote healthy digestive secretions.

1fl oz (30ml) chamomile extract

1fl oz (30ml) hops extract

1fl oz (30ml) fennel extract

Combine the extracts and store in a dark glass bottle. Take half a teaspoon, three times daily, 15 minutes before meals for up to two months.

168
Take time for relaxation

Emotional tension and anxiety make IBS symptoms worse. Try stress-reducing techniques that calm both body and mind, such as meditation, yoga, and focused breathing exercises. Regular daily exercise such as walking also alleviates stress and encourages healthy bowel rhythms.

169
Drink peppermint tea

Peppermint contains potent essential oils with antispasmodic properties and helps ease intestinal cramping and gas.

1 cup (250ml) boiling water

1 teaspoon dried peppermint

Pour the boiling water over the peppermint in a teapot. Cover, steep for 10 minutes, and strain. Drink three cups throughout the day.

Constipation

Insufficient dietary fiber and fluids and not enough exercise are the primary causes of constipation. Eating more whole grains, vegetables, and fruits, drinking plenty of water, and exercising daily will resolve most cases of sluggish bowels. To avoid weakening the intestinal tract, don't rely on laxatives—even herbal laxatives—for more than occasional relief from constipation.

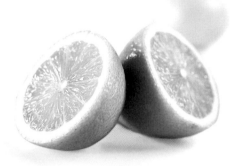
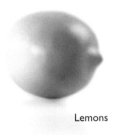

Lemons

170
Herbal relief for constipation

Cascara sagrada is an effective and gentle herbal intestinal stimulant and is a popular ingredient in over-the-counter and prescription laxatives. Ginger and fennel mask its bitter taste and help relieve gas and intestinal cramps.

1 teaspoon dried cascara sagrada bark

½ teaspoon fresh or dried ginger root

½ teaspoon fennel seeds

2 cups (500ml) water

Simmer the herbs and water in a covered pot for 10 minutes. Remove from the heat and allow to steep for an additional 10 minutes. Strain, add sweetener if desired, and drink one cup (250ml) before bed and another cup in the morning if necessary. If you prefer, you can take cascara sagrada extract; dilute half a teaspoon in a small amount of warm water.

171
Lemon reliever

To relieve mild constipation, drink a glass of warm water mixed with the juice from half a lemon first thing in the morning.

172
Add additional fiber

For stubborn constipation, add additional bulk to your diet in the form of fiber supplements such as psyllium husks. Take one to three teaspoons daily stirred into a glass of warm water, followed by an additional glass of water. Be sure to drink plenty of water throughout the day when taking fiber supplements to avoid constipation.

Diarrhea

Acute diarrhea is the body's attempt to rid itself of toxins, irritants, or infection in the intestinal tract. Diarrhea can be especially serious in young children because it can quickly cause dangerous dehydration.

173

Prevent dehydration

Increasing fluid intake will prevent dehydration. Drink at least eight to 10 glasses of fluids daily. Try one cup (250ml) of apple juice to two cups (500ml) of water—it helps replace lost potassium and is easily absorbed.

174

Eat a brown apple

To help stop an attack of diarrhea, shred a peeled apple on to a plate, let it turn brown, and eat it. Apples contain pectin, which helps bind loose stools.

175

Eat bananas and carob

Bananas and carob are both rich in pectin, which binds loose stools. Eat a banana mashed with a tablespoon or two of carob powder. One serving may take care of the problem, or you may need more. This is an especially good remedy for children.

176

Herbal tea

Catnip eases abdominal cramps and the emotional tension that may contribute to diarrhea. Peppermint helps expel gas and calms intestinal spasms. Raspberry leaf contains astringent compounds called tannins, which soothe intestinal inflammation.

2 cups (500ml) boiling water
2 teaspoons dried catnip
2 teaspoons dried peppermint
2 teaspoons dried raspberry leaf

Pour the water over the herbs. Cover, and steep for 15 minutes. Strain, sweeten if desired, and drink half a cup (125ml) every hour.

177

Traveler's diarrhea

Protect yourself from harmful germs by drinking only bottled water, eating properly cooked foods, washing your hands before eating, and only eating raw foods that can be peeled. If you do come down with diarrhea, try goldenseal. Take half a teaspoon of extract or two 500–600mg capsules three times daily, about 15 minutes before eating. ***Caution:*** Do not take goldenseal if you have high blood pressure or are pregnant.

178

Restore intestinal flora

To reestablish healthy intestinal flora, take a *Lactobacillus acidophilus* supplement for a couple of weeks following a bout of diarrhea.

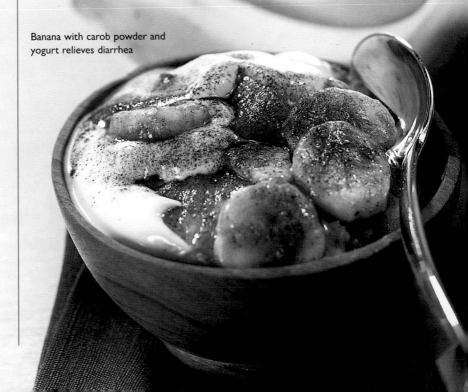

Banana with carob powder and yogurt relieves diarrhea

Nausea

Nausea can be brought on by various causes, incuding motion sickness, pregnancy, an adverse reaction to food, nervous tension, a virus, or migraine headache.

179
Ginger calmer

To help prevent motion sickness, take six 500mg capsules of powdered ginger about 45 minutes before departing on your journey.

180
Chew candied ginger

Ginger is a proven antinausea aid and has no harmful side effects. Chewing on a piece of candied ginger root can ease mild nausea.

181
Acupressure for nausea

Acupressure wristbands for relieving nausea from motion sickness or morning sickness are available at many natural food stores and pharmacies. To make your own, tape a mustard seed on the inside of each wrist, about 2in (5cm) above the wrist crease and between the two tendons. When an attack of nausea hits, press firmly on your left wrist for one minute, then repeat on your right wrist.

182
Ease morning sickness

While a cup of ginger tea helps ease morning sickness for some women, many find that they need to take larger amounts to alleviate nausea. Powdered ginger in capsules provides a more concentrated dose. Take several 500mg capsules at a time (up to 6g per day) with a little ginger tea.

183
Alleviate nausea

Simmer one or two teaspoons of chopped fresh ginger root in one cup of water in a covered pot for about 10 minutes. Strain, and sweeten if desired. Drink small amounts during the day as often as you wish.

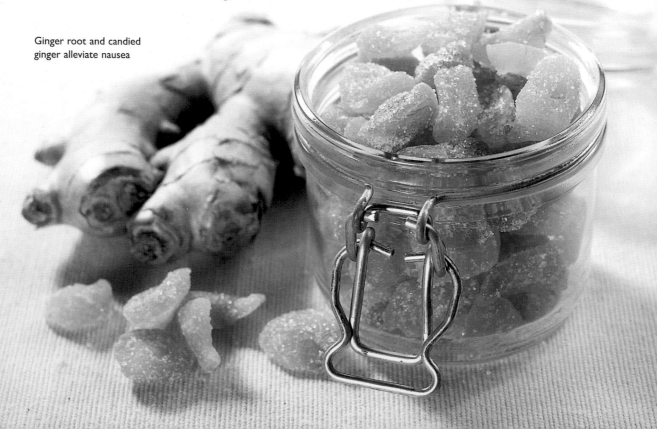

Ginger root and candied ginger alleviate nausea

Indigestion

An attack of indigestion can be triggered by too many fatty or spicy foods; stimulants such as tea, coffee, or alcohol; or emotional upset. Digestion also tends to slow a bit with age, causing bloating, indigestion, gas, and fatigue. Herbal remedies ease symptoms and help improve digestion.

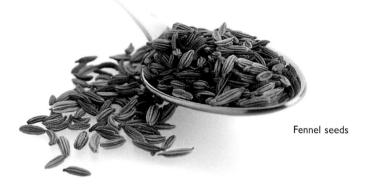

Fennel seeds

184
Herbal tea for indigestion

Fennel seed, ginger, and peppermint are all excellent as mild aids to the process of digestion. The fragrant essential oils that give them their characteristic flavors and aromas stimulate the flow of digestive juices, relieve indigestion, and help ease the pains associated with gas.

1 teaspoon fresh chopped ginger root
½ teaspoon fennel seed
1 cup (250ml) water
½ teaspoon dried peppermint

Simmer the ginger and fennel in the water in a covered pot for about five minutes. Remove from the heat and add the peppermint. Cover, and steep for an additional 10 minutes. Strain the tea, sweeten it with honey if you desire, and sip while warm.

185
Herbal digestive tonic

Herbal digestive tonics include bitter herbs such as dandelion and gentian, which stimulate digestive fluids. Herbs such as fennel and ginger ease gas pains. Licorice soothes the intestinal tract and sweetens the tonic.

½ oz (15g) dried dandelion root
¼ oz (7.5g) dried gentian root
¼ oz (7.5g) dried licorice root
¼ oz (7.5g) dried fennel seeds
¼ oz (7.5g) ginger root
1 bottle vodka

Grind the herbs into a coarse powder in a blender. Place in a wide-mouthed glass jar and cover the herbs with vodka, plus an additional 2in (5cm) of vodka. Stir well, cover, and place in a warm, dark place. Shake the jar every day to keep the herbs from settling. After two weeks, strain the liquid from the herbs through several layers of cheesecloth, reserving the liquid (tonic). Store the bitters tonic in a dark glass container in a cool, dark place. It will remain potent for at least three years. Take half a teaspoon in a quarter of a cup (60ml) of warm water about 15 minutes before meals to get your digestive juices flowing.

186
Cultivate a taste for bitter foods

Bitter flavors trigger the flow of digestive fluids. Eating a salad that contains a handful of greens (such as arugula, dandelion, or radicchio) before lunch or dinner is an easy way to get a tasty ration of bitters.

187
Chew food thoroughly

Digestive enzymes are secreted in your saliva, and the production of stomach juices is triggered when you begin to eat. The more thoroughly you chew your food, the easier you make it on the rest of your digestive system. Plus, slowing down relaxes your stomach and digestive organs, which helps them work properly.

188
Digestion enhancer

Drinking a small amount of liquid facilitates digestion, but gulping large amounts dilutes stomach juices and can cause bloating and indigestion. Try sipping a small cup of digestion-enhancing ginger or peppermint tea during a meal.

Ulcers

Many duodenal and gastric ulcers appear to be caused by the *Helicobacter pylori* bacterium; medical treatment generally involves taking antibiotics to eradicate the bacteria. Other factors, however, including stress and diet, also play a role in the development of ulcers.

189
Avoid dietary irritants

Because an ulcer is basically an open wound in the stomach, protecting the lining of the stomach is important. Avoid aspirin, ibuprofen, tobacco, coffee, and alcohol. They are all serious gastrointestinal irritants. But don't avoid spicy foods (unless they bother you). It's a myth that spicy foods cause ulcers—in fact, cayenne helps relieve inflammation and can stop the bleeding that may occur with ulcers.

190
Abstain from antacids

Don't take antacids for ulcers. They can cause the stomach to produce extra acid, a phenomenon known as rebound acid production. Don't drink milk, either, to soothe ulcer pain. Although milk initially has a mild antacid effect, it causes the stomach to produce extra acid.

191
Heal ulcers with licorice

Licorice root possesses antibacterial properties, increases the production of protective mucus in the stomach, and helps ulcers heal more quickly.

You can buy chewable tablets of deglycyrrhizinated licorice (DGL), which has had the compound glycyrrhizic acid removed because it can cause water retention and high blood pressure. Take two 380mg tablets three times a day, 20 minutes before meals. It may take up to three months for the full benefits of licorice to take effect.

192
Practice managing your stress

Because emotional stress causes the stomach to secrete excessive amounts of acid, it is important to learn to manage it and to alleviate tension. To help you do this, practice some deep-breathing exercises, yoga, tai chi, or another form of relaxation therapy daily.

Menstrual Cramps

Caused by contractions of the uterus, menstrual cramps are often accompanied by nausea, headache, and backache. Inflammatory hormonelike substances trigger cramping; dietary changes and herbs can help balance hormones and encourage production of the body's natural pain-relieving chemicals.

193
Dietary relief for cramps

Omega-3 fatty acids promote the production of pain-relieving chemicals. Include foods rich in omega-3 fats in your daily diet: cold-water fish, such as mackerel, salmon, and sardines; and fresh walnuts and flaxseeds. You can also supplement your diet by taking one tablespoon of cold-pressed flaxseed oil, or one tablespoon of freshly ground flaxseeds, each day. Avoid eating hydrogenated oils, saturated fats, polyunsaturated oils, and red meat, all of which stimulate the production of hormones that cause inflammation.

194
Tea for mild cramps

To relieve mild menstrual cramps, drink a tea made from ginger and chamomile. Ginger eases cramping, and chamomile promotes relaxation.

1 teaspoon fresh chopped ginger root
1 cup (250ml) water
1 teaspoon dried chamomile

Simmer the ginger root in the water in a covered pot for five minutes. Remove from the heat and add the chamomile. Cover, and let the tea steep for 10 minutes. Strain, sweeten with honey if you desire, and drink up to three cups each day.

195
Cramp bark relaxant

Cramp bark has sedative properties and helps relax the uterine muscle. Valerian eases overall tension. Ginger is antispasmodic and helps relieve stagnation in the uterus (that can contribute to cramping) by gently stimulating menstrual flow.

1fl oz (30ml) cramp bark extract
½fl oz (15ml) valerian extract
½ teaspoon ginger root extract

Mix the extracts together in a dark glass bottle. Shake well, and take half to one teaspoon of extract in a small amount of warm water three to four times daily as needed.

196
Relax to ease cramps

Because emotional and physical stressors contribute to menstrual cramps, taking time out for relaxation is important. Lie down, place a hot-water bottle over your abdomen to relax the uterine muscle, and rest for at least 30 minutes.

197
Eliminate caffeine

Most menstrual cramps are caused by too much estrogen and too little progesterone. Caffeine interferes with the proper metabolism of estrogen; it also causes fluctuations in blood-sugar levels, which exacerbate menstrual cramps. Avoid coffee, black tea, colas, chocolate, and any over-the-counter medications (e.g. menstrual pain-relief formulas) that contain caffeine.

Premenstrual Syndrome

Hormonal imbalances—particularly an excess of estrogen in relation to progesterone—cause the physical and emotional discomfort of premenstrual syndrome (PMS); symptoms include mood swings, fatigue, fluid retention, breast tenderness, and headaches. Herbs and lifestyle adjustments provide relief from symptoms and help balance hormones.

198
Eating to balance your hormones

Caffeine, unhealthful fats (saturated, polyunsaturated, and hydrogenated fats), red meat, alcohol, and sugar all stimulate excess estrogen production and exacerbate the symptoms of premenstrual syndrome. Help your body eliminate excess estrogen by eating plenty of high-fiber foods—fresh vegetables and fruits, whole grains, legumes, nuts, and seeds.

199
Balance your hormones with the right fats

Although saturated, hydrogenated, and polyunsaturated fats and oils contribute to hormonal imbalances, foods rich in essential fatty acids help balance hormone levels. Eat at least one serving daily of a food rich in omega-3 essential fatty acids. Choose from cold-water fish, such as salmon, sardines, and trout, and walnuts and flaxseeds. Gamma-linolenic acid (GLA), which is found in evening primrose, blackcurrant, and borage oils, may also help balance the hormones; take enough capsules to equal 240mg of GLA daily.

200
Take extra vitamin B₆ for water retention

Vitamin B₆ helps relieve the water retention that is associated with the symptoms of premenstrual syndrome such as swollen breasts, mood swings, and headaches. Take 50 to 100mg daily along with a high-potency vitamin-B complex.

201
Exercise to alleviate mood swings

Regular exercise, which means at least 30 minutes a day, helps lower estrogen levels and is a great antidote for the mood swings, depression, and anxiety that often accompany premenstrual syndrome.

202
Herbal help for PMS

Chaste-tree berries have sedative and antispasmodic properties and help to balance hormone levels. Take half a teaspoon of chaste-tree berry extract three times a day in a small amount of warm water. For best results, take the extract for at least six months (it can be taken indefinitely).

203
Relieve water retention with dandelion

Dandelion leaf is a gentle diuretic that safely helps relieve premenstrual water retention.

1 cup (250ml) boiling water
1 teaspoon dried dandelion leaf

Pour the boiling water over the dandelion leaf. Cover, steep for 10 minutes, and strain. Drink as needed, up to three cups a day.

Dandelion

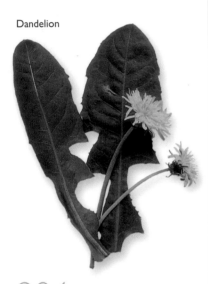

204
Aromatherapy bath for PMS

A warm bath with Epsom salts and clary sage and lavender essential oils helps ease emotional tension.

2 cups (250g) Epsom salts
10 drops lavender essential oil
5 drops clary sage essential oil

Mix the Epsom salts and essential oils and add to a bathtub of warm water. Soak in the bath for 20 minutes.

Menopause

Menopause, which is triggered by decreasing hormones, is often accompanied by physical and emotional symptoms—hot flashes, irregular menstruation, vaginal dryness, and mood swings. Heart disease and osteoporosis are also linked to lower estrogen levels. Natural therapies help relieve symptoms and prevent degenerative diseases that can occur after menopause.

205
Avoid dietary stressors

Avoid refined carbohydrates and sugar, which contribute to mood swings and depression. Limit your intake of alcohol and caffeine, which can trigger hot flashes. Eat small, high-protein meals and snacks through the day to help keep blood-sugar levels balanced and energy levels steady, and to strengthen the adrenal glands.

206
Eat to keep bones strong

To keep bones strong and prevent osteoporosis, eat at least two servings a day of low-fat dairy products, dark leafy greens, and canned sardines with bones. All are excellent sources of calcium. In addition, take a daily calcium–magnesium supplement that supplies at least 1,000mg of calcium and 500mg of magnesium.

207
Herbal help for menopause

Although the ovaries stop producing hormones after menopause, other endocrine glands, such as the adrenal glands, take over the production of estrogen and other hormones to some extent. To support adrenal function, take Siberian ginseng daily for at least three months. Either take half a teaspoon of a liquid ginseng extract once a day; or take 250mg twice a day of an extract that has been standardized for eleutherosides, regarded as the primary active ingredients of ginseng. Siberian ginseng is safe to take for up to six weeks. **Caution:** If you suffer from high blood pressure (hypertension), consult your doctor before using any type of ginseng.

208
Regular exercise

Exercising regularly can relieve many of the uncomfortable symptoms of menopause. Regular aerobic exercise decreases the risk of heart disease and provides an outlet for relieving emotional tension. Aim for at least 30 minutes each day, four days a week. In addition, to maintain bone density, include at least two 30-minute sessions a week of strengthening exercises, such as working out with weights or doing heavy gardening.

209
Comfrey salve for vaginal dryness

Vaginal dryness creates a perfect environment for chronic vaginal infections and makes sexual activity painful. A salve made from comfrey lubricates and heals vaginal tissues. Comfrey contains allantoin, which stimulates healthy new cell growth. Apply about half a teaspoon of comfrey salve to vaginal tissues daily, after bathing, until they heal.

210
Facial mist

Make a soothing aromatherapy facial mist to cool hot flashes.

4fl oz (125ml) rose water
10 drops lavender essential oil

Combine the ingredients in a spray bottle. Shake well, and store in the refrigerator for extra cooling benefits. Spray your face whenever you need.

Lavender

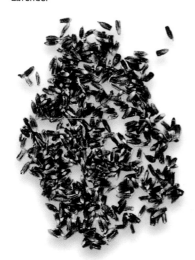

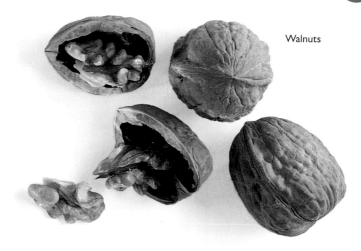

Walnuts

211
Cooling hot flashes

Hot flashes are the most common symptom of menopause. A tea made from sage can help relieve the flashes; the strong astringent properties of sage reduce perspiration by up to 50 percent.

1 cup (250ml) boiling water
2 teaspoons dried sage

Pour the boiling water over the sage. Cover, steep for 10 minutes, and strain. Sweeten if desired, and drink a cup before bedtime or as needed throughout the day.

212
Eat plenty of healthful fats

If you experience vaginal dryness, make sure you're getting enough essential fatty acids. Flaxseeds, walnuts, and fatty fish such as salmon and sardines are excellent sources of omega-3 fatty acids. To keep skin, hair, and body tissues healthy and pliable, eat fish several times a week, or take one tablespoon of flaxseed oil, or one tablespoon of ground flaxseeds, every day. You may also find it helpful to take a daily supplement of 240mg of gamma-linolenic acid (GLA). This is an essential fatty acid which is found in evening primrose, borage, and black currant oils.

213
Eat soy foods

Soy foods such as tofu, tempeh, and soybeans contain phytoestrogens. These compounds, which are like natural estrogens, help balance hormones. Eat about 2oz (60g) of soy foods daily.

214
Balance estrogen levels with black cohosh

Black cohosh helps balance estrogen levels and is excellent for relieving hot flashes, vaginal thinning, and mood swings. Take half a teaspoon of liquid black cohosh extract twice a day for at least three months.

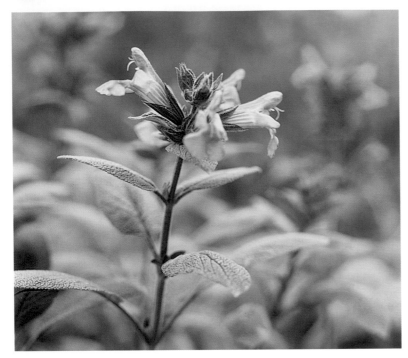

Purple sage has antimicrobial properties

Yeast Infection

Yeast infections are characterized by vaginal itching, irritation, and inflammation accompanied by a white discharge. These common infections are caused by an overgrowth of *Candida albicans*, fungi that normally inhabit the vagina. Overgrowth is often caused by a general systemic weakness brought on by stress, a high-sugar diet, or hormonal fluctuations, which upset the normal acidic balance of the vagina.

215
Starve the fungi

Help prevent vaginal yeast infections by avoiding sugars and refined foods, which feed the *Candida albicans* organism. Take supplements of *Lactobacillus acidophilus*, one with each meal for one month, to help repopulate the healthy intestinal flora that keep fungi in check.

216
Restore healthy vaginal flora

After a yeast infection, help restore the healthy flora in the vagina by inserting a capsule of *Lactobacillus acidophilus* into the vagina at night before sleeping. Repeat each night for two weeks. The capsule will dissolve during the night.

217
Preventing yeast infections

To prevent yeast infections, avoid tight-fitting clothing and synthetic underwear, which encourage the proliferation of yeast organisms. Stay away from scented toilet paper, deodorant soaps, and deodorant tampons and menstrual pads. All contain chemicals that dry out sensitive vaginal tissues and lay the groundwork for infectious microorganisms to breed.

218
Herbal vagina rinse

A strong infusion of thyme, rosemary, and sage is a potent infection fighter. It has antimicrobial properties which inhibit the overgrowth of the fungi, and astringent properties which soothe irritated tissues.

1½ cups (375ml) boiling water

2 teaspoons dried thyme

1 teaspoon dried rosemary

1 teaspoon dried sage

Pour the water over the herbs, cover, and steep for 20 minutes. Strain, and use as a vaginal wash twice daily.

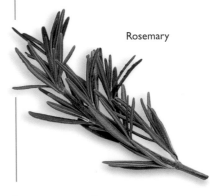

Rosemary

Prostate Enlargement

After the age of 40, many men are diagnosed with benign prostatic hyperplasia (BPH), also known as prostate enlargement. Symptoms include an increased need to urinate and a decreased force in the urine stream. Prostate enlargement is caused by hormonal changes associated with aging. Dietary changes and herbal remedies are often effective treatments. As with all medical conditions, see your doctor for an accurate diagnosis.

219
Eat healthful fats

A diet high in cholesterol and fat increases production of the hormone dihydrotestosterone, which stimulates prostate growth. Reduce all the saturated fats, hydrogenated fats, and polyunsaturated oils in your diet, and substitute the healthful fats found in extra-virgin olive oil, raw nuts and seeds, avocados, and cold-water fish such as salmon and trout.

220
Pumpkin seeds for a healthy prostate gland

Pumpkin seeds are an especially rich source of zinc, an essential nutrient for maintaining healthy prostate function. Eat a quarter of a cup (35g) of raw seeds and take 30mg of supplemental zinc every day.

221
Take saw palmetto

Saw palmetto is an herb that alleviates prostate enlargement by blocking the formation of the hormone dihydrotestosterone. Take 160mg twice daily of a saw palmetto extract that has been standardized to contain 85 percent fatty acids and sterols, the active ingredients. It takes about six weeks of continual use to see results.

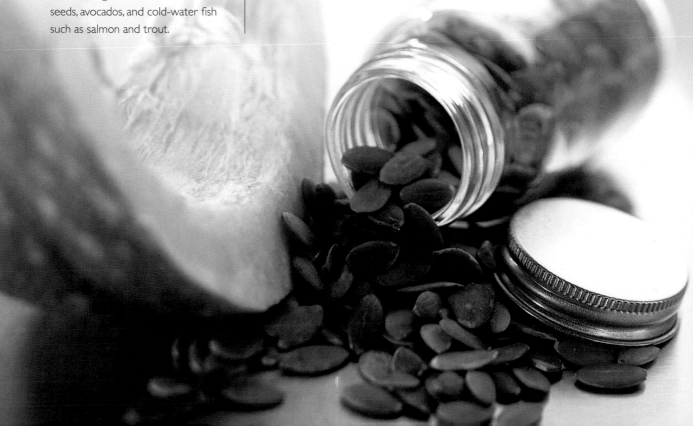

Pumpkin seeds keep the prostate gland healthy

Urinary Tract Infections

Infections of the urinary tract are commonly known as cystitis in women and urethritis in men. It is important to catch these infections at the very first sign (often a burning sensation and an increased need to urinate) to prevent a more serious infection. Consult your doctor for any type of urinary tract infection, or if you have a fever or blood in your urine.

222
Drink cranberry juice

Cranberry juice helps prevent and treat bladder infections. It makes the walls of the bladder slippery and prevents bacteria from gaining a hold.

2fl oz (60ml) water
4fl oz (125ml) unsweetened
     cranberry juice
2fl oz (60ml) unsweetened apple juice

Combine the ingredients in a glass. Drink six glasses daily at the first sign of a bladder infection. If you're prone to such infections, drink two glasses every day as a preventive measure.

Cranberry and apple juice

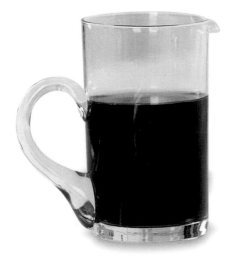

223
Flush out bacteria

Drinking plenty of water—at least six glasses daily—flushes the bladder of problem-causing bacteria and can help prevent bladder infections.

224
Drink parsley tea

Parsley has natural diuretic properties and helps cleanse the bladder of infectious organisms.

$1/2$ cup (20g) coarsely chopped fresh
     parsley
2 quarts (2.5 liters) water

Simmer the parsley and the water for five minutes in a covered pot, steep for 15 minutes, and strain. Drink the tea over a period of three hours to flush out the bladder.

225
Drink uva ursi tea

Uva ursi contains a potent antiseptic that combats urinary tract infections.

1 cup (250ml) boiling water
1 teaspoon dried uva ursi leaves

Pour the boiling water over the leaves. Cover, steep for 15 minutes, and strain. Drink three cups daily at the first sign of infection. Continue for three days after the symptoms have subsided. Alternatively, take half a teaspoon of uva ursi tincture three times a day in a small amount of warm water. Don't drink cranberry juice while you are taking uva ursi because the herb works best in an alkaline environment.

226
Fight the infection

Uva ursi, echinacea, and goldenseal make a powerful infection-fighting formula for urinary tract infections.

1fl oz (30ml) uva ursi extract
$1/2$fl oz (15ml) echinacea extract
$1/2$fl oz (15ml) goldenseal extract

Combine extracts in a dark glass bottle. Shake well, and take one teaspoon in a small amount of warm water four times a day. *Caution:* Avoid goldenseal if you have high blood pressure or are pregnant.

227
Ease discomfort with a sandalwood bath

An aromatherapy bath can help to ease the pelvic discomfort that often accompanies a bladder infection. Sandalwood is used in Ayurvedic medicine for treating urinary tract infections. Add 10 drops of sandalwood essential oil to a bath of comfortably warm water and soak for 20 minutes to ease the pelvic discomfort. Repeat daily until the infection has subsided.

Colic & Diaper Rash

Colic in young babies is characterized by gas pains, abdominal distension, flatulence, and irritability. For the usual diaper rash (rough, red, and covering the entire diapered area) use an herbal salve to heal and protect delicate skin. For the rarer diaper rash caused by *Candida albicans* (fiery red and in the creases of the legs and buttocks) avoid salves, and dust with herbal powder.

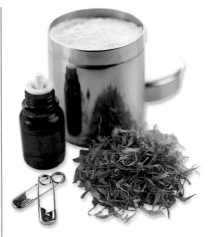

Herbal baby powder prevents diaper rash

228
Foods to avoid to combat colic

Cow's milk is a primary cause of colic in bottle-fed infants; but even breast-fed babies can suffer from colic if the mother has eaten something that the baby's sensitive digestive tract cannot tolerate. As a result, nursing mothers should avoid cow's milk products, spicy foods, and caffeine (found in tea, coffee, chocolate, and caffeinated soft drinks). Other dietary offenders that may cause colic include cabbage, cauliflower, garlic, wheat, citrus fruits, soy products, corn, and eggs.

229
Ease colic cramps with chamomile

Chamomile is an antispasmodic and a gentle sedative; it soothes both the physical and emotional tension caused by colic. There are two ways you can use chamomile to ease your baby's colic. Put two drops of chamomile essential oil in a small tub of warm water and gently bathe the infant. Or you can add five drops of chamomile essential oil to one ounce (30g) of almond oil and gently massage the baby's abdomen.

230
Herbal relief for colic

Chamomile and fennel promote digestion and help expel gas.

- 1 cup (250ml) boiling water
- 1 teaspoon dried chamomile
- 1 teaspoon fennel seeds

Pour the water over the herbs. Cover, and steep for 10 minutes. Strain, and give the baby a dropperful as often as needed.

231
Warm relief for colic

To ease colic pains, place a warm hot-water bottle on the baby's abdomen for a few minutes.

232
Bath for irritated skin

Oatmeal contains soothing mucilage, which helps calm irritated skin. Grind half a cup (100g) of rolled oats into a fine powder in a blender; add to a lukewarm bath along with three drops of lavender essential oil, which has anti-inflammatory properties. Bathe the baby gently. Avoid using soap; it further irritates tender skin.

233
Herbal baby powder to prevent chafing

Herbal baby powder can absorb excess moisture and help prevent diaper rash. Calendula has antifungal properties, and lavender essential oil soothes irritated skin.

- ½ cup (15g) dried calendula flowers
- 1 cup (100g) arrowroot powder
- ¼ teaspoon lavender essential oil

Pull the petals off the calendula flowers and grind them into a fine powder in a clean coffee grinder. Stir into the arrowroot, then add the lavender oil drop by drop, mixing it thoroughly into the powder with your fingertips. Powder your baby's skin at every diaper change.

234
Calendula healer

To protect your baby's tender skin from chafing and to help heal irritated skin, apply a salve containing calendula at every diaper change.

Arthritis

Arthritis is an inflammation of the joints and cartilage that can affect any part of the body. The main symptoms of osteoarthritis, the most common form of arthritis, are pain and stiffness; they are generally relieved by resting the affected joint. Rheumatoid arthritis is an inflammatory disease that affects people of all ages and is thought to be an autoimmune disorder that causes the body to attack its own tissues. The primary symptom is painful, stiff joints that become swollen, tender, and deformed. Fatigue, a low-grade fever, and depression may accompany rheumatoid arthritis.

Cayenne peppers

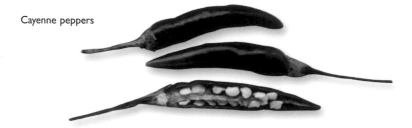

235
Avoid dietary allergens

People with rheumatoid arthritis often have food allergies and may benefit from consulting with a health practitioner for guidance. Eliminating the most common food allergens (wheat, corn, beef, and dairy products) is a good place to begin. Avoiding foods from the nightshade family (tomatoes, potatoes, eggplant, and peppers) is also helpful.

236
Relieve inflammation with healthful fats

To relieve inflammation, avoid saturated animal fats and eliminate polyunsaturated, hydrogenated, and partially hydrogenated oils from your diet. Beneficial fats that alleviate inflammation include extra-virgin olive oil and omega-3 fatty acids found in cold-water fish (such as salmon, sardines, or herring), and walnuts and flaxseeds. Use olive oil as your primary source of fat, and eat one to two servings daily of foods rich in omega-3 fats.

237
Supplements for arthritis

For osteoarthritis, take 500mg of glucosamine sulfate, three times a day, to help relieve pain and inflammation and to stimulate regeneration of cartilage. For rheumatoid arthritis, take 400mg of bromelain between meals, three times a day, to help reduce joint swelling.

238
Herbal anti-inflammatories

Ginger and turmeric help reduce the inflammation associated with rheumatoid arthritis. Include both frequently in cooking, and take either one 500mg capsule of powdered ginger, or one 400mg capsule of curcumin (the active ingredient in turmeric), three times daily.

239
Cayenne cream

To ease the pain of arthritis, apply a cream containing capsaicin, the active ingredient in cayenne pepper, to painful areas.

240
Aromatherapy pain relief

A hot bath with eucalyptus and rosemary essential oils helps ease painful, stiff joints. Add five drops of each to a bathtub of hot water and soak for 15 minutes.

241
Keep exercising for mobility

Gentle exercise, such as walking, tai chi, yoga, and swimming, improves circulation to the joints, slows down cartilage loss, and improves range of motion. Aim for at least 30 minutes of exercise daily, and be sure to include stretching as well as some aerobic activity.

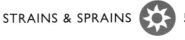

Strains & Sprains

Strains occur when muscles are overstretched. Sprains affect ligaments and usually happen when a joint is suddenly wrenched. Symptoms for both include pain, swelling, bruising, and stiffness in the affected area.

242
First aid for a muscle injury

Elevate the affected area immediately, and apply a cold pack to reduce swelling and inflammation. On the first day, apply the cold pack to the injury for 20 minutes each hour for at least six hours. On the second and third days, apply the cold packs at least three times a day for 20 minutes at a time. To minimize the swelling, wrap the injury with an elastic compression bandage.

243
Making a cold pack

To make a homemade cold pack, fill a heavy zipper-lock bag with three parts water and one part rubbing alcohol. Freeze, and use as needed.

244
Exercise to heal faster

Rest the injured part as much as you can for several days. After the initial sharp pain and swelling subside, begin gentle stretching and move normally to prevent continuing stiffness. The stretching helps increase circulation to the injured area and prevents the buildup of scar tissue.

245
Herbal pain relief

Valerian is a potent sedative, ginger is an anti-inflammatory, and white willow bark contains salicin, from which aspirin was originally derived.

1fl oz (30ml) valerian extract
½fl oz (15ml) white willow bark extract
¼fl oz (7.5ml) ginger extract

Mix the extracts and store in a dark glass bottle. Take half to one teaspoon of the mixture in a quarter of a cup (60ml) of warm water up to four times a day as needed.

246
Take turmeric for inflammation

The inflammation that occurs with a muscle injury can be relieved with the aid of turmeric. Take 300mg of turmeric twice daily, or add liberal amounts of powdered turmeric to food—it's great in curries, soups, and egg and vegetable dishes.

247
Encourage healing with arnica

Arnica helps control swelling, bruising, and inflammation. Apply arnica gel liberally to the injured muscle three times a day until the injury has healed. *Caution:* Do not apply arnica to broken skin.

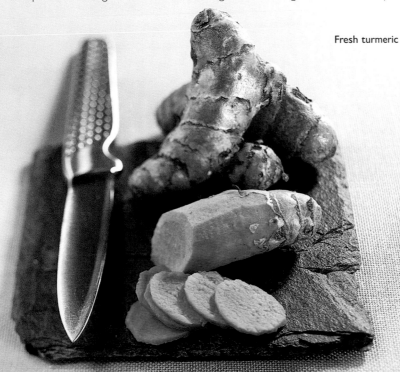

Fresh turmeric

248
Alternate heat and cold to speed recovery

After the swelling and pain have lessened, apply alternating heat and cold to the affected area to increase circulation and speed recovery. Apply a hot pack for five minutes then a cold pack for three minutes. Repeat the sequence three times, ending with the cold pack.

249
Ease pain with a hot salt pack

A hot salt pack can ease pain and stimulate circulation, which in turn speeds healing. Heat one pound (500g) of salt in a heavy pan. Funnel the hot salt into a clean, heavy sock. Do not overfill the sock—it should be pliable, like a beanbag. Pin the end securely and apply the warm sock to the painful muscle area. Leave in place for 30 minutes.

250
Prevent stiffness with aromatherapy massage

Regular massage helps prevent the residual stiffness from a muscle injury. Rosemary and peppermint essential oils improve circulation.

1fl oz (30ml) almond oil

15 drops rosemary essential oil

5 drops peppermint essential oil

Combine the oils in a dark glass bottle. Shake well, and rub a small amount into the injured muscle each day until the muscle heals.

Backache

The most common causes of low back pain are poor posture, lack of exercise, weak abdominal or lower back muscles, and lifting heavy objects improperly. Yoga, acupuncture, or chiropractic treatments are often effective for relieving chronic back pain. In addition, exercises to strengthen your back and abdominal muscles are essential. If back pain is accompanied by numbness in your leg or foot, or loss of bladder or bowel function, see your physician immediately.

251
Help from the freezer

A large package of frozen peas or frozen corn makes a handy substitute for an ice pack.

252
First aid for back pain

At the first sign of back pain or strain, apply a cold pack to your lower back for 20 minutes at a time to calm the inflammation. Repeat as often as desired, taking a 15-minute break in between cold applications. Use an ice pack or a gel-filled cold pack and be sure to wrap it in a towel to prevent freezing the skin.

253
Arnica for soreness

Arnica gel or ointment helps ease muscle pain and soreness and has anti-inflammatory properties. It will

Apply arnica ointment to ease muscle soreness

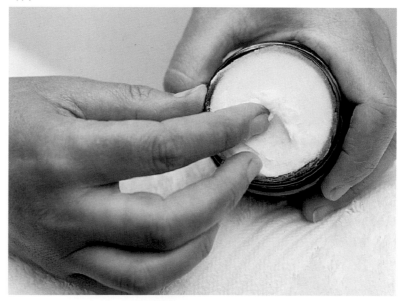

also speed the healing process. Rub a liberal amount into your back three to four times a day until the pain has subsided. **Caution:** Do not apply arnica to broken skin.

254
Ease soreness with aromatherapy

Once the initial inflammation of a backache has subsided, soak in a hot aromatherapy bath to encourage healing and alleviate soreness. Epsom salts promote relaxation; marjoram helps relieve pain and is deeply relaxing; rosemary eases muscle stiffness; and lavender is both a mild antispasmodic and gentle sedative.

2 cups (250g) Epsom salts
5 drops marjoram essential oil
5 drops rosemary essential oil
5 drops lavender essential oil

Mix the Epsom salts and essential oils together and add to a tubful of hot water. Soak for 20 minutes.

255
Herbal relief for muscle spasms

A combination of valerian, skullcap, and cramp bark helps ease muscle spasms and pain.

1fl oz (30ml) valerian extract
1fl oz (30ml) skullcap extract
1fl oz (30ml) cramp bark extract

Combine the extracts together in a dark glass bottle. Shake well, and take half a teaspoon three times a day in a small amount of warm water until the spasms subside.

256
Strengthening exercises to prevent back pain

Strengthening your abdominal muscles is necessary for preventing low back pain. Bent-leg sit-ups are one of the easiest and most effective exercises you can practice. Lie down on your back with your knees bent and your feet flat on the floor. Cross your arms in front of your chest and gently lift your head, shoulders, and upper back off the floor. Keeping your lower back pressed into the floor, concentrate on using your stomach muscles to raise your upper body. Exhale as you come up. Gently roll back down until your upper body is once again flat on the floor. Repeat as many times as you can, working up to five sets of 20 repetitions each. **Caution:** Practice these exercises in your own time and do only what is comfortable for you. Do not strain yourself by trying too hard.

257
Stretch out pain

Gentle stretching helps ease pain and stiffness in your back. Lie flat on your back with one leg straight out in front of you and the other knee bent. Gently pull your bent knee into your chest, keeping your lower back flat by pressing down into the floor. Hold for ten seconds, release, and repeat with the other leg. Work up to three sets of 10 repetitions each.

Carpal Tunnel Syndrome

Constant, repetitive hand movements can cause inflammation and swelling of tissues. This pinches the nerves passing through the narrow opening (the carpal tunnel) in the wrist bones. Symptoms include pain, tingling, numbness, and weakness in the hands; the pain may radiate up the arm and shoulder.

258
Use cold compresses to relieve pain

Applying cold packs to the affected wrist can help shrink the swelling, ease the inflammation, and relieve the pain associated with carpal tunnel syndrome. Place a cold gel pack or ice pack on the affected wrist for 15 minutes and then take a break for 15 minutes. Repeat the sequence as often as desired until the pain has been relieved.

259
Wrist exercises

Gentle wrist exercises can help by opening up the carpal tunnel and taking pressure off the nerve. Bend your elbows, bringing your hands up into the air, and rotate your wrists in circles for one minute. Follow by clenching your fists gently and then spreading your fingers wide apart; repeat 10 times. It's most helpful to repeat these exercises often throughout the day.

Diabetes

Diabetes is a serious disease and treatment should always be supervised by a qualified health-care professional. Type II diabetes (also known as adult-onset diabetes), the most common form, is conventionally treated with drugs that stimulate insulin production and control blood-sugar levels. Mild cases of Type II diabetes can almost always be managed with diet and exercise.

260
Avoid refined carbohydrates

If you eat refined sugars and food products manufactured with white flour, such as breads, pastas, cookies, and pastries, you will flood your bloodstream with excess sugar. The effect of this is to put stress on the organs and glands that regulate the levels of sugar in your blood. Instead, eat complex carbohydrates, such as whole grains, and satisfy your sweet tooth with fresh fruits.

261
Eat to stabilize blood sugar

High-fiber foods, especially lentils and black beans, which contain soluble fiber, can help normalize blood-sugar levels. Protein and healthful fats also help keep blood-sugar levels stable. Eat about 3oz (90g) of lean protein twice a day. Be sure your daily diet also includes foods that contain monounsaturated fats (for example, extra-virgin olive oil, raw nuts and seeds, and avocados) and omega-3 fatty acids (for example, cold-water fish, such as salmon, sardines, and mackerel, and walnuts and flaxseeds).

262
Herbal help for diabetes

The herb gymnema has been used for centuries in Ayurvedic medicine to treat diabetes. Gymnema enhances the production of insulin and helps decrease blood-sugar levels. Take 200mg of gymnema twice a day.
Caution: If you are taking drugs for diabetes, make sure you consult your doctor before taking gymnema.

263
Control blood sugar with chromium

The element chromium can help control the levels of sugar and insulin in the bloodstream. Take 200mcg of a chromium supplement three times a day with meals.

264
Control blood sugar with daily exercise

Regular exercise—a 30-minute walk daily is sufficient—is one of the best ways to help your cells use glucose efficiently and to keep your blood sugar from climbing to dangerous levels. Exercise also helps you lose weight so that your body can use insulin more effectively.

Low Blood Sugar

Symptoms of low blood sugar, also known as hypoglycemia, include fatigue, irritability, headaches, dizziness, nausea, and mental confusion. The symptoms generally appear two to three hours after eating, especially if you've eaten sugar or refined carbohydrates. Dietary changes and herbs can help keep blood sugar and energy levels stable.

265
Exercise regularly

Regular exercise uses energy by burning glucose and so helps your body to maintain a healthy level of sugar in your bloodstream. Try to get into the habit of engaging in at least 30 minutes of moderate aerobic exercise, such as walking, swimming, or biking, every day.

266
Regulate blood sugar with ginseng

Siberian ginseng increases energy and strengthens the adrenal glands, which play an important role in regulating blood sugar. Buy an extract that has been standardized for eleutherosides and take approximately 250mg twice a day. It is safe to take for up to six weeks. **Caution:** If you have high blood pressure, consult your doctor before using any type of ginseng.

267
Dietary suggestions

Cut out sugar, refined carbohydrates, and caffeine to keep blood-sugar levels on an even keel. Make sure that each meal contains protein and fat. Choose healthful fats such as those found in raw nuts, avocados, olive oil, and cold-water fish (for example, salmon, sardines, and mackerel). Eat a small meal or a protein-rich snack every three hours for a steady supply of fuel. In addition, take a high-potency multivitamin and mineral formula that contains 200mcg of chromium picolinate, a trace mineral that helps stabilize blood-sugar levels.

268
Herbal tea for hypoglycemia

Licorice and burdock tea can help stabilize blood-sugar levels. Licorice root strengthens the adrenal glands; burdock root improves liver function. Both play a role in regulating blood sugar. **Caution:** Because licorice may cause water retention in susceptible individuals, people with high blood pressure or kidney disease should consult a doctor or medical herbalist before using it.

3 cups (750ml) water
1 tablespoon dried licorice root
1 tablespoon dried burdock root

Simmer the ingredients in a covered pot for 15 minutes. Strain, and drink up to three cups a day for a month.

Eat avocados to help boost low blood-sugar levels

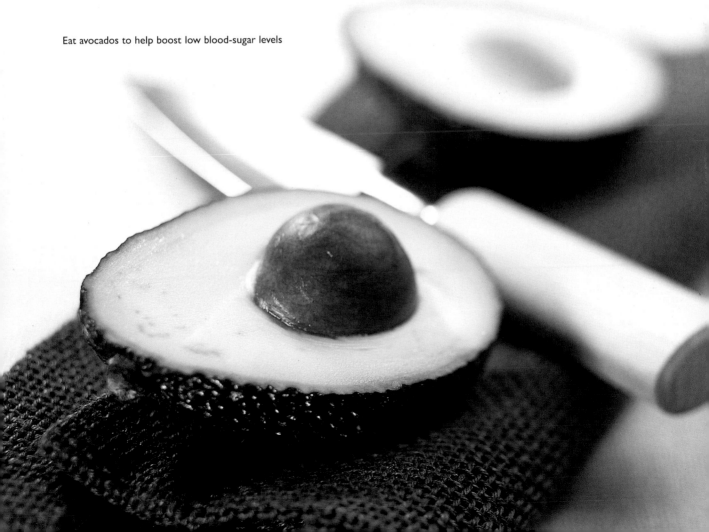

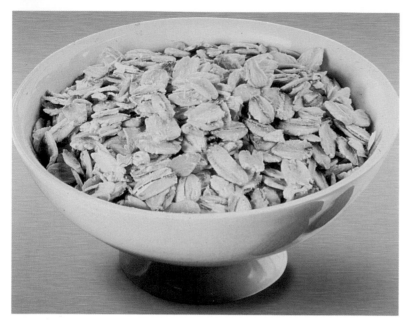

The high fiber in oats can reduce cholesterol

High Cholesterol

High levels of blood cholesterol are a primary factor in heart disease, heart attacks, and strokes. In most people, elevated cholesterol levels are caused by a diet high in saturated and hydrogenated fats, and by a sedentary lifestyle. Simple dietary changes and exercise are usually all that's needed to bring cholesterol levels into a healthy range.

269
Eat fiber to lower cholesterol

A diet high in soluble fiber helps to absorb excess cholesterol in the intestinal tract and sweep it out of the body. Oatmeal, oat bran, barley, and cooked dried beans and legumes are some of your best bets for lowering cholesterol. Eat at least one of these foods daily. In addition, eat five servings or more of fresh vegetables, and two servings of fresh fruit every day. Apples, berries, oranges, peaches, bananas, broccoli, carrots, green beans, corn, prunes, spinach, and sweet potatoes are all excellent sources of soluble fiber.

270
Replace unhealthful fats with healthful fats

Saturated fats (found in butter, cheese, and meat) and hydrogenated fats (found in shortening, margarine, and many processed foods) raise blood-cholesterol levels. But healthful fats, such as the monounsaturated fat found in extra-virgin olive oil and the omega-3 fatty acids found in cold-water fish, walnuts, and flaxseeds, do the opposite. They help make arteries more flexible and lower cholesterol levels. Use extra-virgin olive oil for cooking and salads, and eat at least one serving daily of a food rich in omega-3 fats.

271
Eat garlic to lower cholesterol

Garlic not only decreases levels of harmful low-density lipoprotein (LDL) cholesterol, but it also increases levels of beneficial, heart-protective high-density lipoprotein (HDL) cholesterol. Just one clove of garlic daily is usually enough to help regulate cholesterol levels—but the more you can eat, the better.

272
Exercise to prevent high cholesterol

Regular aerobic exercise is essential for preventing and reducing high cholesterol levels. This means you need to exercise at least 30 minutes every day, five days a week. Aerobic exercise lowers damaging low-density lipoprotein (LDL) cholesterol and raises healthful high-density lipoprotein (HDL) cholesterol. Try to exercise outdoors in the fresh air as much as possible; sunlight, in reasonable amounts, helps your body to metabolize cholesterol and to lower cholesterol levels.

High Blood Pressure

High blood pressure (hypertension) is caused by a variety of factors. Hardening of the arteries and emotional stress are often contributing factors. For most people, lifestyle changes bring their blood pressure into a healthy range. Work with your doctor to monitor your blood pressure and track your progress.

273
Eat fresh fruits and vegetables

Fresh fruits and vegetables are rich in potassium, calcium, magnesium, fiber, and vitamin C—all help lower blood pressure. Strive for as many as 10 servings daily: eat vegetables and fruits with every meal and as snacks.

274
Eat celery, garlic, and onions

Celery is a traditional Chinese remedy which is thought to help relax the smooth muscles of the artery walls. Garlic and onions also help relax the blood vessels. Eat four stalks of celery and at least one clove of garlic or half an onion every day.

275
Exercise aerobically to reduce stress

Make sure you do at least 30 minutes of moderate aerobic exercise, such as brisk walking, bicycling, or dancing, five times a week. This will not only improve your cardiovascular health but also help decrease your levels of stress hormones which can otherwise raise your blood pressure.

276
Relax to lower blood pressure

Emotional stress is often a factor in hypertension. Eliminate stress triggers if possible, but more importantly, identify and change the way that you respond to stressful situations. Learn to slow down, to relax, and to take life with gentleness and humor. Practice some form of relaxation every day. Meditation, yoga, tai chi, and deep relaxation exercises help regulate breathing and heart rate, relax tense muscles, and reduce stress hormone levels.

277
Reduce blood pressure with herbs

Hawthorn dilates the arteries and so helps lower blood pressure. Linden calms the emotional tension that often underlies high blood pressure. Yarrow dilates the peripheral blood vessels and acts as a mild diuretic.

Caution: Hawthorn is a restricted herb and must be prescribed by a qualified herbalist.

3 cups (750ml) boiling water
3 teaspoons crushed dried hawthorn
    berries
3 teaspoons dried linden
2 teaspoons dried yarrow

Pour the water over the herbs. Cover, and steep for 20 minutes. Strain, and drink three cups a day.

Fresh vegetables and hawthorn berries help lower blood pressure

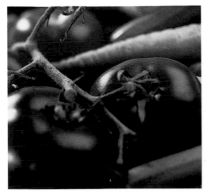 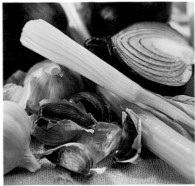 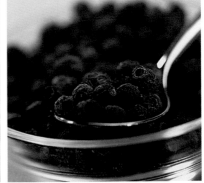

Varicose & Spider Veins

Varicose veins and spider veins are not only unsightly, they can be painful, too. Both are caused by weakened valves in the leg veins that allow blood to pool, forcing the veins to expand. Varicose veins may develop in otherwise healthy people if they stand for long periods without movement.

278
Take anthocyanins to strengthen the veins

Blueberries, cherries, blackberries, and purple grapes are all rich sources of pigments known as anthocyanins. These compounds have been shown to strengthen the veins. Eat at least one cup (120g) daily of anthocyanin-rich fruit to prevent and treat varicose veins.

Blueberries, cherries, blackberries, and purple grapes contain anthocyanins

279
Preventing varicose veins

Avoid anything that puts stress on the veins: sitting or standing for a long time, constipation, excess weight, or tight clothing that constricts blood flow. Regular exercise such as walking is also helpful; the contraction of the leg muscles pushes the blood through the veins and keeps it from pooling in the legs.

280
Eat high-fiber foods

A diet rich in fiber helps prevent constipation, a primary contributing factor to varicose veins. Eat plenty of fresh vegetables, fruits, whole grains, legumes, nuts, and seeds daily. For an extra fiber boost, each morning take one tablespoon of powdered psyllium husks stirred into a glass of water. Follow with another glass of water.

281
Spice up your diet

Garlic, onions, ginger, and cayenne help your body break down fibrin, the protein that creates the hard, lumpy tissue surrounding varicose veins. Include at least one or two fibrin-fighting foods in your daily diet to help relieve varicose veins.

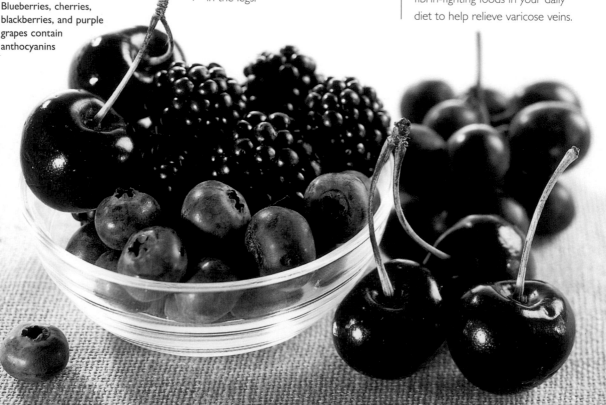

282
Supplement with grape-seed extract

Grape-seed extract is a good source of antioxidants, which can strengthen veins and capillaries. Each day take 300mg of a standardized extract of grape-seed containing 85 to 95 percent procyanidins, regarded as the primary active compounds.

283
Take horse chestnut

Horse chestnut improves circulation in the legs, reduces inflammation, and strengthens capillaries and veins. Take 300mg twice daily of an extract standardized for aescin, regarded as the primary active compound in horse chestnut. It may take three months to see results. **Caution:** Do not exceed the daily recommended dose. While this dose can be taken safely for an indefinite period of time, larger doses can be toxic.

284
Soothing aromatherapy lotion

Witch hazel extract and the essential oils of cypress and yarrow can help to reduce the swelling of varicose veins and soothe inflammation.

4fl oz (125ml) distilled witch hazel
    extract
10 drops cypress essential oil
10 drops yarrow essential oil

Mix the ingredients in a bottle and shake well. Apply to your legs as often as desired.

Hemorrhoids

Hemorrhoids are anal varicose veins and are most often caused by constipation or straining during elimination. Dietary changes relieve constipation, and herbal remedies provide relief from pain.

285
Calendula salve

Calendula promotes healing and soothes irritation. Apply calendula salve to the swollen veins twice every day until they subside.

286
Dietary suggestions for constipation

To prevent constipation, include several servings of fiber-rich foods in your daily diet—fresh vegetables, fruits, whole grains, and nuts. In addition, drink at least six glasses of water a day. A diet that is rich in both fiber and water creates bulkier, softer bowel movements.

287
Ease discomfort with witch hazel

To help relieve discomfort and shrink hemorrhoids, apply cotton pads soaked with witch hazel extract several times daily. Leave in place for 10 minutes whenever possible. Witch hazel has both astringent and cooling properties.

Dried and fresh bark

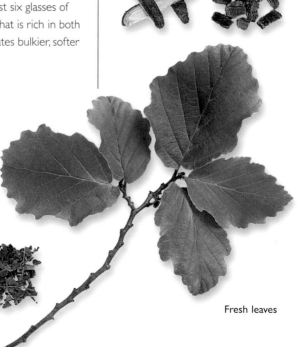

Witch hazel has astringent properties

Dried leaves

Fresh leaves

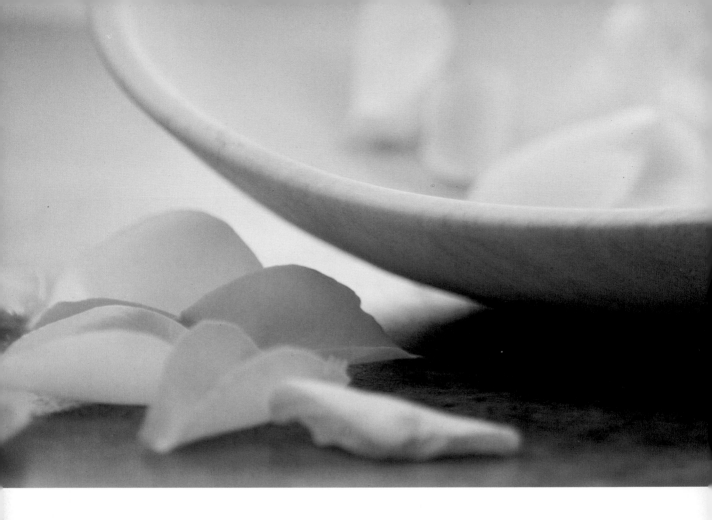

NATURAL
BEAUTY

· ·

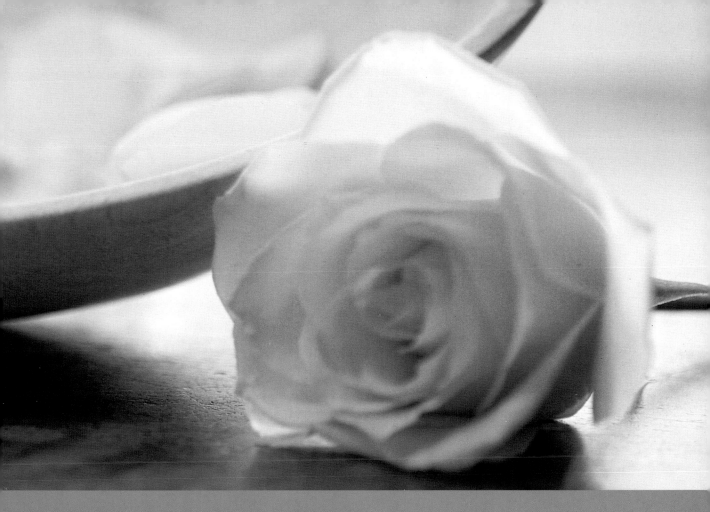

Real beauty doesn't come from a bottle or a jar— it comes from within us. There is just no substitute for the healthy glow that comes from taking care of yourself naturally, with a nutritious diet, regular exercise, and plenty of relaxation, rest, and play. At the same time, natural beauty and body-care treatments can help you look good and feel your best.

In this chapter, you will find hundreds of simple recipes, handy tips, and nourishing remedies for caring for your body from head to toe—from skin and hair to eyes, lips, hands, elbows, knees, nails, and feet. Spending time making and using these special beauty treatments is a wonderful way to unwind.

The skin-care products are easy to make, inexpensive, and provide your skin with all the moisture and nourishment it needs to look great. The shampoos, conditioners, and other hair-care products are specifically organized by hair type—discover your own and enjoy the fragrant benefits that herbs and essential oils can bring.

What better way to end the chapter than with recipes for heavenly baths. Soaking in a luxurious bath is the ultimate at-home spa experience and a terrific way to indulge in a little self-nurturing. Depending on which herbs and essential oils you choose, and the water temperature you select, baths are wonderfully versatile. They are able to soothe, detoxify, and energize your body, mind, and spirit.

Nutrients for Great Skin

The following nutrients are essential for healthy skin. Many are antioxidants, which neutralize the free radicals that damage skin and cause aging. Don't forget to drink at least eight glasses of water daily, and to reduce your intake of alcohol and caffeine.

288
Vitamin A

Vitamin A helps rebuild tissue and reduce excess production of sebum (oil). Beta-carotene, a compound stored in the skin and used by the body to produce vitamin A, is an antioxidant. Foods rich in vitamin A and beta-carotene include yellow and orange fruits and vegetables, and dark leafy greens such as kale and collards. Supplement your diet with 4,000 IU of vitamin A daily. **Caution:** If you are pregnant or trying to conceive, don't take more than 4,000 IU a day. Higher doses can increase the risk of birth defects.

289
Vitamin C

This potent antioxidant and immune system booster is also used to make collagen, a component of your body's connective tissue. Citrus fruits, red and green peppers, and broccoli are rich in vitamin C. Supplement your diet with one 250 to 500mg tablet of vitamin C daily.

290
Vitamin E

Vitamin E scavenges your body for damaging free radicals. Increase your intake of vitamin E by eating nuts, seeds, avocados, and extra-virgin olive oil daily. It's hard to get enough of this powerful antioxidant without supplementing your diet so take one 400 IU capsule daily.

Red peppers and broccoli contain vitamin C

291
Omega-3 fatty acids

These "good" fats fight inflammation of the skin and increase resiliency and lubrication of your body's tissues. You can find omega-3 fatty acids in cold-water fish, such as salmon, or in flaxseed oil or ground flaxseeds. An easy way to supplement your diet is to take one tablespoon of flaxseed oil every day.

Facial Skin Care Basics

Whatever your skin type—normal, dry, or oily—you need a regular routine to help give your complexion a fresh, healthy glow. Follow a daily program of proper cleansing, toning, and moisturizing, and treat your skin to weekly or monthly facials.

292
Facial cleansers

Everyone should clean their face at least once daily (twice if necessary) with warm water and a cleanser specific to their skin type. Soaps are generally too harsh to use on facial skin: they strip away natural, moisture-retaining oils and cause dryness. Gentle ingredients, such as herbs, milk, yogurt, and vegetable glycerin, clean skin without drying.

293
Astringents and toners

Use astringents and toners after face cleaning to help restore a healthy pH balance to the skin. Astringents work best for skin that tends to be oily or blemished—they remove excess oil and temporarily tighten enlarged pores. Natural astringents include witch hazel, peppermint, yarrow, and sage. Toners are gentler and rely on soothing ingredients such as rose water, aloe, chamomile, and lavender.

294
Moisturizers

Moisturize your skin immediately after applying toner, while your face is still damp. Water helps keep your skin plump and moist. Choose a natural moisturizer appropriate for your skin type. Dry skin responds well to moisturizers such as cocoa butter, which contain rich plant oils. Oily skin benefits more from lighter moisturizers such as aloe. Adding vitamin E and grapefruit-seed extract to your homemade remedies helps to prevent bacterial growth.

295
Skin-refining scrubs and exfoliants

Facial exfoliants remove accumulated dead cells that make skin look flaky or dull. The simplest are made from finely ground grains and nuts, such as oatmeal, cornmeal, almonds, and walnuts. Use a gentle facial scrub daily for oily or normal skin, and twice a week for dry skin. Enzyme exfoliants rely on papain, a protein-dissolving enzyme that comes from papayas. Leave them on the skin for up to 15 minutes, then rinse them off with warm water. Use enzyme exfoliants once or twice a week, no matter what your skin type.

296
Facial saunas

Deep-cleaning facial saunas bring a healthy glow to the complexion. Warm steam opens pores, washes away impurities, and hydrates skin. Herbs and essential oils increase the cleansing benefits. To keep skin in top condition, use a facial sauna twice a month—weekly if you have oily or blemished skin.

297
Facial masks

In as little as 15 minutes, a facial mask tightens pores, stimulates circulation, or deep-moisturizes the skin. Use clay-based masks for cleansing and tightening, and masks rich in natural plant oils for moisturizing. Herbs and essential oils provide a variety of skin-nourishing benefits. Treat yourself to a facial mask designed for your skin type at least once a week.

298
Healing sleep

Dull skin and circles and bags under the eyes are telltale signs of sleep deprivation. For your skin to look its best, try to sleep for seven to eight hours a night.

299
Lavender glow

If you cleanse your face thoroughly before going to bed, you do not need to wash it with soap in the morning. Instead, dip a washcloth in a basin of warm water mixed with a couple of drops of lavender essential oil. Wring out the cloth and hold it to your face for a few seconds. Repeat ten times each morning and wake up to a healthy glow.

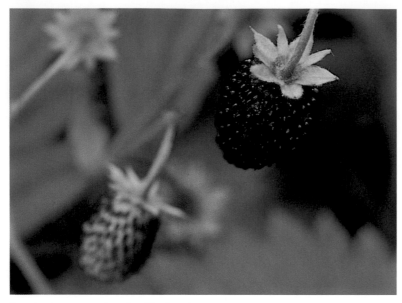

Strawberries are excellent for skin-cleansing

Caring for Normal Skin

Normal skin is clear, smooth, finely textured, and has just the right amount of natural moisture. Use a gentle cleanser, toner, and moisturizer daily, and treat yourself to regular exfoliating treatments and facials to keep your skin looking its best.

300
Simple yogurt cleanser

Yogurt and strawberries are gentle cleansers, and lavender soothes skin.

1 fresh strawberry
1 tablespoon plain whole-milk yogurt
1 drop lavender essential oil

Crush the fresh strawberry and combine the yogurt and the juice (approximately one teaspoon). Add the lavender essential oil and mix together well. Dampen your face with warm water and massage the yogurt mixture into your skin for a minute. Rinse well with warm water.

301
Herbal lotion for cleansing the face

This mild lotion can be used on most skin types. Witch hazel is a gentle astringent. Rose water, elderflower, calendula, and chamomile soothe and clean. Vegetable glycerin helps to soften and moisturize skin.

¼ cup (60ml) rose water
1 teaspoon dried elderflower
1 teaspoon dried calendula
1 teaspoon dried chamomile
¼ cup (60ml) distilled witch hazel extract
¼ cup (60ml) vegetable glycerin

Steep the herbs in witch hazel and rose water in a covered glass jar for one week. Strain, pour into a clean bottle, add the glycerin, and shake well. To use, dampen skin with warm water and gently massage lotion into the skin. Rinse with lukewarm water.

302
Aromatherapy cleanser

Rose water and aloe vera are gentle cleansers. Vegetable glycerin softens the skin, and lavender helps balance the production of oil.

¼ cup (60ml) rose water
¼ cup (60ml) vegetable glycerin
¼ cup (60ml) aloe vera gel
10 drops lavender essential oil

Mix the ingredients in a bottle and shake well. To use the cleanser, dampen your skin with warm water and gently massage the lotion in. Rinse with lukewarm water.

303
Herbal cleansing milk

An herbal skin wash made with whole milk, calendula, chamomile, and rose petals cleans normal skin without drying it out.

1 cup (250ml) whole milk
1 tablespoon dried calendula
1 tablespoon dried chamomile
1 tablespoon dried rose petals

Combine the ingredients in a glass jar. Steep the mixture overnight in the refrigerator. Strain, rebottle, and store in the refrigerator for up to one week. To cleanse your face, dampen your skin with warm water. Soak a cotton cosmetic pad in the cleansing milk and gently wipe your face. Repeat until your skin is clean. Rinse with warm water, apply toner, and follow with a moisturizer.

304
Herbal toner

This toner, which contains beneficial herbs that are soothing and healing, is excellent for normal skin. Witch hazel is mildly astringent.

1 cup (250ml) distilled witch hazel
1 teaspoon dried chamomile
1 teaspoon dried calendula
1 teaspoon dried comfrey leaf
1 teaspoon dried elderflower
1 teaspoon dried rose petals

Mix the witch hazel with the dried herbs in a glass jar. Cover with a lid and allow to steep for two weeks in a warm, dark place. Gently shake the jar every day to keep the herbs from settling. Strain, and store in a clean bottle. To use, apply to your skin with a cotton cosmetic pad after washing your face—or use as a quick skin-freshener after exercising.

305
Simple skin toner

To make a simple toner for normal skin, mix one teaspoon of distilled witch hazel with 10 drops of lavender essential oil in a 4fl oz (125ml) bottle. Shake vigorously to mix the oil with the witch hazel, then fill the bottle with distilled water. Saturate a cotton ball with toner and gently wipe it over your skin.

306
Simple moisturizer

To make a simple facial moisturizer, add 10 drops of lavender essential oil to one ounce of jojoba oil in a glass pharmacy bottle with a dropper and shake well. After cleansing your face and applying toner, massage a few drops of the oil onto your skin.

307
Aromatherapy moisturizing oil

Jojoba is moisturizing, while lavender and geranium are soothing.

1fl oz (30ml) jojoba oil
7 drops lavender essential oil
3 drops geranium essential oil

Combine the ingredients in a small glass pharmacy bottle with a dropper.

After cleansing, and while your skin is still damp, gently massage in several drops of the oil.

308
Citrus and lavender moisturizing cream

This rich cream is good in very cold or dry weather. Lavender soothes and grapefruit refreshes. Grape-seed oil is an antioxidant and aloe is healing. Jojoba and beeswax are moisturizing. Vitamin E helps preserve the cream.

2 tablespoons grape-seed oil
2 tablespoons jojoba oil
1 tablespoon grated beeswax
1 400-IU capsule vitamin E oil
¼ cup (60ml) aloe vera juice
3 drops grapefruit-seed extract
5 drops lavender essential oil
5 drops grapefruit essential oil

Essential oils are beneficial for all skin types

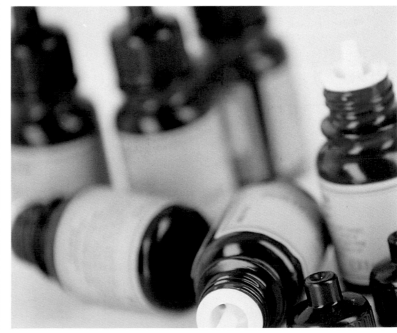

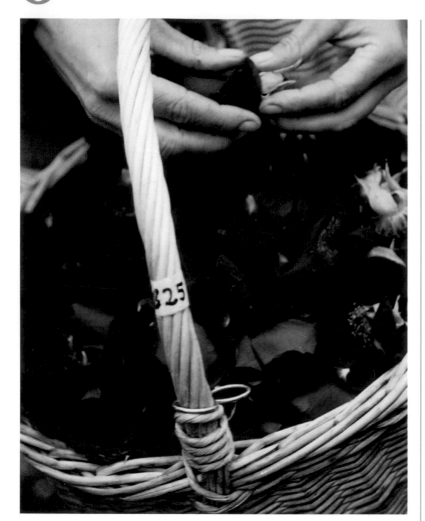

Rose petals are soothing for the skin

Warm the grape-seed oil, jojoba oil, and beeswax gently over a low heat until the wax melts. Remove from the heat. Add the capsule's contents. Warm the aloe vera juice over a low heat. Remove from the heat. When the liquids are lukewarm, slowly pour the aloe into the oil, beating steadily with a wire whisk or an electric mixer set on the lowest speed until cool, thick, and smooth. Stir in the grapefruit-seed extract and essential oils. Spoon into a clean jar and cool

completely before covering. Store in a cool place. Use the cream sparingly.

309
Simple facial scrub

Mix two parts of rolled oats with one part almond meal, both finely ground. Mix two teaspoons of the scrub with enough warm water to make a paste. Gently massage onto damp skin. Rinse your face with warm water and follow with a toner and moisturizer.

310
Facial sauna

Calendula, chamomile, rose petals, and lavender make a sweetly scented steam for normal skin.

2 quarts (2.5 liters) water
2 tablespoons dried calendula
2 tablespoons dried chamomile
2 tablespoons dried rose petals
2 tablespoons dried lavender

Bring the water and herbs to a boil in a large covered pot. Remove from the heat and allow the herbs to steep for five minutes. Place the pot on a table, remove the lid, and make a towel tent over your head and the steaming pot of herbs. Stay under the tent for 10 minutes, taking care to not burn yourself. Finish by rinsing your face with warm water and applying a toner. You could use a facial mask instead of a toner, if desired.

311
Honey and yogurt facial scrub

This scrub can be used on all skin types. Yogurt contains skin-smoothing lactic acid, honey is moisturizing and healing, finely ground almonds and oats add gentle exfoliating action, and lavender essential oil is balancing for all skin types.

1 teaspoon finely ground almonds
2 teaspoons finely ground oats
1 tablespoon plain low-fat yogurt
1 teaspoon honey
1 drop lavender essential oil

Mix all the ingredients together. To use, dampen your skin with warm water, then gently massage the scrub onto your damp skin. Rinse your face with warm water and follow with a toner and moisturizer.

312

Aromatherapy hot-towel treatment

When you don't have time for a facial sauna, try this quick cleansing treatment. Begin by washing your skin as usual. Add two drops of geranium essential oil to a basin of hot water. Soak a washcloth in the scented hot water, wring out, and apply to your face for two minutes.

313

Quick facial sauna

Pour four cups (1 liter) of boiling water over one tea bag each of chamomile and peppermint in a large heatproof bowl. Let it steep uncovered for two minutes, and then make a towel tent over your head and the bowl to capture the steam. Stay under the tent for 10 minutes, taking care to not burn yourself.

314

Aromatherapy facial steam

Pour 3 pints (1.8 liters) of boiling water into a large, heat-proof bowl. Add two drops of lavender essential oil and make a tent over your head and the bowl with a large towel. Breathe deeply, and stay under the towel for 10 minutes. Finish by rinsing your face with lukewarm water and applying moisturizer.

315

Aromatherapy facial mask

Yogurt smooths the skin's texture, cosmetic clay draws out impurities, and lavender and geranium essential oils help keep skin healthy and the complexion glowing.

2 teaspoons plain whole-milk yogurt

½ teaspoon cosmetic clay

2 drops lavender essential oil

1 drop geranium essential oil

Combine all the ingredients and mix well. Smooth the mask onto clean skin. Remove after 15 minutes with a warm, wet washcloth.

316

Honey and lavender facial mask

Honey is an excellent moisturizer for all skin types. It draws moisture into the skin, but doesn't leave skin feeling oily. Lavender essential oil is balancing for all skin types.

1 tablespoon raw honey

3 drops lavender essential oil

Combine the ingredients. Dampen your face and neck with warm water. Smooth on the honey and lavender mixture. Allow the mask to remain on your skin for 15 minutes, then rinse off with warm water.

Caring for Dry Skin

Dry skin needs plenty of moisture and protection from indoor heating, air conditioning, cold weather, and wind. Avoid harsh soaps and cleansers. Use warm, not hot, water for cleaning. Rich cleansers, toners, and moisturizers keep skin supple; mild exfoliation and facials smooth and soften rough, dry skin.

317

Pure water

Drink at least 3 pints (1.8 liters) of pure water daily to provide your skin with the moisture it needs to stay healthy. To make plain water more refreshing, add slices of lemon, lime, or orange, and a sprig of fresh mint.

318

Boost your oil intake

Dry skin is often caused by not eating enough essential fatty acids. Include healthy fats, such as extra-virgin olive oil, avocados, and walnuts, in your daily diet, and take one tablespoon of flaxseed oil daily as a supplement.

319

Simple creamy cleanser

Cream is soothing and sandalwood essential oil is moisturizing. Herbal cleansing milk (see *No. 303*) is also a good daily cleanser for dry skin.

1 tablespoon heavy cream

1 drop sandalwood essential oil

Mix the ingredients together. Dampen your face with warm water and

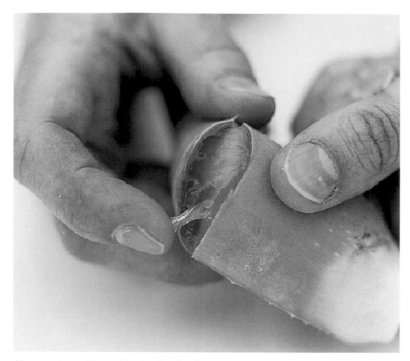

Aloe vera is soothing and healing for the skin

massage the cleanser into your skin with your fingertips for one minute. Rinse with warm water.

320
Cleansing oil

This gentle oil is good for removing makeup. Jojoba and vitamin E oils moisturize while almond oil cleanses the skin.

2fl oz (60ml) jojoba oil
2fl oz (60ml) almond oil
1 400-IU capsule vitamin E oil
10 drops carrot-seed essential oil

Mix the oils together in a small glass bottle. Shake well before using. To use, apply the cleansing oil with a cotton cosmetic pad. Follow by cleansing your skin with your choice of facial cleanser.

321
Aromatherapy cleansing lotion

Palmarosa and rose essential oils help nourish dry skin and rejuvenate mature complexions. The vegetable glycerin helps prevent the skin from losing moisture, and aloe gel is both soothing and healing.

¼ cup (60ml) rose water
¼ cup (60ml) vegetable glycerin
¼ cup (60ml) aloe vera gel
5 drops palmarosa essential oil
2 drops rose essential oil

Mix the ingredients thoroughly together in a bottle and shake well before using. Dampen your skin with warm water and gently massage some of the lotion in. Rinse with lukewarm water.

322
Herbal toner

Chamomile, calendula, comfrey, and rose soothe dry skin. Witch hazel is healing, and vegetable glycerin helps the skin retain moisture.

½ cup (125ml) distilled witch hazel
½ cup (125ml) rose water
2 teaspoons dried comfrey leaf
1 teaspoon dried chamomile
1 teaspoon dried calendula
1 teaspoon dried rose petals
1 teaspoon vegetable glycerin

Combine the ingredients in a glass jar with a tight-fitting lid. Steep the mixture for two weeks in a warm, dark place. Gently shake the jar every day to keep the herbs from settling. Strain, and store in a clean bottle. To use, saturate a cotton cosmetic pad with the toner and gently wipe over your skin.

323
Aromatherapy toner

Witch hazel has healing effects and sandalwood is moisturizing. Rose water soothes dry skin, and vegetable glycerin helps draw moisture into the skin.

20 drops sandalwood essential oil
1 teaspoon distilled witch hazel
1 teaspoon vegetable glycerin
1 cup (250ml) rose water

Combine the sandalwood essential oil and witch hazel in a bottle and shake well. Add the vegetable glycerin and rose water and shake again. Saturate a cotton cosmetic pad with the toner and gently wipe over your skin.

324
Herbal scrub

Almonds and oats nourish dry skin and slough off dead skin cells. Rose petals, calendula, and comfrey soothe and heal.

2 cups (200g) rolled oats
½ cup (75g) almonds
2 tablespoons dried calendula
2 tablespoons dried rose petals
2 tablespoons dried comfrey leaf
½ teaspoon almond oil

In separate batches, finely grind the oats, almonds, and herbs in a coffee grinder or blender. Mix well, and store in a covered container in a cool, dry place. To use, mix a heaped teaspoon of cleansing grains with half a teaspoon almond oil and enough warm water to make a paste. Gently massage the mixture onto your skin, then rinse well with warm water. Use this scrub once or twice a week.

325
Aromatherapy moisturizing oil

Jojoba oil and sandalwood essential oil moisturize dry skin. Palmarosa essential oil balances the production of oil in your skin.

1fl oz (30ml) jojoba oil
7 drops sandalwood essential oil
3 drops palmarosa essential oil

Combine the ingredients thoroughly in a small glass pharmacy bottle with a dropper. After cleansing your skin, gently massage several drops of the oil onto your damp skin with your fingertips.

326
Rose moisturizing cream

Jojoba and beeswax moisturize, rose soothes and heals, and almond oil cleanses. Vitamin E and grapefruit-seed help preserve the cream.

2 tablespoons jojoba oil
2 tablespoons almond oil
1 tablespoon grated beeswax
1 400-IU capsule vitamin E oil
¼ cup (60ml) rose water
5 drops rose essential oil
3 drops grapefruit-seed extract

Warm the jojoba and almond oils with the beeswax in a pot over a low heat until the wax melts. Add the contents of the capsule. Warm the rose water over a low heat. When the liquids are lukewarm, slowly pour the rose water into the oil, beating steadily until cool, thick, and smooth. Stir in the rose essential oil and grapefruit-seed extract. Spoon into a clean jar and cool completely before covering. Store in a cool place. Apply this rich cream sparingly.

327
Avocado mask

Mash a quarter of a ripe avocado, mix with a teaspoon of plain whole-milk yogurt into a paste, and apply to

Avocado

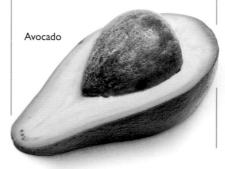

clean skin for 15 minutes. Remove with a warm, wet washcloth. Use weekly for soft, smooth skin.

328
Aromatherapy facial mask

Yogurt and jojoba oil moisturize while sandalwood and rose essential oils soothe irritation and nourish the skin.

2 teaspoons plain whole-milk yogurt
½ teaspoon jojoba oil
½ teaspoon cosmetic clay
2 drops sandalwood essential oil
1 drop rose essential oil

Mix the ingredients well and apply to clean skin. Remove after 15 minutes with a warm, wet washcloth.

329
Facial sauna

Chamomile, rose petals, elderflower, and comfrey create a beneficial steam for dry skin. Almond oil moisturizes.

2 quarts (2.5 liters) water
2 tablespoons dried chamomile
2 tablespoons dried rose petals
2 tablespoons dried elderflower
2 tablespoons dried comfrey leaf
1 teaspoon almond oil

Bring the water and herbs to a boil in a large covered pot. Let the herbs steep for five minutes. Add the almond oil. Place the pot on a table, remove the lid, and make a towel tent over your head and the pot. Remain for 10 minutes, taking care to not burn yourself. Rinse your face with warm water, and apply a toner or a facial mask if desired.

Caring for Oily Skin

Oily skin needs thorough cleansing to remove excess oil. Avoid harsh astringents that can leave skin overly dry. Gentle herbal astringents help control oiliness and temporarily tighten pores. Herbal scrubs, steams, and masks are especially helpful for deep cleansing oily skin and can be used twice a week.

Yogurt, lavender, and peppermint

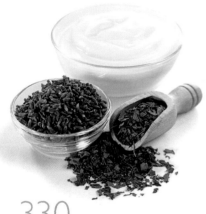

330
Herbal cleansing milk

This lavender and peppermint skin wash cleanses oily skin without causing dryness.

½ cup (125ml) plain low-fat yogurt
½ cup (125ml) water
2 tablespoons dried lavender
1 tablespoon dried peppermint

Mix the ingredients together in a pint-(half-liter-) sized glass jar and steep the mixture overnight in the refrigerator. Strain, rebottle, and refrigerate for up to one week. To cleanse your face, first dampen your skin with warm water. Soak a cotton cosmetic pad in the cleansing milk and gently wipe your face. Repeat until your skin is clean. Rinse with warm water, apply a toner, and follow with a moisturizer.

331
Simple yogurt cleanser

Yogurt, lemon juice, and rosemary essential oil make a quick and simple cleanser for oily skin.

1 tablespoon plain low-fat yogurt
1 teaspoon lemon juice
1 drop rosemary essential oil

Mix the ingredients together. Dampen your face with warm water and apply cleanser with your fingertips. Massage onto your skin for one minute, then rinse off with warm water.

332
Aromatherapy cleanser

This gentle cleanser refreshes oily skin. Witch hazel is mildly drying and lemon and grapefruit are fragrant astringents. Aloe is a soothing toner.

¼ cup (60ml) distilled witch hazel
¼ cup (60ml) vegetable glycerin
¼ cup (60ml) aloe vera gel
1 tablespoon apple cider vinegar
5 drops grapefruit essential oil
2 drops lemon essential oil

Mix the ingredients in a bottle and shake well. Dampen your skin with warm water and gently massage in the lotion. Rinse your skin with lukewarm water.

333
Aromatherapy astringent

Witch hazel and juniper are mild astringents and reduce excess oil from the skin. Lavender helps normalize oil production.

1 cup (250ml) distilled witch hazel
10 drops juniper essential oil
10 drops lavender essential oil

Combine the ingredients in a bottle and shake well. To use, saturate a cotton cosmetic pad with astringent and gently wipe over skin.

334
Quick skin refresher

Place your toner or astringent into a small spray bottle so you can carry it around with you and mist your skin throughout the day.

335
Herbal astringent

Witch hazel, yarrow, and sage are mild astringents. Peppermint refreshes and is antibacterial. Comfrey leaves help heal eruptions of the skin.

1 cup (250ml) distilled witch hazel
2 teaspoons dried yarrow
1 teaspoon dried sage
1 teaspoon dried peppermint
1 teaspoon dried comfrey leaf

Combine the ingredients in a glass jar with a tight-fitting lid. Allow the mixture to steep for two weeks in a warm, dark place. Gently shake the jar every day to keep the herbs from settling. Strain, and store in a clean

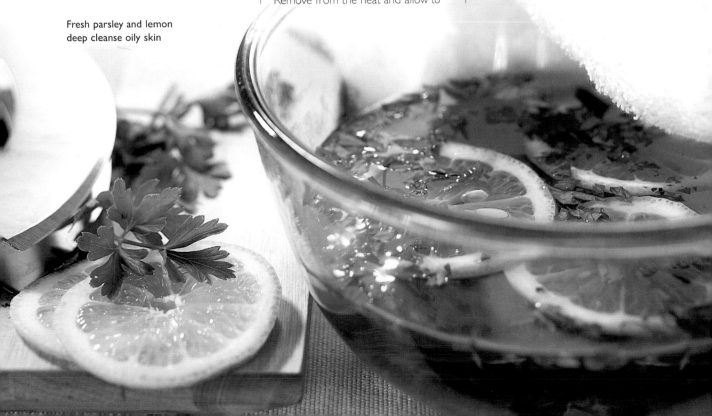

bottle. To use, saturate a cotton cosmetic pad with astringent and gently wipe over the skin.

336
Aloe vera gel

As soon as you have cleansed your skin and applied a toner, smooth on a layer of refreshing aloe vera gel as a moisturizer.

337
Aromatherapy moisturizing oil

Cypress and grapefruit essential oils are mild astringents and help regulate the production of oil in the skin.

1 fl oz (30ml) jojoba oil
5 drops cypress essential oil
5 drops grapefruit essential oil

Fresh parsley and lemon deep cleanse oily skin

Mix the ingredients in a small glass pharmacy bottle with a dropper. After cleansing your skin, gently massage two to three drops of the oil onto your damp skin with your fingertips.

338
Fresh parsley and lemon facial sauna

Oily or problem skin can be deep-cleaned and invigorated with this facial sauna made from fresh parsley, peppermint, and lemon.

2 quarts (2.5 liters) water
½ cup (20g) fresh parsley, chopped
¼ cup (10g) fresh peppermint, chopped
½ lemon, sliced

Bring the water, parsley, peppermint, and lemon to a boil in a covered pot. Remove from the heat and allow to

steep for five minutes. Place the pot on a table, remove the lid, and make a towel tent over your head and the pot to capture the steam. Stay under the tent for 10 minutes, taking care to not burn yourself. Finish by cleansing your skin with a facial scrub and warm water or applying a deep-cleansing mask.

339
Facial sauna

An herbal combination of rosemary, lavender, yarrow, and peppermint makes a refreshing, cleansing facial steam for oily skin.

2 quarts (2.5 liters) water
2 tablespoons dried rosemary
2 tablespoons dried lavender
2 tablespoons dried yarrow
1 tablespoon dried peppermint

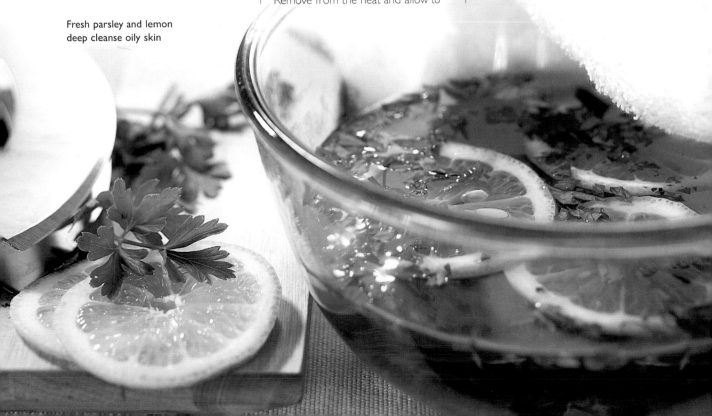

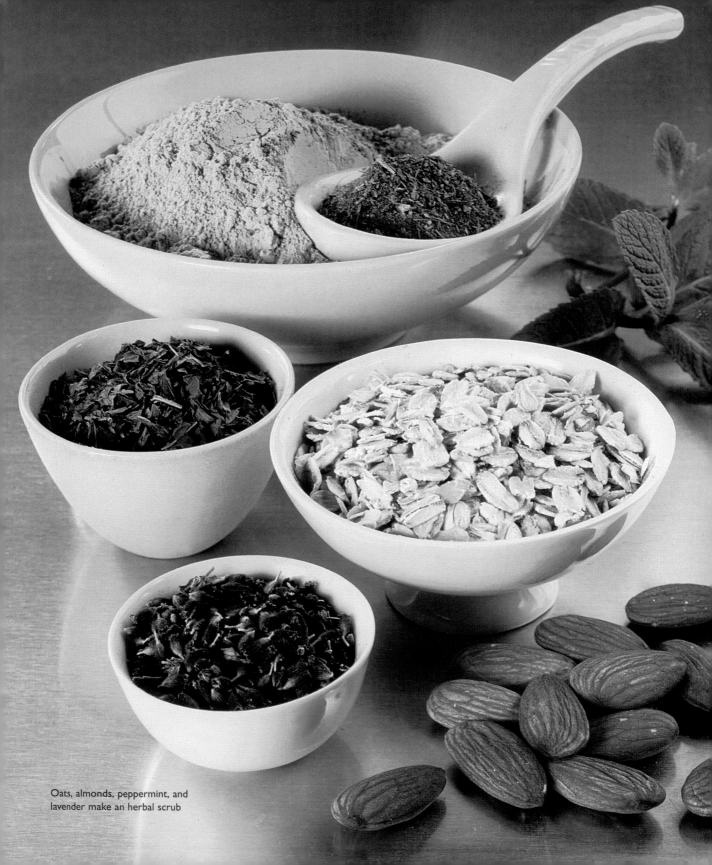

Oats, almonds, peppermint, and lavender make an herbal scrub

Bring the water and herbs to a boil in a large covered pot. Remove from the heat and allow the herbs to steep for five minutes. Place the pot on a table, remove the lid, and make a towel tent over your head and the steaming pot of herbs. Stay under the tent for 10 minutes, taking care to not burn yourself with the steam. Finish by rinsing your face with warm water; apply a toner or a deep-cleansing facial mask if desired.

340
Herbal scrub

Apply this herbal scrub each day to help unclog pores and smooth the texture of your skin. Cosmetic clay absorbs excess oil produced by the skin while finely ground oats and almonds gently exfoliate your skin. Lavender, peppermint, and comfrey all have antibacterial and astringent properties. The lavender essential oil will also help balance the production of oil in the skin.

2 cups (200g) rolled oats
½ cup (75g) almonds
2 tablespoons dried lavender
1 tablespoon dried peppermint
1 tablespoon dried comfrey leaf
½ cup (60g) cosmetic clay
(To make and use, see below)

341
Removing blackheads easily

To ease the removal of blackheads from your face, massage a small amount of jojoba oil into your skin before treating yourself to a facial sauna (see No. 338). The jojoba oil helps soften the debris and hardened sebum, or oil, that clog up the pores.

342
Aromatherapy facial mask

Cucumber cleans and refreshes oily skin, while cosmetic clay absorbs excess oil produced by the skin. Juniper and lavender essential oils are purifying and help normalize the production of oil.

2 teaspoons plain low-fat yogurt
1 tablespoon finely chopped
    cucumber pulp
2 teaspoons cosmetic clay
2 drops lavender essential oil
1 drop juniper essential oil

Combine all the ingredients together and mix them thoroughly into a paste. Cleanse your face and then smooth on the aromatherapy mask. Relax for 15 minutes. Afterward, remove the paste with a warm, wet washcloth.

MAKING AND USING AN HERBAL SCRUB

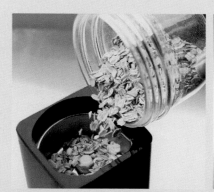

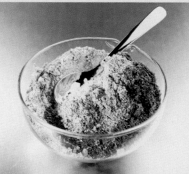

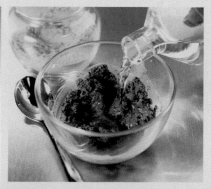

1 In separate batches, finely grind the rolled oats, almonds, and mixed dried herbs in a coffee grinder or blender. Thoroughly combine the three batches into a mixture of cleansing grains.

2 Add the cosmetic clay to the mixture of cleansing grains and combine thoroughly. Store the resulting herbal scrub in a covered container and keep in a cool, dry place.

3 To use, mix a heaped teaspoon of the herbal scrub with enough warm water to make a paste. Gently massage the mixture onto your skin, then rinse well with warm water.

Caring for Sensitive Skin

Sensitive skin needs an especially gentle touch. Use only the purest natural products, cleanse skin with lukewarm water, and apply toners and moisturizers as protection from the elements. Herbs and essential oils with anti-inflammatory properties help calm the irritation and redness characteristic of sensitive skin.

343
Rose water and glycerin cleanser

Dry and sensitive skin will especially benefit from this gentle cleansing lotion. Rose water is a mild cleanser, vegetable glycerin helps the skin retain moisture, and rose essential oil is soothing.

½ cup (125ml) rose water
½ cup (125ml) vegetable glycerin
2 drops rose essential oil

Combine the ingredients in a bottle and shake well. Dampen skin with warm water and gently massage the lotion in with your fingertips. Then rinse your skin with warm water.

344
Aromatherapy toner

Lavender and rose essential oils are both gentle toners for sensitive skin and help calm skin irritation. Witch hazel is mildly astringent, and rose water is cleansing.

1 teaspoon distilled witch hazel
5 drops lavender essential oil
5 drops rose essential oil
1 cup (250ml) rose water

Combine the witch hazel and essential oils in a bottle and shake well. Add the rose water and shake again. Saturate a cotton cosmetic pad with the toner and gently wipe over your skin.

345
Creamy scrub for dry and delicate skin

Adding cream to a facial scrub makes an especially rich and gentle facial exfoliant for dry and delicate skin. Rose essential oil gives the scrub a rich aroma.

½ cup (50g) rolled oats
2 tablespoons almonds
1 drop rose essential oil
1 tablespoon heavy cream

Finely grind the oats and almonds in separate batches in a clean coffee grinder or blender. Mix the batches together and store in a covered container. Add one drop of rose essential oil to scent the blend, if desired. To use, combine one tablespoon of scrub mixture with one tablespoon of heavy cream. Dampen your face with warm water, and massage the cream gently onto your skin with your fingertips. Rinse well with warm water.

346
Moisturizing oil

Chamomile and neroli essential oils soothe even the most sensitive skin.

1fl oz (30ml) jojoba oil
3 drops chamomile essential oil
3 drops neroli essential oil

Combine all ingredients in a small bottle. A glass pharmacy bottle with a dropper works well for dispensing drops of oil. After cleansing your skin, gently massage several drops of the moisturizing oil onto your damp skin with your fingertips.

Moisturizing oils protect sensitive skin

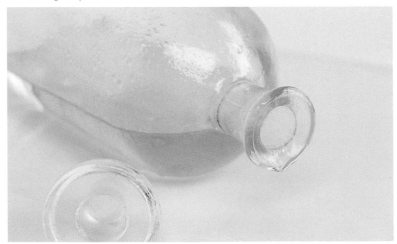

347

Chamomile cream

Chamomile and rose essential oils combine to make a gentle, healing cream for sensitive skin. Grape-seed oil has antioxidant actions and rose water has soothing properties. Vitamin E and grapefruit-seed extract are added to prevent bacterial growth and preserve the cream.

2 tablespoons grape-seed oil
2 tablespoons jojoba oil
1 tablespoon grated beeswax
1 400-IU capsule vitamin E oil
¼ cup (60ml) rose water
5 drops chamomile essential oil
5 drops rose essential oil
3 drops grapefruit-seed extract

Honey, yogurt, and oats soothe sensitive skin

Gently warm the grape-seed and jojoba oils with the beeswax over a low heat until the wax melts. Remove from the heat. Add the contents of the vitamin E capsule. Warm the rose water over a low heat. Remove from the heat. When both liquids are lukewarm, slowly pour the rose water into the oil, beating steadily with a wire whisk or an electric mixer set on the lowest speed until cool, thick, and smooth. Stir in the chamomile and rose essential oils and then the grapefruit-seed extract. Spoon the chamomile cream into a clean jar and cool it completely before covering. Store in a cool place. Apply the cream sparingly to the skin after cleansing and toning.

348

Aromatherapy facial mask

Yogurt, honey, and oats can soothe skin irritation. Chamomile essential oil is an anti-inflammatory and a source of healing for sensitive skin.

2 teaspoons rolled oats
2 teaspoons plain whole-milk yogurt
½ teaspoon honey
1 drop chamomile essential oil

Grind the oats into a fine powder in a clean blender or coffee grinder. Combine all ingredients and mix well. Smooth the mask onto clean skin and then remove after 15 minutes with a warm, wet washcloth.

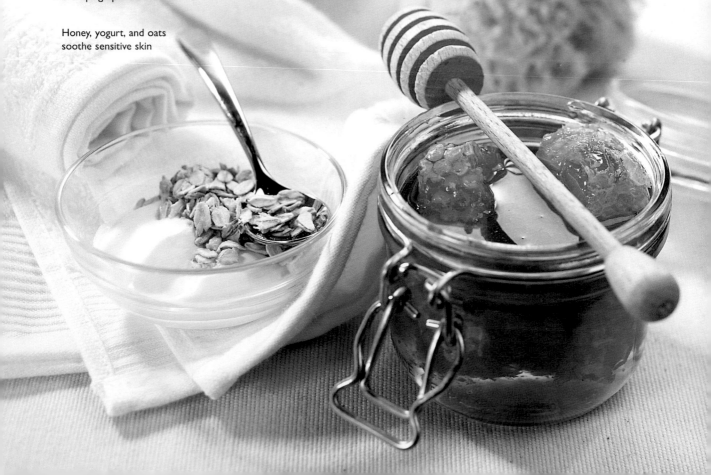

Caring for Mature Skin

Mature skin benefits from rich moisturizing treatments and cell-regenerating essential oils. Scrubs and facial masks help exfoliate skin and stimulate rejuvenation. Cleansers, toners, and moisturizers listed under dry skin (*see pages 67–69*) are also appropriate for mature skin care.

349
Regular sleep

Go to bed at the same time every night and try to sleep for at least eight hours. This encourages rapid eye movement (REM) sleep, during which your body repairs and regenerates tissue. Avoid caffeine or alcohol close to bedtime, because they can disrupt the sleep cycle.

350
Take exercise

Vigorous exercise is as beneficial for your complexion as it is for your muscle tone. Exercise increases circulation and stimulates skin cleansing through perspiration.

351
Aromatherapy moisturizing oil

Frankincense and rose essential oils make an excellent blend for stimulating cellular rejuvenation.

1 fl oz (30ml) jojoba oil
7 drops frankincense essential oil
3 drops rose essential oil

Combine the ingredients in a small glass pharmacy bottle with a dropper and shake well. After cleansing your skin, gently massage several drops of the moisturizing oil onto your damp skin with your fingertips.

352
Orange blossom cleansing cream

This rich cream is suitable for dry and mature skin types. Neroli and palmarosa essential oils rejuvenate mature skin. Vitamin E and grapefruit-seed extract serve as preservatives.

2 tablespoons jojoba oil
1 tablespoon almond oil
1 tablespoon coconut oil
1 tablespoon grated beeswax
1 400-IU capsule vitamin E oil
4 tablespoons rose water
3 drops neroli essential oil
3 drops palmarosa essential oil
3 drops grapefruit-seed extract

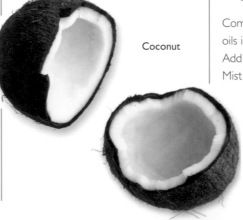

Coconut

Gently warm the jojoba, almond, and coconut oils with the beeswax over a low heat until the wax melts. Remove from the heat. Add the contents of the vitamin E capsule. Warm the rose water over a low heat. Remove from the heat. When both liquids are lukewarm, slowly pour the rose water into the oil, beating steadily with a wire whisk or electric mixer set on the lowest speed until cool, thick, and smooth. Stir in the essential oils and grapefruit-seed extract. Spoon into a clean jar and cool completely before covering. Store in a cool place. Apply the cream sparingly to your skin, wipe off with a damp cotton cosmetic pad, and rinse thoroughly with warm water. Follow with a toner.

353
Aloe and lavender facial mist

Aloe vera juice, and lavender and frankincense essential oils have cell-renewing properties and make a wonderfully fragrant facial mist.

1 teaspoon distilled witch hazel
10 drops lavender essential oil
10 drops frankincense essential oil
1 cup (250ml) aloe vera juice

Combine the witch hazel with the oils in a spray bottle. Shake vigorously. Add the aloe juice and shake again. Mist your skin as often as desired.

354
Revitalizing cream

This rich cream contains frankincense, neroli, and sandalwood essential oils to nourish and rejuvenate mature skin and complexions. Vitamin E and grapefruit-seed extract are added to the cream to act as preservatives and help prevent bacterial growth. Rose water is a gentle cleanser.

3 tablespoons almond oil

1 tablespoon coconut oil

1 tablespoon grated beeswax

1 400-IU capsule vitamin E oil

¼ cup (60ml) rose water

3 drops frankincense essential oil

3 drops neroli essential oil

3 drops sandalwood essential oil

3 drops grapefruit-seed extract

Warm the almond oil, coconut oil, and beeswax gently over a low heat until the wax melts. Remove from the heat. Add the contents of the vitamin E capsule. Warm the rose water over a low heat. When both liquids are lukewarm, slowly pour the rose water into the oil, beating steadily with a wire whisk or an electric mixer set on the lowest speed until the cream is cool, thick, and smooth. Stir in the frankincense, neroli, and sandalwood essential oils together with the grapefruit-seed extract. Spoon the cream into a clean jar and cool completely before covering. Store in a cool place. Apply this cream sparingly after cleansing and toning skin.

355
Daily moisturizer

To keep your skin youthful, use a moisturizer every day. Dry skin wrinkles more easily than moist skin, and chronically dry skin is more likely to develop permanent wrinkles than skin that is kept moisturized.

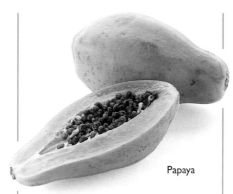

Papaya

356
Papaya exfoliating mask

Papaya contains protein-digesting enzymes that gently remove dead skin cells. Frankincense and comfrey stimulate the production of new skin cells, and honey moisturizes the skin.

2 tablespoons mashed papaya

1 teaspoon honey

2 drops frankincense essential oil

1 tablespoon or more powdered comfrey leaf

Mix the mashed papaya, honey, and frankincense essential oil. Add enough comfrey to make a thick, spreadable mask and smooth onto clean, damp skin. Leave on for 15 minutes, then remove with warm water.

357
Skin renewer

To renew your skin, apply the Papaya exfoliating mask (above) once a day for several days in a row, leaving it on your face for about 30 minutes each time. You can expect to have softer, smoother, and fresher-looking skin after this gentle but intensive series of exfoliating treatments.

358
Aromatherapy facial mask

Whole-milk yogurt smooths the skin, honey adds moisture, and the finely ground almonds gently exfoliate dead cells. Frankincense and neroli essential oils stimulate cell renewal and regeneration.

1 teaspoon finely ground almond meal

2 teaspoons plain whole-milk yogurt

½ teaspoon cosmetic clay

½ teaspoon honey

2 drops frankincense essential oil

1 drop neroli essential oil

To make almond meal, grind chopped almonds in a clean blender or coffee grinder. Combine all ingredients and mix well. Smooth the mask onto clean skin. Remove after 15 minutes with a warm, wet washcloth.

359
Fruit enzyme mask

The natural alpha-hydroxy acids in apples and strawberries help to slough off dead skin cells.

¼ cup (30g) diced apple

2 strawberries, sliced

2 tablespoons plain whole-milk yogurt

1 teaspoon honey

2 teaspoons cosmetic clay (or more as needed)

Blend the fruit, yogurt, and honey until smooth. Mix in enough clay to make a spreadable mask. Wash your face and neck with warm water, and apply the mask. Relax for 20 minutes, remove the mask with warm water, and apply a toner and moisturizer.

Acne & Blemished Skin

Everyone gets a few blemishes, but acne or frequent breakouts call for special attention. Your body needs help with detoxing so drink at least eight glasses of pure water daily and eat plenty of high-fiber foods. Use natural treatments to deep-clean your skin and antimicrobial herbs and essential oils to heal blemishes.

360
Tea for clear skin

Burdock root, dandelion root, and red clover blossoms improve liver, kidney, and intestine function and so may help clear the skin.

2 teaspoons dried burdock root
2 teaspoons dried dandelion root
3 cups (750ml) water
2 teaspoons dried red clover blossoms

Simmer the burdock and dandelion roots in the water in a covered pot for 20 minutes. Remove from the heat and add the clover blossoms. Steep the mixture for an additional 10 minutes. Strain, and drink up to three cups of the tea each day.

361
Herbal cleansing lotion

Thyme and lavender are antimicrobial herbs, while calendula and comfrey help heal blemishes. Witch hazel and rose water are gentle astringents and remove excess oil. Vegetable glycerin provides moisturizing benefits without making the skin oily.

1 teaspoon dried thyme
1 teaspoon dried lavender
1 teaspoon dried calendula
1 teaspoon dried comfrey leaf
¼ cup (60ml) distilled witch hazel
¼ cup (60ml) rose water
2 tablespoons vegetable glycerin

Steep the herbs in witch hazel and rose water in a glass jar with a tight-fitting lid for one week. Strain and pour the liquid into a clean bottle, and add the vegetable glycerin. Shake well. To use, saturate a cotton cosmetic pad with the cleansing lotion and gently wipe over your face. Repeat as necessary until your skin is thoroughly cleansed.

362
Herbal cleansing milk

A gentle skin wash made with yogurt smooths blemished skin. Calendula and thyme are antimicrobial and help cleanse the skin of the bacteria that contribute to blemishes. Comfrey promotes healing.

½ cup (125ml) plain low-fat yogurt
½ cup (125ml) water
1 tablespoon dried calendula
1 tablespoon dried thyme
2 tablespoons dried comfrey leaf

Combine all the ingredients in a glass jar with a tight-fitting lid. Steep the mixture overnight in the refrigerator. Strain, rebottle, and store in the refrigerator for up to one week. To cleanse your face, dampen your skin with warm water. Soak a cotton cosmetic pad in the cleansing milk

A purifying tea can improve blemished skin

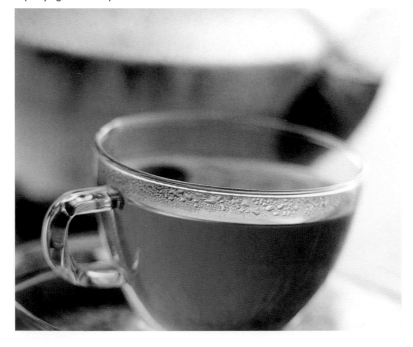

and gently wipe your face. Repeat until your skin is clean. Rinse with warm water, apply toner, and follow with a moisturizer.

363
Herbal astringent

Witch hazel and yarrow are gentle astringents, peppermint is refreshing and antibacterial, and comfrey helps heal skin eruptions.

1 cup (250ml) distilled witch hazel
2 teaspoons dried yarrow
1 teaspoon dried peppermint
1 teaspoon dried comfrey leaf

Combine all ingredients in a glass jar with a tight-fitting lid. Allow the mixture to steep for two weeks. Strain, and pour into a clean bottle. Apply liberally to your face with a cotton cosmetic pad.

364
All-around face treatment

Yogurt both softens and smooths troubled skin, comfrey helps heal blemishes, honey moisturizes, and the cosmetic clay helps draw impurities out of the skin.

1 tablespoon plain low-fat yogurt
1 tablespoon dried comfrey leaf
1 teaspoon honey
1 teaspoon cosmetic clay

Grind the comfrey into a powder in a coffee grinder. Mix the ingredients into a spreadable mask. Smooth the mask over freshly cleansed skin and relax for 15 minutes. Remove with a warm, wet washcloth.

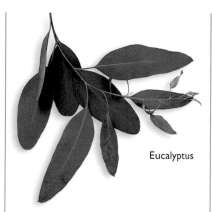
Eucalyptus

365
Aromatherapy facial mask

Yogurt smooths skin, oats soothe and gently exfoliate, and cosmetic clay cleans pores. Lavender and eucalyptus essential oils fight the bacteria that contribute to breakouts.

1 tablespoon finely ground rolled oats
1 tablespoon plain low-fat yogurt
1 teaspoon cosmetic clay
2 drops lavender essential oil
1 drop eucalyptus essential oil

Grind the rolled oats into a fine meal in a blender or clean coffee grinder. Combine the ingredients and mix well. Smooth the mask onto clean skin and remove after 15 minutes with a warm, wet washcloth.

366
Overnight paste

Mix together two drops of tea tree essential oil, half a teaspoon of cosmetic clay, and a few drops of water—just enough to make a thick paste. Dab the mixture onto the blemishes and leave it on overnight to help heal and dry breakouts.

367
How to treat a blemish

Don't squeeze pimples. Instead, apply a sequence of alternating warm and cold, clean washcloths (a minute of warm, then a minute of cold) several times a day. This heals the skin by boosting the circulation. Follow with a dab of tea tree essential oil.

368
Honey mask

Raw, unprocessed honey is excellent for oily, blemished skin because of its antibacterial properties and its ability to moisturize the skin without making it oily. Cosmetic clay absorbs excess oil from the skin and draws toxins out of the skin. Lavender essential oil calms and soothes skin inflammation and helps heal blemishes.

2 tablespoons raw unprocessed honey
1 teaspoon cosmetic clay
2 drops lavender essential oil

Combine the ingredients and mix into a thin paste (adding more cosmetic clay if necessary). Spread over clean, damp skin. Remove after 15 minutes with warm water.

369
Aromatherapy blemish treatment

Dab a mixture of equal parts of tea tree and lavender essential oils directly onto the blemishes twice a day. Tea tree oil fights the bacteria that cause breakouts. Lavender helps heal blemishes and masks the medicinal smell of tea tree oil.

Solutions for Age Spots

Brown spots, or age spots, that appear on the face, neck, and the backs of the hands are caused by excessive exposure to the sun. To prevent them, apply daily a sunscreen that protects against both UVA and UVB rays. Sunscreens with micronized titanium dioxide do not cause the skin irritation associated with many chemical sunscreens. To lighten existing spots, try the following.

370
Strawberry mask

A strawberry and yogurt mask is an effective, yet gentle treatment for lightening freckles and age spots. Frankincense essential oil stimulates skin rejuvenation.

1 fresh strawberry
2 teaspoons plain whole-milk yogurt
2 drops frankincense essential oil
½ teaspoon cosmetic clay

Mash the strawberry and mix the juice (approximately one teaspoon) with the yogurt, frankincense essential oil, and clay. Apply the mixture to freshly washed skin. Leave the mask in place for 20 minutes, then remove with a warm, wet washcloth. Follow with a moisturizer. For best results, use this mask daily if you have oily or normal skin—twice a week if your skin is dry.

371
Yogurt mask for age spots

Yogurt has mild bleaching effects and can help lighten age spots and skin discolorations. Wash your skin with warm water, pat dry, and spread on a layer of thick, plain, whole-milk yogurt.

Leave on for 30 minutes, then rinse off with warm water. You have to apply the mask daily for at least a couple of months to notice any difference. Even if your age spots don't disappear, your skin will be noticeably smoother and softer.

372
Fade dark age spots

Paint your age spots with undiluted lemon juice daily (use a soft-bristled artist's paint brush). Lemon is a powerful bleaching agent. You should see a difference within three months.

373
Bleach pigmented skin

For dark, stubborn age spots, try a hydroquinone cream. This is a safe and natural way to bleach unwanted skin pigmentation. You should see a difference within three months.

A strawberry and yogurt mask lightens age spots

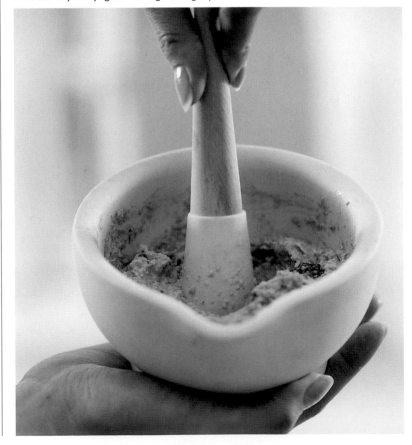

Sunburn Remedies

Spending an hour in the early morning or late afternoon sun is healthy for your body and spirit. But too much sun can damage the skin. Wear a sunscreen and protective clothing between 10 a.m. and 4 p.m. when the sun's rays are strongest. The following remedies can ease the pain of sunburn and speed healing.

374
Cooling facial mist

Witch hazel, aloe vera, lavender, and rose water make a cooling and healing lotion for sunburned skin.

1 teaspoon distilled witch hazel
20 drops lavender essential oil
¼ cup (60ml) rose water
¾ cup (180ml) aloe vera juice

Mix the witch hazel and lavender in a spray bottle. Shake vigorously. Add the rose water and aloe vera and shake again. Store in the refrigerator, and mist skin as often as desired.

375
Yogurt mask

Yogurt and lavender essential oil calm sunburned or windburned skin.

1 tablespoon plain whole-milk yogurt
1 drop lavender essential oil

Mix the ingredients into a paste and smooth over your skin. Wash off with lukewarm water after 15 minutes.

376
Cooling the skin

Mix a drop of lavender essential oil with a tablespoon of aloe vera gel. Spread gently over your burned skin.

377
Honey mask

As honey moisturizes, aloe vera helps cool and heal burned skin. Lavender essential oil heals burns and helps the production of healthy skin cells.

2 teaspoons raw honey
2 teaspoons aloe vera gel
2 drops lavender essential oil

Mix the ingredients. Dampen your face with cool water, apply the mask to your skin and leave for 20 minutes. Rinse with lukewarm water.

378
Eyelid soother

Close swollen, sunburned eyelids and cover with cucumber slices or cool tea bags for 15 minutes.

379
Baking soda bath

The quickest way to cool sunburn is by soaking in a tub of lukewarm water. Baking soda and lavender essential oil draw out heat and calm inflammation.

2 cups (250g) baking soda
10 drops lavender essential oil

Add ingredients to a tub of lukewarm water, and stir to dissolve. Soak for up to 20 minutes. Avoid soap as it dries and irritates tender, burned skin. Pat yourself dry gently. Apply a soothing body lotion to seal in moisture.

380
Healing bath

Green tea's potent antioxidants help neutralize cell damage. Chamomile and calendula provide additional skin-soothing and healing compounds.

2 quarts (2.5 liters) water
⅓ cup (10g) dried green tea
⅓ cup (10g) dried chamomile
⅓ cup (10g) dried calendula

Bring the water and herbs to a boil in a covered pot. Remove from the heat and steep until cool. Strain, and add the tea to a lukewarm bath. Soak daily for 20 minutes until your sunburn heals.

381
Green tea healer

Drink three cups (750ml) of green tea daily to provide extra antioxidants to help your sunburned skin heal.

382
Cooling sunburn spray

Green tea, aloe juice, and lavender essential oil will help cool sunburn and promote skin healing.

¼ cup (60ml) brewed green tea
¼ cup (60ml) aloe vera juice
¼ teaspoon lavender essential oil

Mix the ingredients in a spray bottle. Shake well. Spray liberally over your burned skin. Refrigerate, and use within two weeks.

Eye Care

Take short breaks during the day to relax your eyes, either with a relaxation exercise or cool herbal compresses. Eyes show age more quickly than the rest of the face because the skin beneath them is thin and lacks oil glands. Treat the skin around your eyes gently. Use a light moisturizer daily to keep skin smooth.

383
Refreshing tired eyes

If your eyes are irritated from smog, dust, or allergies, or if you need a break from staring at a computer screen or doing other close-up work, try this 10-minute routine to relax and soothe your eyes. Splash your eyes several times with cold water over a sink. Place a hot washcloth over your closed eyelids, gently pressing your eyes with your fingertips. Alternate the cold-water splash and the hot washcloth several times, ending with the cold-water splash. Pat your eyes dry with a soft towel. Finish by lying on your back with your feet slightly elevated. Place a slice of chilled cucumber over each closed eye and rest for five minutes or longer.

384
Herbal help for bags under the eyes

A cold chamomile tea eye compress is excellent for soothing tired eyes and helps alleviate puffiness.

1 heaped tablespoon dried chamomile
1 cup (250ml) boiling water

Pour the water over the chamomile. Cover, and steep for 20 minutes. Strain, and refrigerate. To use, soak two cotton cosmetic squares in the chilled tea, lie down, and apply to your closed eyelids for 10 minutes.

385
Combat puffiness

When fatigue or allergies make your eyes puffy, place cold, wet, black tea bags on your closed eyelids for 10 minutes. Black tea contains tannins, which shrink swollen tissues.

386
Soothing eye relaxation

This exercise soothes tired eyes and helps relax your entire body. Practice it when you want. Sit comfortably with your feet flat on the floor. Rub your palms together briskly until they feel warm. Close your eyes, and cup your hands over your eyes, fingers pointing upward. Adjust your palms to create complete darkness. Breathe deeply and rhythmically for at least a minute, allowing the velvety blackness to soothe and refresh your eyes.

387
Rose refresher

Keep a bottle of rose water in your refrigerator. Dilute two tablespoons of chilled rose water with an equal amount of cold water. Soak cotton cosmetic squares in the solution and apply to your closed eyelids.

388
Herbal eye freshener

Chamomile, fennel, and elderflower refresh tired or puffy eyes.

2 cups (500ml) boiling water
1 tablespoon dried chamomile
1 tablespoon fennel seed, crushed
1 tablespoon dried elderflower

Pour the water over the herbs, cover, and steep until cool. Strain, and chill in the refrigerator. Soak a washcloth in the mixture, wringing it out slightly. Lie down, place the cloth over your eyes, and relax for 10 minutes.

389
Aromatherapy eye oil

Chamomile and rose essential oils moisturize the area under the eyes.

5 drops chamomile essential oil
5 drops rose essential oil
1fl oz (30ml) jojoba oil

Mix the ingredients and store in a small glass bottle with a dropper. Cleanse your face, apply two drops around the eyes with your fingertips and gently tap into the skin.

390
Eyebrow care

After tweezing your brows, apply an astringent such as witch hazel with a cotton ball. Smooth on a thin coat of honey with your fingers. Rinse off with warm water after a few minutes.

Lip Care

Because your lips have no oil glands, it's important to protect them from the elements, such as the sun, wind, and cold weather. Try these easy-to-make lip balms.

391

Honey lip balm

Almond oil and beeswax create a barrier against wind and cold. Honey helps the lips retain moisture.

4 tablespoons almond oil
1 tablespoon grated beeswax
1 teaspoon honey

Warm the almond oil and beeswax in a small pan over a very low heat until the wax melts. Remove from heat, add honey, and stir thoroughly.

Honey lip balm keeps lips smooth

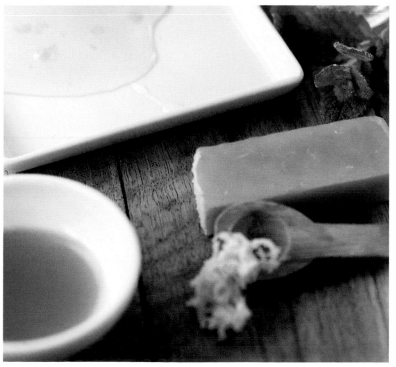

Pour into a small, wide-mouthed glass jar. Allow to cool, stirring occasionally to keep the mixture from separating. Store in a cool place. Apply a small amount to lips as often as desired.

392

Peppermint lip balm

For a refreshing lip balm, follow the recipe for Honey lip balm (see No. 391), stirring in 10 drops of peppermint essential oil after mixing in the honey.

393

Grapefruit and lavender lip balm

For a sweet citrus lip balm, follow the recipe for Honey lip balm (see No. 391), stirring in 10 drops of grapefruit essential oil and five drops of lavender essential oil after mixing in the honey.

394

Chamomile and orange blossom lip balm

For a soothing lip balm with the scent of orange blossoms, follow the recipe for Honey lip balm (see No. 391), stirring in five drops of chamomile and 10 drops of neroli essential oils after mixing in the honey.

395

Rose lip balm

For a fragrant, delicate balm for sensitive lips, follow the recipe for Honey lip balm (see No. 391), stirring in 10 drops of rose essential oil after mixing in the honey.

396

Healing balm for chapped lips

Vitamin E together with tea tree and lavender essential oils help soothe and heal dry, chapped lips. Follow the recipe for Honey lip balm (see No. 391). Add the contents of a 400-IU vitamin E capsule with the honey and stir thoroughly. Then add 10 drops of tea tree and five drops of lavender essential oils. Stir again.

Healthy Teeth & Gums

Vitamin C, coenzyme Q10, calcium, magnesium, and daily brushing and flossing are essential for healthy teeth and gums. To clean your teeth, nothing is more effective than baking soda. It polishes and whitens teeth naturally and gently. Herbal mouthwashes are quick to make, are beneficial for your gums, and freshen your breath as well.

397
Vitamin C

The antioxidant vitamin C reduces inflammation. It boosts the immune system to help fight the bacteria that cause infection and to heal gums. Eat foods that are rich in vitamin C, such as citrus fruits and green leafy vegetables (for example, spinach and broccoli), and supplement your diet with 250 to 500mg a day.

398
Coenzyme Q10

Coenzyme Q10 is a powerful antioxidant that reduces the number of gum-damaging free radicals. Your body makes it naturally, but less so as you age. Consider supplementing your diet with 60 to 100mg daily.

399
Calcium

A deficiency of the element calcium can weaken both your teeth and the bone that holds them in place. Increase your intake by eating dark leafy greens, tofu, and low-fat dairy products, and by supplementing your diet with 1,200mg daily, taken in two separate doses.

400
Magnesium

The element magnesium works with calcium to keep teeth and bones strong. Eat magnesium-rich foods, such as nuts, seeds, legumes, and dark leafy greens, and supplement your diet with a 400mg capsule daily.

401
Brush teeth and gums

With a soft-bristled brush, gently brush away from your gums, cleaning carefully along the gum line where food particles and bacteria collect. Use a natural toothpaste: some have immune-boosters to keep gums healthy and minimize inflammation. If you cannot brush after meals, at least rinse your mouth with water to flush out sugars and food particles.

402
Daily flossing

Flossing is an essential daily habit for keeping gums and teeth healthy. Use a fresh piece of floss each time, and gently guide it between the teeth and below the gum next to each tooth.

403
Herbal tooth powder

Baking soda whitens your teeth and freshens your breath. Sea salt tightens the gums. Peppermint oil and ginger fight bacteria and provide flavor.

2 tablespoons baking soda
½ teaspoon finely ground sea salt
¼ teaspoon dried powdered ginger
3 drops peppermint essential oil

Mix the ingredients and store in an airtight container. Use half a teaspoon of the powder each time you brush.

404
Brush your tongue

A build-up of bacteria in the crevices on the tongue can cause bad breath. Gently brush the top of your tongue each time you brush your teeth.

405
Breath fresheners

To quickly freshen your breath, chew on a few fennel seeds or eat a sprig of parsley.

406
Whitening your teeth

Mix a teaspoon each of baking soda and 3 percent hydrogen peroxide. Dip your toothbrush into the mixture and brush for three minutes, then rinse thoroughly. Follow with regular toothpaste or an herbal mouth rinse.

407
Strawberry whitener

To lighten tooth stains and whiten your teeth, crush a fresh strawberry and rub it onto your teeth. Follow by rinsing with water.

408
Daily herbal mouthwash

Rinsing vigorously with a mouthwash for one minute a day can prevent plaque buildup, which contributes to gum inflammation and cavities. Look for brands with antiseptic ingredients such as tea tree essential oil and the disinfectant herb myrrh.

409
Mint mouthwash

Peppermint essential oil helps fight odor-causing bacteria, and aloe vera soothes gums.

1 cup (250ml) water
1 teaspoon vegetable glycerin
1 teaspoon aloe vera juice
6 drops peppermint essential oil

Mix the ingredients together and store in a covered container. Shake well and use within a few days.

410
Herbal mouthwash for healthy gums

Peppermint and aniseed freshen breath. Myrrh helps strengthen gums and is an antiseptic and preservative.

1 cup (250ml) boiling water
2 teaspoons dried peppermint
1 teaspoon aniseed
½ teaspoon myrrh tincture

Pour the boiling water over the peppermint and aniseed. Cover, and steep until cool. Strain, and add the myrrh. Store the mouthwash in a bottle and shake before using.

Aniseed freshens the breath

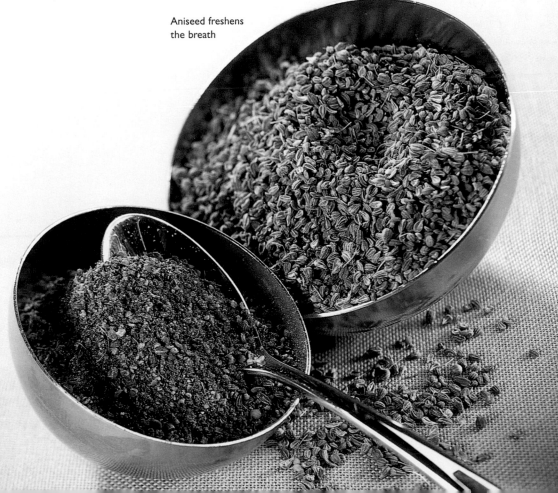

Body Lotions & Moisturizers

Regularly moisturizing your body helps keep skin supple and youthful. Moisturizers protect skin by creating a barrier that guards against moisture loss and the damaging effects of wind, heat, and a dry environment.

411
Moisturizing oil for mature skin

Jojoba is richly moisturizing, and frankincense and palmarosa essential oils stimulate skin rejuvenation.

2fl oz (60ml) jojoba oil
15 drops frankincense essential oil
10 drops palmarosa essential oil

Mix the jojoba oil and essential oils in a small bottle. Apply several drops to damp skin immediately after bathing or showering.

Frankincense

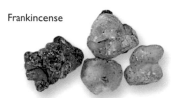

412
Aromatherapy moisturizing oil

A combination of jojoba oil and lavender and grapefruit essential oils makes a sweetly scented moisturizer.

2fl oz (60ml) jojoba oil
15 drops lavender essential oil
10 drops grapefruit essential oil

Combine the jojoba oil and essential oils in a small bottle. Immediately after showering or bathing, smooth a few drops onto your damp skin.

413
Sandalwood moisturizing lotion

To make a simple and fragrant moisturizer, add a few drops of sandalwood essential oil to one tablespoon of natural body lotion. Massage the resulting mixture into your damp skin immediately after showering or bathing.

414
Sandalwood and rose body cream

Sandalwood and rose essential oils both moisturize and soothe dry skin. Together, they impart a a lasting fragrance to this rich body cream. Coconut oil and beeswax are rich moisturizers. Grape-seed oil has antioxidant actions that help protect the skin, and rose water is soothing. Vitamin E oil and grapefruit-seed extract are added to preserve the cream.

3 tablespoons grape-seed oil
1 tablespoon coconut oil
1 tablespoon grated beeswax
1 400-IU capsule vitamin E oil
¼ cup (60ml) rose water
5 drops sandalwood essential oil
5 drops rose essential oil
3 drops grapefruit-seed extract

Mix the grape-seed oil, coconut oil, and beeswax in a pot and warm gently over a low heat until the wax melts. Remove from the heat. Add the contents of the vitamin E capsule. Warm the rose water over a low heat and then remove from the heat. When both liquids are lukewarm, slowly pour the rose water into the oil, beating steadily with a wire whisk or an electric mixer set on the lowest speed until cool, thick, and smooth. Stir in the sandalwood and rose essential oils and also the grapefruit-seed extract. Spoon the cream into a clean jar and let it cool completely before covering. Store in a cool place. Apply the cream sparingly.

415
Orange-flower body cream

This rich cream has the fragrance of orange flowers and is nourishing for allover body care. Frankincense and neroli essential oils rejuvenate the skin. Follow the recipe for Sandalwood and rose body cream (see No. 414), substituting the sandalwood and rose oils with five drops of frankincense essential oil and five drops of neroli essential oil. Apply this cream sparingly to your skin.

416
Prevent moisture from evaporating

Apply a body oil or a moisturizer immediately after taking a shower or bath—preferably while your skin is still damp—to help prevent moisture from evaporating from your skin.

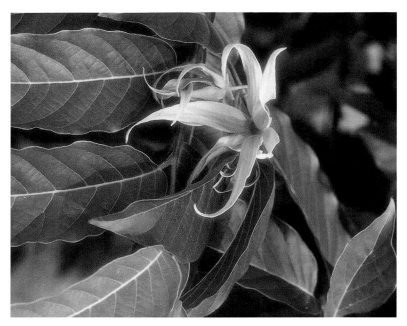

Ylang ylang adds an exotic scent to body care products

Body Powders

Body powders are great for absorbing excess perspiration and reducing chafing and irritation. Most commercial brands contain talc—a lung irritant which is often contaminated with asbestos. Excellent, inexpensive, and natural alternatives are cornstarch, arrowroot, and white cosmetic clay.

417
Simple body powder

To make a simple body powder, scent one cup of cornstarch with 10–30 drops of an essential oil of your choice. Mix in thoroughly with your fingertips and use at once.

418
Uplifting body powder

Lavender and grapefruit essential oils have a refreshing, uplifting scent that is perfect for hot summer days. The arrowroot (or cornstarch) and clay absorb excess perspiration.

½ cup (50g) arrowroot or cornstarch
2 tablespoons white cosmetic clay
7 drops lavender essential oil
7 drops grapefruit essential oil

Mix the arrowroot or cornstarch with the cosmetic clay. Add the essential oils drop by drop to the powder, mixing well with your fingers. Store in a tightly covered container. Let the mixture sit for a couple of days before using to allow the oils to fully scent the powder.

419
Soothing body powder

Rose, lavender, and ylang ylang create a soothing, floral-scented powder. Arrowroot (or cornstarch) and clay help keep perspiration in check.

2 tablespoons dried fragrant rose petals
½ cup (50g) arrowroot or cornstarch
2 tablespoons white cosmetic clay
8 drops lavender essential oil
5 drops rose essential oil
1 drop ylang ylang essential oil

Grind the rose petals into a powder in a clean coffee grinder, then mix with the arrowroot or cornstarch and cosmetic clay. Add the oils drop by drop, mixing them thoroughly into the powder with your fingers. Store in a tightly covered container. Let the mixture sit for a couple of days before using to allow the essential oils to fully scent the powder.

420
Warming body powder

For a good body powder for fall and winter, follow the recipe for Uplifting body powder (see *No. 418*) and substitute 12 drops of sandalwood, three drops of ginger, and one drop of patchouli essential oils.

421
Calming body powder

To make a calming body powder with a lasting scent, follow the recipe for Uplifting body powder (see *No. 418*), substituting 10 drops of sandalwood, three drops of lavender, and three drops of clary sage essential oils.

Hands & Nails

Hands, cuticles, and nails take a beating from daily tasks. Cold weather and too much sun can make hands and cuticles rough and dry. Use a rich moisturizing cream daily, and treat yourself to a weekly natural manicure. Begin with an herbal hand soak; then a rejuvenating hand pack, mask, or scrub; and, finally, a nail oil or cream massaged into your cuticles and nails.

422
Moisturize dry hands

To quickly soften and moisturize dry hands, add five drops of lavender essential oil and one teaspoon of almond oil to a basin of warm water and soak your hands for 10 minutes. Follow with a rich hand cream to seal in moisture.

423
Comfrey hand soak for rough hands

A simple treatment for rough or chapped skin is to soak your hands in warm comfrey tea. Comfrey contains allantoin, which stimulates the growth of healthy new skin cells.

3 tablespoons dried comfrey root
3 cups (750ml) water

Simmer the comfrey and water in a covered pot for 10 minutes. Remove from heat and allow it to steep until lukewarm. (Dried comfrey leaf has only half as much allantoin—pour three cups (750ml) of boiling water over six tablespoons of dried leaf and steep until lukewarm.) Strain, and soak your hands in the warm tea for about 15 minutes. Pat your hands dry, and apply a moisturizing cream or oil.

424
Herbal hand soak

This soak cleans and softens the hands, making it easy to shape nails and cuticles. Almond oil moisturizes and chamomile, calendula, and lavender soothe and heal.

2 cups (500ml) water
1 tablespoon dried calendula
1 tablespoon dried chamomile
1 tablespoon dried lavender
1 teaspoon almond oil

Bring the water and herbs to a boil in a pot. Cover, remove from heat, and let steep for 10 minutes. Strain into a bowl and add almond oil. Soak your hands in the warm solution for 10 minutes. Clean under your nails and push back the cuticles while your hands are damp, then massage moisturizer into your hands and nails.

425
Gentle hand scrub

Almonds and oats make a gentle exfoliant that buffs away dry skin and leaves hands soft and smooth.

1 tablespoon almonds
1 tablespoon rolled oats
1 teaspoon almond oil

Grind the almonds and oats into a coarse powder in a clean coffee grinder. Mix with the almond oil. Dampen your hands with warm water and massage in the scrub for a couple of minutes. Rinse well with warm water and pat dry.

426
Yogurt hand mask

A combination of honey, lemon, oats, and yogurt smooths and softens the hands. Frankincense essential oil adds skin-rejuvenating properties.

1 tablespoon rolled oats
1 tablespoon plain whole-milk yogurt
1 teaspoon almond oil
1 teaspoon lemon juice
1 teaspoon honey
2 drops frankincense essential oil

Grind the oats into a coarse powder in a clean coffee grinder. Add the rest of the ingredients and mix well. Apply mask to the backs of freshly washed, damp hands. Relax for 20 minutes, then rinse off the mask with warm water and apply a moisturizing cream.

427
Soothing hand mask

Honey and almond oil moisturize dry hands while lavender essential oil soothes the skin.

1 teaspoon almond oil
1 teaspoon honey
2 drops lavender essential oil

Mix the ingredients and massage into freshly washed, damp hands. Relax for 15 minutes, then rinse the hands with warm water and apply a moisturizer.

428
Almond and honey pack

Chapped hands are a common and painful problem in winter. Try this soothing pack to restore moisture to dry hands. All ingredients are prized for their healing, moisturizing actions.

1 tablespoon almonds
1 tablespoon rolled oats
1 teaspoon honey
1 teaspoon almond oil
Buttermilk or plain whole-milk yogurt

Grind the almonds and oats into a coarse powder in a coffee grinder. Mix with honey, almond oil, and enough buttermilk or yogurt to make a thick paste. Apply to your hands—it will be easier if you have someone help you. Pull on a pair of loose-fitting thick cotton gloves. Leave on for a couple of hours. Rinse off with warm water and apply a moisturizing cream.

429
Comfrey hand pack

This hand pack is messy, but it's great when your hands need an intensive healing treatment. Oats, yogurt, and honey soften and smooth damaged skin. Comfrey contains allantoin, which stimulates skin regeneration, and lavender soothes irritation.

2 tablespoons rolled oats
2 tablespoons dried comfrey leaf
1 tablespoon plain whole-milk yogurt
1 tablespoon honey
5 drops lavender essential oil

Grind the rolled oats and comfrey into a powder in a clean coffee grinder. Add the remaining ingredients and stir the mixture into a thick, spreadable paste. Smooth onto your hands—ask someone to help you. Pull on a pair of loose-fitting thick cotton gloves. Leave on for at least a couple of hours, then rinse your hands with warm water and apply a moisturizing hand cream.

430
Aromatherapy cuticle oil

Jojoba oil is moisturizing, and vitamin E, lavender, and frankincense help heal ragged cuticles.

1 fl oz (30ml) jojoba oil
2 400-IU capsules vitamin E oil
5 drops lavender essential oil
5 drops frankincense essential oil

Comfrey helps heal damaged skin

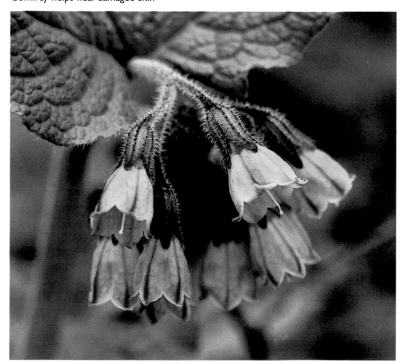

Combine the ingredients in a small bottle and shake well. Massage a few drops of the oil into your nails and cuticles every night before bed.

431
Warm oil for cuticles

Rough cuticles respond quickly to a warm oil soak. Olive oil and lavender and lemon essential oils help heal and smooth cuticles.

¼ cup (60ml) extra-virgin olive oil
5 drops lavender essential oil
2 drops lemon essential oil

Warm the olive oil to a comfortable temperature and stir in the essential oils. Soak your fingertips in the warm oil for 10 minutes. This mixture can be reused several times; store in a cool place and reheat as needed.

432
Nourishing nail oil

Nails become brittle and dry when exposed to hot water, soaps, and nail polishes and removers. This mixture of oils will help you restore them.

1 teaspoon jojoba oil

1 teaspoon apricot-seed oil

1 teaspoon almond oil

1 400-IU capsule vitamin E oil

Mix the ingredients in a small bottle. Shake well to blend. Massage several drops into nails and cuticles in the morning and evening. Buff with a chamois buffer if desired to heighten the natural shine of your nails.

433
Rich nail butter

Jojoba oil, cocoa butter, and beeswax are deep-penetrating moisturizers. Lemon essential oil brings strength to brittle nails and sandalwood essential oil moisturizes dry cuticles.

2 tablespoons jojoba oil

1 tablespoon cocoa butter

1 tablespoon grated beeswax

10 drops sandalwood essential oil

5 drops lemon essential oil

Combine the jojoba oil, cocoa butter, and beeswax in a small pot and warm gently over very low heat until the cocoa butter and beeswax melt. Remove the pot from the heat. Stir in the sandalwood and lemon essential oils. Pour the mixture into a small, glass jar with a wide mouth and allow it to cool completely before covering. Rub a small amount of this protective butter into your nails each day.

434
Aromatherapy hand cream

Coconut oil and beeswax are rich moisturizers. Grape-seed oil has antioxidant actions, while sandalwood and rose essential oils are healing for dry skin. Vitamin E oil and grapefruit-seed extract preserve the cream.

3 tablespoons grape-seed oil

1 tablespoon coconut oil

1 tablespoon grated beeswax

1 400-IU capsule vitamin E oil

¼ cup (60ml) rose water

5 drops rose essential oil

5 drops sandalwood essential oil

3 drops grapefruit-seed extract

Mix the grape-seed and coconut oils with the beeswax in a pot and warm gently over a low heat until the wax melts. Remove from the heat. Add the contents of the vitamin E capsule. Warm the rose water over low heat. Remove from heat. When both the liquids are lukewarm, slowly pour the rose water into the oil, beating steadily with a wire whisk or an

Aromatherapy cream moisturizes hands

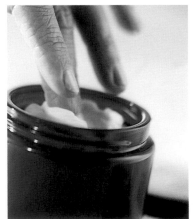

electric mixer set on the lowest speed until cool, thick, and smooth. Stir in the essential oils and grapefruit-seed extract. Spoon the cream into a clean jar and cool completely before covering. Store in a cool place. Use daily to keep hands soft and smooth.

435
Healing hand cream

This hand cream is excellent for rough, dry, and cracked hands. Jojoba and coconut oils and beeswax are rich moisturizers. Aloe gel and tea tree and lavender essential oils encourage healing. Vitamin E and grapefruit-seed extract are included to preserve the cream.

3 tablespoons jojoba oil

1 tablespoon coconut oil

1 tablespoon grated beeswax

1 400-IU capsule vitamin E oil

¼ cup (60ml) aloe vera gel

5 drops tea tree essential oil

5 drops lavender essential oil

3 drops grapefruit-seed extract

Mix the jojoba and coconut oils with the beeswax in a pot. Warm gently over a low heat until the wax melts. Remove from the heat. Add the contents of the capsule. Warm the aloe gel over a low heat. Remove from the heat. When both mixtures are lukewarm, slowly pour the gel into the oil, beating steadily with a wire whisk or an electric mixer set on the lowest speed until cool, thick, and smooth. Stir in the essential oils and grapefruit-seed extract. Spoon the cream into a clean jar and cool completely before covering. Store the cream in a cool place.

Foot Care

Calluses, corns, and aching feet are often the result of poorly fitting shoes so choose shoes with plenty of toe room and arch support. Massage your feet nightly with a rich moisturizing cream; cool and deodorize them with refreshing foot sprays; and rejuvenate them when they're tired with wonderful foot baths.

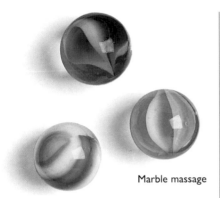

Marble massage

436
Relaxing foot bath for tired feet

Lavender is relaxing and rosemary stimulates circulation. Add five drops of lavender essential oil and two drops of rosemary essential oil to a basin of warm water and mix the oils into the water with your hand. At the end of a long day, soak your tired feet for 15 minutes, and finish with a cold-water rinse.

437
Cooling foot bath

For a refreshing foot bath on a hot summer's day, add five drops of lavender essential oil and two drops of peppermint essential oil to a basin of cool water. Mix the oils into the water with your hand, and soak your feet for 15 minutes.

438
Marble massage

Add a layer of marbles to any foot bath of your choice and enjoy rolling your feet on the marbles while you soak them.

439
Odor-fighting foot bath

Cypress, lavender, and patchouli essential oils fight the bacteria that cause foot odor and leave your feet feeling clean and refreshed.

5 drops lavender essential oil
3 drops cypress essential oil
2 drops patchouli essential oil

Add the oils to a basin of warm water. Mix the oils into the water with your hand, and soak your feet for 15 minutes.

440
Stimulate circulation

To rest and rejuvenate aching feet, lie on the floor and place your feet on a chair so that they are higher than your head. Relax in this position for ten minutes. Lying with your feet higher than your head stimulates circulation and relieves stagnation in the legs and feet.

441
Aromatherapy foot soak

Baking soda and borax soften rough skin, and almond oil is moisturizing. Lavender and grapefruit essential oils clean and refresh feet.

1 cup (125g) baking soda
½ cup (60g) borax
5 drops lavender essential oil
2 drops grapefruit essential oil
1 teaspoon almond oil

Add hot water to a plastic tub large enough to hold both of your feet comfortably. Add the baking soda and borax and stir to dissolve. Mix the lavender and grapefruit essential oils with the almond oil and add to the foot bath. Soak your feet for 10 minutes or longer. While your feet are still damp, gently remove calluses with a pumice stone or callus file.

442
Invigorating foot scrub

Cornmeal and sea salt buff away rough skin. Peppermint essential oil is cooling and energizing. Almond oil is moisturizing.

¼ cup (45g) finely ground cornmeal
1 tablespoon sea salt
1 teaspoon almond oil
3 drops peppermint essential oil

Mix the ingredients together in a small plastic tub and add enough warm water to make a thick paste. Sit on the edge of the bathtub and massage your clean, damp feet with the scrub, paying attention to rough, callused areas. Rinse your feet well with warm, soapy water.

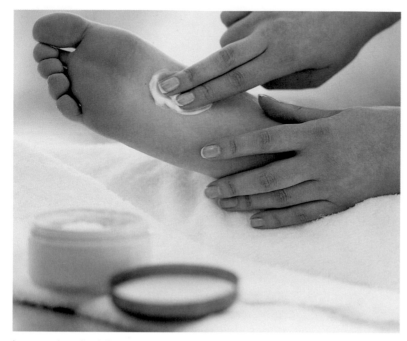

Lemon and patchouli foot cream softens calluses

443

Lemon and patchouli foot cream

Lemon essential oil softens calluses, while patchouli essential oil heals cracked skin. Cocoa butter is an excellent moisturizer.

¼ cup (60g) cocoa butter
10 drops lemon essential oil
5 drops patchouli essential oil

Put the cocoa butter in a small heavy saucepan and warm over a low heat until it melts. Remove the saucepan from the heat and stir the lemon and patchouli essential oils into the melted butter. Pour the mixture into a glass jar and allow to cool. Massage the cream into your feet before going to bed at night. To avoid staining your sheets, slip on a pair of cotton socks before climbing into bed.

444

Aromatherapy foot powder

Arrowroot, cornstarch, and clay absorb excess perspiration. Cypress, lavender, and patchouli essential oils prevent foot odor.

½ cup (50g) arrowroot or cornstarch
2 tablespoons white cosmetic clay
10 drops cypress essential oil
10 drops lavender essential oil
3 drops patchouli essential oil

Mix the arrowroot or cornstarch with the cosmetic clay. Add the essential oils drop by drop, mixing the oils into the powder with your fingers. Store in a covered container, and let the powder sit for a couple of days to allow the oils to completely scent the powder. Dust the powder onto your feet once or twice daily.

445

Refreshing foot spray

Witch hazel extract and lavender and peppermint essential oils make a cooling foot spray.

4fl oz (125ml) distilled witch hazel
15 drops lavender essential oil
5 drops peppermint essential oil

Combine the ingredients in a spray bottle and shake well. Spray liberally on your feet as often as desired.

446

Aromatherapy foot spray

Lavender, cypress, and patchouli not only freshen the feet but have potent antimicrobial properties which help eliminate odor-causing bacteria. Witch hazel is cooling and astringent.

4fl oz (125ml) distilled witch hazel
30 drops lavender essential oil
10 drops cypress or patchouli
    essential oil

Combine the witch hazel with the essential oils. Shake well, and spray on your feet twice daily.

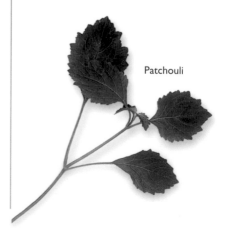

Patchouli

Elbows & Knees

The skin covering elbows and knees lacks oil glands and easily becomes rough, scaly, and darkened. Regular moisturizers do little to improve the skin's leathery appearance, but a few sessions of special exfoliating treatments and rich moisturizers will produce quick results.

447
Rich elbow and knee cream

This rich cream is good for very dry areas of the body, such as the elbows and knees. Avocado oil, coconut oil, and beeswax are all moisturizing. Patchouli essential oil helps heal cracked skin and lemon essential oil softens rough skin. Vitamin E and grapefruit-seed extract are added to the cream as preservatives and to help prevent bacterial growth.

2 tablespoons avocado oil

2 tablespoons coconut oil

1 tablespoon grated beeswax

1 400-IU capsule vitamin E oil

2 tablespoons lemon juice, strained

2 tablespoons filtered water

5 drops patchouli essential oil

2 drops lemon essential oil

3 drops grapefruit-seed extract

Place the avocado oil, coconut oil, and beeswax in a small saucepan and warm gently over a low heat until the beeswax melts. Remove from the heat. Add the contents of the vitamin E capsule. Warm the lemon juice and water over a low heat. Remove this from the heat. When both mixtures are lukewarm, slowly pour the lemon water into the oil, beating steadily with a wire whisk or an electric mixer set on the lowest speed until cool, thick, and smooth. Stir in the patchouli and lemon essential oils as well as the grapefruit-seed extract. Spoon the resulting cream into a clean jar and cool completely before covering. Store in a cool place. Massage a small amount of cream into your elbows and knees as often as you desire.

448
Elbow or knee bleaching treatment

This treatment will help soften and bleach the skin of your elbows or knees. Cut a lemon in half and sprinkle each half with one teaspoon of sugar. Rub the lemon halves into each elbow or knee for a couple of minutes. Rinse your skin well, and apply a rich moisturizing cream (see No. 447).

449
Avocado and lemon treatment

Save your avocado peels for softening the rough skin on your elbows and knees. Halve the avocado and scoop out most of the flesh, leaving a shell. Sprinkle a bit of lemon juice on the inside of the shell. Rub the inside of the shell on each elbow or knee for a couple of minutes. Rinse your skin with warm water.

450
Honey and lemon skin-smoother

Honey and almond oil are both excellent moisturizers. Lemon juice contains natural fruit acids that can help soften the scaly skin on your elbows and knees.

2 teaspoons almond oil

2 teaspoons honey

2 teaspoons lemon juice

Mix the ingredients together and massage the mixture into your elbows and knees for a couple of minutes. Rinse with warm water and apply a moisturizer (see No. 447). Repeat as often as you desire.

Honey and lemon soften rough skin

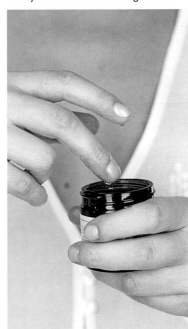

Natural Deodorants

Body odor occurs when sweat comes into contact with bacteria on the skin. Most cases of body odor are simple to cure: bathe or shower daily, and use a natural deodorant to check the growth of odor-causing bacteria.

451
Aromatherapy deodorant

Cypress and lavender essential oils combined with grapefruit-seed extract help stop the growth of odor-causing bacteria. Witch hazel has an astringent action.

2fl oz (60ml) distilled witch hazel
10 drops grapefruit-seed extract
10 drops cypress essential oil
10 drops lavender essential oil

Mix the ingredients in a small spray bottle and shake well before using. Spray under your arms as needed.

452
Citrus and lavender deodorant

Lavender and grapefruit essential oils are light and refreshing natural deodorants. Witch hazel is a gentle astringent and grapefruit-seed is antimicrobial and helps fight the bacteria that cause body odor.

2fl oz (60ml) distilled witch hazel
10 drops grapefruit-seed extract
10 drops lavender essential oil
10 drops grapefruit essential oil

Mix the ingredients in a small spray bottle and shake well before using. Spray under your arms as needed.

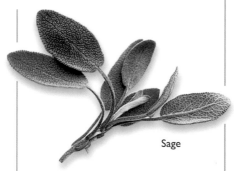

Sage

453
Sage deodorant

Sage is strongly astringent and helps reduce excessive perspiration. Witch hazel is cleansing and cooling, while grapefruit-seed extract fights odor-causing bacteria. Clary sage and patchouli are effective deodorants.

2fl oz (60ml) distilled witch hazel
1fl oz (30ml) sage herbal extract
　　(alcohol-based)
10 drops grapefruit-seed extract
10 drops clary sage essential oil
5 drops patchouli essential oil

Mix the ingredients in a small spray bottle and shake well before using. Spray under your arms as needed.

454
Gentle herbal deodorant

Thyme, sage, lavender, and lemon peel make a refreshing deodorant. Apple cider vinegar helps fight the odor-causing bacteria, and witch hazel is mildly astringent.

2 tablespoons dried thyme
2 tablespoons dried sage
2 tablespoons dried lavender
1 tablespoon chopped fresh lemon peel
1 cup (250ml) distilled witch hazel
2 tablespoons apple cider vinegar

Steep the dried thyme, sage, and lavender with the lemon peel and witch hazel in a covered jar for one week. Strain the liquid, and pour into a clean spray bottle. Add the apple cider vinegar and shake well. Spray under your arms as needed.

455
Deodorant body powder

The arrowroot and cosmetic clay in this light deodorant body powder absorb the excess perspiration from your skin. A combination of clary sage, lavender, and patchouli essential oils helps neutralize the odor-causing bacteria.

½ cup (50g) arrowroot
2 tablespoons white cosmetic clay
7 drops lavender essential oil
5 drops clary sage essential oil
2 drops patchouli essential oil

Mix together the arrowroot and the cosmetic clay. Add the lavender, clary sage, and patchouli essential oils drop by drop to the powder, mixing well with your fingers. Store the powder in a tightly covered container. Let the powder sit untouched for a couple of days before using to allow the essential oils to completely permeate the powder. Use the powder as often as you desire.

Skin-soothing Aftershaves

Shaving and waxing are two of the most common methods of removing unwanted hair. Although quick and efficient, both can cause skin irritation and rashes. A brief warm shower softens hair and makes it easier to remove; applying a soothing herbal aftershave helps calm inflammation and irritation.

456
Herbal aftershave body lotion

Chamomile, calendula, lavender, and rose soothe skin inflammation and promote healing. Witch hazel is a gentle astringent, and vegetable glycerin moisturizes skin.

2 tablespoons dried chamomile

2 tablespoons dried calendula

½ cup (125ml) distilled witch hazel

½ cup (125ml) rose water

1 teaspoon vegetable glycerin

10 drops lavender essential oil

5 drops rose essential oil

Steep the chamomile and calendula in the witch hazel and rose water in a covered jar for two weeks. Strain, and add the vegetable glycerin and essential oils. Shake well, and smooth into your skin after shaving or waxing to prevent skin irritation.

457
Soothe irritated skin with chamomile tea

Cold chamomile tea provides quick relief for skin irritation caused by waxing or shaving. Chamomile contains azulene, a potent anti-inflammatory. For small areas of skin, such as the bikini line or upper lip, use wet, chilled chamomile tea bags. For larger areas of skin, such as the legs, prepare chamomile tea by pouring two cups (500ml) of boiling water over four tablespoons of the dried herb. Cover, and steep until cool. Strain, and refrigerate for up to one week. After shaving or waxing, soak a clean washcloth in the cold tea and apply the wet cloth to the irritated area for 10 minutes.

458
Soothing lavender spray

In an 8fl oz (250ml) spray bottle, mix 30 drops of lavender essential oil with one tablespoon of distilled witch hazel. Shake well, fill the bottle with filtered water, and shake again. Spray liberally on irritated skin as often as desired. To enhance the cooling properties, store in the refrigerator.

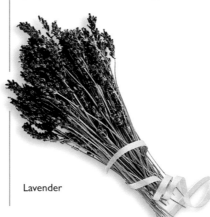

Lavender

459
Prevent razor burn

Razor burn plagues many men, especially those with sensitive skin or coarse, thick facial hair. If you prepare your skin first, you can enjoy a smooth, close shave without irritation. First, soften your beard with hot compresses. Soak a washcloth in a basin of hot water to which one drop of lavender essential oil has been added. Wring out the cloth and apply it to your face and neck, repeating the process several times. Next, apply a thin layer of moisturizing oil (such as jojoba or avocado oil) to your skin. Use a rich shaving cream, and rinse your face thoroughly with warm water after shaving.

460
Herbal aftershave lotion for men

Comfrey and calendula help heal skin irritation and tiny cuts caused by shaving. Witch hazel is a mild astringent and sandalwood calms inflammation. Vegetable glycerin helps moisturize skin.

2 tablespoons dried comfrey leaf

1 tablespoon dried calendula

1 cup (250ml) distilled witch hazel

½ teaspoon vegetable glycerin

20 drops sandalwood essential oil

Steep the comfrey and calendula in the witch hazel in a covered jar for two weeks. Strain, and add the vegetable glycerin and sandalwood essential oil. Shake well, and apply to your skin after shaving.

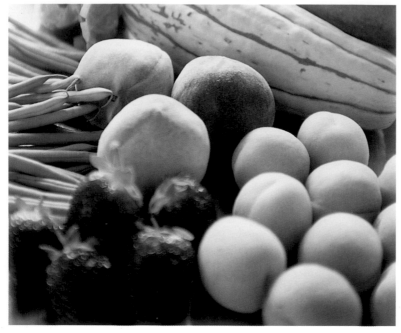

Fresh fruit and vegetables provide essential nutrients for beauty

Natural Hair Care

A nutrient-rich diet creates healthy, strong, and shiny hair. Protein, healthful fats, and a daily intake of vitamin A, vitamin B complex, and iron are essential. Choose hair-care products specifically for your hair type, and enjoy the fragrant benefits that herbs and essential oils add to natural hair-care treatments.

461
Vitamin A

Vitamin A keeps the scalp healthy and helps rebuild tissue. Foods rich in vitamin A and beta-carotene—a vegetable form of vitamin A—include dark leafy greens and yellow and orange vegetables and fruits. The foods richest in beta-carotene include carrots and sweet potatoes. You can supplement your diet with 4,000 IU of vitamin A daily. *Caution:* If you are pregnant or trying to conceive,

do not take more than 4,000 IU because of the risk of birth defects.

462
Vitamin B complex

The vitamin B complex keeps hair strong and the scalp healthy. Increase your intake of whole grains, dark leafy greens, nuts, seafood, and soy foods. Take a supplement which has at least 50mcg each of vitamin B_{12} and biotin, 400mcg of folic acid, and 50mg of other B vitamins.

463
Iron-rich diet

Low iron intake is a main cause of hair loss among women who are not menopausal. Iron-rich foods include dark leafy greens, dried fruits, nuts, whole grains, and legumes. *Caution:* If you are a man or a menopausal woman, consult your doctor before taking an iron supplement because excess iron increases your risk for heart disease.

464
Cleansing and conditioning

To clean your hair and scalp, first rinse with warm water, then apply a small amount of shampoo and massage well into your scalp with your fingertips. Rinse out the shampoo with warm water. There's no need to lather twice. Apply a conditioner and massage it into your hair and scalp. If your scalp tends to be oily, apply conditioner only to the ends of your hair. Rinse thoroughly with warm water.

465
Herbal hair rinses

An herbal hair rinse removes shampoo residue, helps restore healthy pH balance to the scalp, and brings out the natural highlights in your hair. Scalp rinses can also help heal inflammation and irritation caused by heat and chemical hair treatments. Apply an herbal rinse either before or after conditioning.

466
Scalp massage

Massaging the scalp stimulates blood circulation to the scalp, helps get rid of debris that can clog hair follicles, and encourages hair growth. Each day, spend a couple of minutes massaging your scalp with an aromatherapy scalp massage lotion—either before going to bed or prior to shampooing your hair.

467
Deep conditioning your hair

To keep your hair in top condition, use a deep-conditioning pack once a month. The rich oils in the packs soften dry and damaged hair. You can also apply a pack each week to help you restore luster and manageability to your hair.

470
Herbal shampoo for dark hair

Lavender, rosemary, and cloves bring out highlights in dark hair.

$^1/_2$ cup (125ml) water
1 teaspoon dried lavender
1 teaspoon dried rosemary
$^1/_2$ teaspoon whole cloves
2 tablespoons unscented natural
    shampoo

Bring the water and herbs to a boil in a small covered pot. Remove from the heat and let the mixture steep for 30 minutes. Strain, and pour into a clean bottle. Add the unscented shampoo and shake well. Use within one week or refrigerate for up to one month.

Caring for Normal Hair

To keep normal hair healthy and manageable, shampoo daily (or as often as needed) with a gentle natural shampoo. Avoid those with synthetic detergents such as sodium lauryl sulfate, which can irritate the scalp. An herbal rinse removes shampoo residue, softens hair, and brings out a healthy shine. Treat your hair and scalp occasionally to a deep-conditioning hair pack (*see No. 490*).

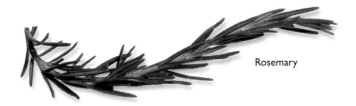

Rosemary

471
Herbal shampoo for blonde hair

To bring out the highlights in blonde hair, follow instructions for Herbal shampoo for dark hair (*see No. 470*), substituting one teaspoon each of dried calendula and chamomile, and one teaspoon chopped lemon peel for lavender, rosemary, and cloves.

468
Aromatherapy shampoo

Lavender and rosemary essential oils may be used in a simple shampoo appropriate for all hair types.

$^1/_4$ cup (60ml) unscented natural
    shampoo
$^1/_4$ cup (60ml) spring water
20 drops lavender essential oil
10 drops rosemary essential oil

Combine the ingredients in a clean bottle and shake well before using.

469
Protect your hair

To protect your hair from damage caused by sun and wind, use a leave-in hair conditioner or wear a hat if you're outdoors for long periods of time. If you are a swimmer, wear a swim cap. Shampoo and condition your hair after a swim in chlorinated or saltwater. Avoid hot blow-dryers and curling irons. If you must use a hair dryer, run it on a cool setting and use a leave-in conditioner.

472
Herbal shampoo for red hair

To bring out highlights in red hair, follow the instructions for Herbal shampoo for dark hair (*see No. 470*), substituting one teaspoon each of dried hibiscus and calendula, and half a teaspoon ground cinnamon for lavender, rosemary, and cloves.

473
Herbal vinegar hair rinse

Apple cider vinegar cuts through the dulling residue left by styling products and shampoos. Lavender, chamomile, and rosemary are beneficial for all hair types.

1 tablespoon dried lavender
1 tablespoon dried chamomile
1 tablespoon dried rosemary
1 cup (250ml) apple cider vinegar

Steep the lavender, chamomile, and rosemary in the apple cider vinegar in a covered glass jar for two weeks. Strain, and pour into a bottle. Add one tablespoon to one cup (250ml) of water and pour through hair as a final rinse after shampooing.

474
Highlight rinse for dark hair

Rosemary, sage, and lavender bring out the highlights in dark hair.

2 tablespoons dried rosemary
2 tablespoons dried sage
2 tablespoons dried lavender
2 cups (500ml) water
1 tablespoon apple cider vinegar

Bring the rosemary, sage, lavender, and water to a boil in a covered pot. Remove from the heat and allow to steep until cool. Strain, pour into a clean container, and add the apple cider vinegar. Shake well. Pour half a cup (125ml) of the rinse through your hair after shampooing. Store the remaining rinse in the refrigerator for up to two weeks.

475
Highlight rinse for blonde hair

Chamomile, calendula, and lemon juice together bring out the highlights in blonde hair.

3 tablespoons dried chamomile
3 tablespoons dried calendula
2 cups (500ml) water
1 tablespoon lemon juice

Bring the chamomile, calendula, and water to a boil in a covered pot. Remove from the heat and allow to steep until cool. Strain, pour into a clean container, and add the lemon juice. Shake well. Pour half a cup (125ml) of the rinse through your hair after shampooing. Store the remaining hair rinse in the refrigerator for up to two weeks.

476
Highlight rinse for red hair

Hibiscus and calendula bring out the highlights in red hair.

3 tablespoons dried hibiscus
3 tablespoons dried calendula
2 cups (500ml) water
1 tablespoon apple cider vinegar

Bring the hibiscus, calendula, and water to a boil in a covered pot. Remove from the heat and allow to steep until cool. Strain, pour into a clean container, and add the apple cider vinegar. Shake well. Pour half a cup (125ml) of the rinse through your hair after shampooing. Store the remaining hair rinse in the refrigerator for up to two weeks.

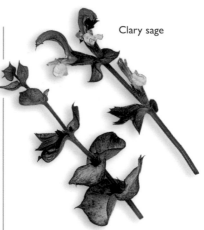

Clary sage

477
Fragrant hair conditioner

Lavender, sandalwood, and clary sage make a richly scented conditioner that smooths flyaway hair.

25 drops lavender essential oil
25 drops sandalwood essential oil
5 drops clary sage essential oil

Combine the oils in a small bottle, shake well, and smooth a few drops onto your hair.

478
Conditioning oil

Use a conditioning oil before you color your hair, both to protect it and to help it absorb color more evenly.

479
Hairbrush oil

Shake a few drops of your favorite essential oil onto your hairbrush to scent your hair and lift your spirits. Experiment with different fragrances. For example, lavender eases tension, rosemary sharpens mental focus, and sandalwood promotes relaxation.

Caring for Oily Hair

Oily hair needs thorough cleansing, but be sure to choose a shampoo that cleanses without overdrying. Shampoos with detergents can stimulate excess oil production; shampoos with built-in conditioners can make hair greasy. Vinegar hair rinses are excellent, as are mildly astringent herbs and essential oils.

480
Herbal shampoo

Yarrow, peppermint, and lemon peel refresh and deep-clean hair and scalp.

1/2 cup (125ml) water
1 teaspoon dried yarrow
1 teaspoon dried peppermint
1 teaspoon chopped fresh lemon peel
2 tablespoons unscented natural shampoo

Bring the water, herbs, and lemon to a boil in a covered pot. Remove from the heat and steep for 30 minutes. Strain, and pour into a clean bottle. Add the shampoo and shake well. Use within a week or store for up to one month in the refrigerator.

481
Aromatherapy shampoo

Juniper and cypress essential oils make a fragrant cleansing shampoo.

1 tablespoon apple cider vinegar
20 drops cypress essential oil
10 drops juniper essential oil
1/4 cup (60ml) unscented natural shampoo
1/4 cup (60ml) spring water

Mix the vinegar and oils and then add the shampoo and water. Shake well.

482
Herbal rinse

Yarrow and lavender are gentle astringents that help reduce oiliness.

2 tablespoons dried yarrow
2 tablespoons dried lavender
2 tablespoons dried peppermint
2 cups (500ml) water
2 tablespoons apple cider vinegar

Bring herbs and water to a boil in a covered pot. Steep until cool. Strain, pour into a clean container, and add the vinegar. Shake well. Pour half a cup (125ml) of rinse through your hair after shampooing. Store the rinse in a refrigerator for up to two weeks.

483
Herbal vinegar rinse

Peppermint, lavender, and juniper make a refreshing rinse for oily hair.

1 tablespoon dried peppermint
1 tablespoon dried lavender
1 tablespoon crushed juniper berries
1 cup (250ml) apple cider vinegar

Steep the herbs and berries in the vinegar in a covered glass jar for two weeks. Strain, and pour into a bottle. Add a tablespoon to a cup (250ml) of water and pour through your hair as a final rinse after shampooing.

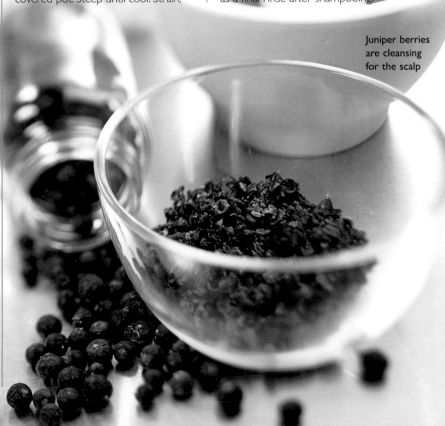

Juniper berries are cleansing for the scalp

Caring for Dry Hair

Dry hair doesn't need to be shampooed daily; instead, simply rinse it under a warm shower on the days you don't shampoo. Use a vinegar and herb rinse after shampooing to restore a healthy pH balance to your scalp and to relieve itching. Once a week, apply a deep-conditioning hair pack to restore luster.

484
Herbal shampoo

Elderflower, marshmallow root, and rose petals help soften and condition dry hair.

1 teaspoon dried elderflower
1 teaspoon dried marshmallow root
1 teaspoon dried rose petals
½ cup (125ml) water
2 tablespoons unscented natural shampoo

Bring the elderflowers, marshmallow root, rose petals, and water to a boil in a small covered pot. Remove from heat and let steep for 30 minutes. Strain, and pour into a clean bottle. Add the unscented shampoo to the herbal liquid and shake well. Either use the shampoo within one week or store it for up to one month in the refrigerator.

485
Aromatherapy shampoo

Sandalwood and palmarosa essential oils combined with vegetable glycerin help moisturize dry hair.

20 drops sandalwood essential oil
10 drops palmarosa essential oil
1 tablespoon vegetable glycerin
¼ cup (60ml) unscented natural shampoo
¼ cup (60ml) spring water

Combine the sandalwood and palmarosa essential oils with the vegetable glycerin in a bottle and shake well. Add the unscented shampoo and spring water to the mixture and then shake again. Either use the shampoo within one week or store it for up to one month in the refrigerator.

486
Herbal rinse

As with the herbal shampoo, rose petals, chamomile, and marshmallow root are beneficial for dry hair.

2 tablespoons dried chamomile
2 tablespoons dried rose petals
2 tablespoons dried marshmallow root
2 cups (500ml) water

Bring the chamomile, rose petals, marshmallow root, and water to a boil in a covered pot. Remove from the heat and allow to steep until cool. Strain, pour the liquid into a clean

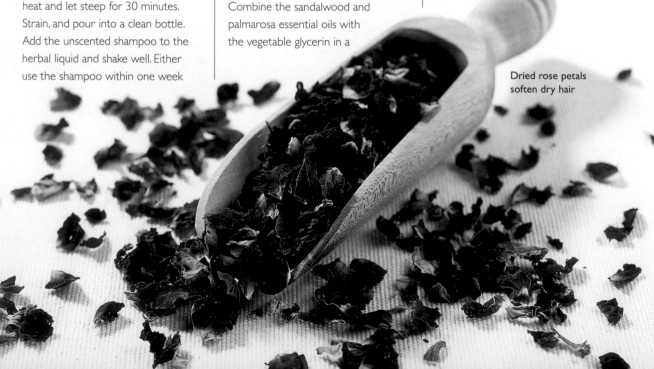

Dried rose petals soften dry hair

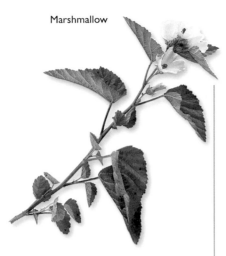

Marshmallow

container, and shake well. Pour half a cup (125ml) of the rinse through your hair after shampooing. Store the remaining hair rinse in the refrigerator for up to two weeks.

487
Comfrey scalp healing rinse

Chemical treatments such as perms and coloring can irritate and inflame the scalp. An herbal scalp rinse made from comfrey, nettle, and rosemary is antiseptic, astringent, and healing.

2 tablespoons dried nettle

2 tablespoons dried rosemary

2 tablespoons dried comfrey leaf

2 cups (500ml) water

2 tablespoons apple cider vinegar

Bring the herbs and water to a boil in a covered pot. Remove from the heat and allow to steep for one hour. Strain, and add the apple cider vinegar. Apply half a cup (125ml) or more to your scalp after shampooing and rinsing. Store the remaining herbal rinse in the refrigerator for up to two weeks.

488
Herbal vinegar rinse

Apple cider vinegar helps restore a healthy pH balance to dry hair.

1 tablespoon dried chamomile

1 tablespoon dried rose petals

1 tablespoon dried marshmallow root

1 cup (250ml) apple cider vinegar

Steep the herbs in the apple cider vinegar in a covered glass jar for two weeks. Strain, and pour into a clean bottle. Add one tablespoon of the rinse to one cup (250ml) of water and pour through your hair as a final rinse after shampooing.

489
Avocado moisturizing hair pack

The natural oils in avocado make an excellent moisturizing treatment for dry hair.

1 large ripe avocado

1 tablespoon honey

Mash the avocado into a smooth purée and stir in the honey. Dampen your hair with warm water and massage the avocado mixture into the hair. Cover with a plastic shower cap and leave in place for 30 minutes. Rinse well and shampoo.

490
Fragrant oil deep-conditioning treatment

Once a week, deep condition your hair and scalp to combat the damage caused by overcleansing, heat, and chemical treatments. Sandalwood

essential oil helps revitalize dry hair. To make the deep conditioner, mix a tablespoon of jojoba or almond oil with five drops of sandalwood essential oil in a small container. (If you have long hair, you may need to double the amounts). Dampen your hair with warm water and massage the oil mixture into your scalp and hair with your fingertips. If your scalp tends to be oily, apply the treatment only to the ends of your hair. Put on a shower cap and allow the oils to remain in your hair for 30 minutes. Shampoo your hair to remove the oil treatment, rinse well, and apply a conditioner if necessary.

491
Honey conditioning hair pack

Honey, egg yolks, and almond oil create a rich moisturizing treatment for damaged hair. Add rosemary and lavender essential oils for their scalp-soothing properties.

2 tablespoons honey

1 tablespoon almond oil

1 egg yolk

3 drops rosemary essential oil

3 drops lavender essential oil

Beat together the honey, almond oil, and egg yolk. Stir in the rosemary and lavender essential oils. Dampen your hair with warm water and massage the conditioning treatment into the hair with your fingers. Cover your hair with a plastic shower cap and leave the conditioning pack in place for about 30 minutes. Rinse your hair well with lukewarm water and then shampoo to remove the conditioner.

Solutions for Hair Loss

Thinning hair is often caused by an underfunctioning thyroid gland, poor nutrient absorption, a lack of essential nutrients, or a hormonal imbalance. If you are experiencing severe or sustained hair loss, consult your doctor for a proper diagnosis and treatment.

492
Feed your hair with protein and minerals

New hair needs protein and minerals. Good sources of these nutrients include tofu and tempeh; cold-water fish, such as salmon, tuna, mackerel, and sardines; and eggs. Consider supplementing your diet with a high-potency multimineral, and take it in divided doses with food.

493
Get your blood moving with exercise

Exercising aerobically for at least 30 minutes, three to four times a week, helps improve blood circulation throughout your body. To increase blood flow specifically to your scalp, end your shower by rinsing your scalp with cold water for one minute.

494
Control stress

Stress causes a tightening of muscles, which can inhibit blood circulation to your scalp. Practice relaxation techniques, deep-breathing exercises, or yoga to relieve stress, and take a high-potency B-complex vitamin to help your body handle stress.

495
Massage your scalp

Aromatherapy essential oils and scalp massage encourage your hair to grow by increasing the blood circulation to the scalp follicles. This, in turn, helps to stimulate the production of stronger, healthier hair.

Witch hazel and essential oils

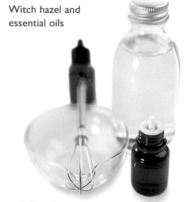

496
Stimulating scalp massage

Rosemary essential oil has been used for centuries to stimulate scalp circulation; lavender oil is soothing, and witch hazel is mildly astringent.

3 drops rosemary essential oil
3 drops lavender essential oil
1 tablespoon distilled witch hazel

Mix the ingredients and massage vigorously into your scalp once a day.

497
Aromatherapy hair growth formula

A combination of rosemary and cedarwood essential oils helps promote hair growth. Jojoba oil and aloe vera gel keep the hair follicles in the scalp healthy.

1 teaspoon jojoba oil
15 drops rosemary essential oil
10 drops cedarwood essential oil
¼ cup (60ml) aloe vera gel

Combine the jojoba oil with the rosemary and cedarwood essential oils. Mix in the aloe vera gel and blend thoroughly. Store in a bottle. Massage one tablespoon of the mixture into your scalp each night before going to bed.

498
Shampoo for hair loss

Shampooing with a mixture of essential oils can help stimulate hair growth. Rosemary, thyme, and lavender essential oils are all regarded as beneficial for hair growth.

8fl oz (250ml) unscented natural shampoo
30 drops rosemary essential oil
10 drops thyme essential oil
10 drops lavender essential oil

Mix the shampoo with the rosemary, thyme, and lavender essential oils in a plastic bottle. Massage a small amount of the mixture into your scalp when shampooing. Keep the shampoo out of your eyes. Let the mixture sit in your hair for three minutes, then rinse thoroughly.

Solutions for Dandruff

Everyone sheds millions of scalp cells daily, but if the white flakes conspicuously dust your shoulders, you may have an overabundant population of a microscopic fungus living on your scalp. An herbal shampoo, rinse, and scalp treatment can help control the fungus while improving your scalp health.

499
Herbal antidandruff shampoo

Eucalyptus, lavender, and tea tree essential oils have antimicrobial properties and help clean and heal the scalp.

1 tablespoon apple cider vinegar
15 drops eucalyptus essential oil
15 drops lavender essential oil
10 drops tea tree essential oil
¼ cup (60ml) mild natural shampoo
¼ cup (60ml) water

Combine the apple cider vinegar with the eucalyptus, lavender, and tea tree essential oils. Shake well. Add the natural shampoo and the water, and shake again.

500
Simple tea tree oil shampoo

To make yourself a simple shampoo to combat dandruff, squeeze a single application of mild natural shampoo into your hand and add four drops of tea tree essential oil. Tea tree is a potent antiseptic and antifungal. Mix well and massage into your scalp with your fingertips. Allow the shampoo to remain on your hair for five minutes, then rinse well.

501
Antidandruff hair rinse

A combination of antimicrobial herbs such as thyme, rosemary, and sage, and essential oils, such as eucalyptus and lavender, fight the microorganisms that cause dandruff. Vinegar restores a healthy pH balance to the scalp.

1 teaspoon dried thyme
1 teaspoon dried rosemary
1 teaspoon dried sage
1 cup (250ml) boiling water
¼ cup (60ml) apple cider vinegar
10 drops eucalyptus essential oil
10 drops lavender essential oil

Pour the water over the herbs and cover. Cool the mixture to room temperature and strain. Combine with the apple cider vinegar. Add the essential oils and shake well. Massage approximately a quarter of a cup (60ml) into your scalp after shampooing and rinsing your hair. Refrigerate the remaining hair rinse and use within one month.

502
Antiseptic scalp treatment

Antiseptic essential oils, such as eucalyptus, rosemary, and lavender, can help eliminate the fungus that causes dandruff. Witch hazel is mildly astringent and healing.

½ cup (125ml) distilled witch hazel
20 drops eucalyptus essential oil
20 drops rosemary essential oil
20 drops lavender essential oil

Combine the witch hazel with the eucalyptus, rosemary, and lavender essential oils. Massage approximately one tablespoon of the mixture into your scalp every night before going to bed. Continue with the treatment until the dandruff clears up.

503
Deep-conditioning treatment for dandruff

Once a week, deep condition your hair and scalp to alleviate scalp dryness and dandruff. Eucalyptus, rosemary, and lavender essential oils help combat dandruff. Jojoba oil helps keep the hair follicles in the scalp healthy.

1 tablespoon jojoba oil
2 drops eucalyptus essential oil
3 drops rosemary essential oil
3 drops lavender essential oil

Combine the jojoba oil with the eucalyptus, rosemary, and lavender essential oils in a small container. (If you have long hair, you may need to double the amounts in the recipe.) Dampen your hair with warm water and massage the oil mixture into your scalp and hair with your fingertips. Put on a shower cap and allow the oils to remain in your hair for 30 minutes. Shampoo your hair to remove the oil treatment, rinse well, and apply a conditioner if necessary.

Herbal Baths

Herbal baths provide gentle healing benefits for the body and mind. Depending on the herbs you choose, an herbal bath can relax or energize you, soften your skin, or ease muscle tension and soreness. Relaxing bath herbs include chamomile, lavender, passionflower, and rose. Energizing bath herbs include lemon, eucalyptus, grapefruit, peppermint, and thyme.

504
Relaxing herbal bath

Chamomile, lavender, and linden can help ease physical and emotional tension. Mix three tablespoons each of dried chamomile, lavender, and linden. Place the mixture of herbs in a double layer of cheesecloth, tie with a string, and toss into the bath as the tub is filling. Soak for 20 minutes. To enhance the relaxing effect of the bath, sip a cup of chamomile or linden tea while soaking in the tub.

Herbal baths provide many healthy benefits

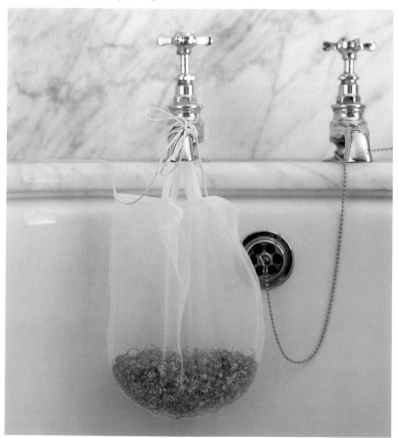

505
Energizing herbal bath

For a refreshing and energizing bath, mix three tablespoons each of dried peppermint, rosemary, and lavender. Place the mixture in a double layer of cheesecloth, tie with a string, and toss into the bath as the tub is filling.

506
Herbal bath for dry skin

Comfrey and marshmallow root help soften dry skin. Chamomile and rose petals add skin-soothing fragrance. Mix two tablespoons each of dried comfrey leaf, marshmallow root, rose petals, and chamomile. Place the mix in a double layer of cheesecloth, tie with a string, and toss into the bath as the tub is filling.

507
Herbal body lotion

Soak in a warm bath for 20 minutes to increase the moisture in your skin. Lightly pat your skin dry and at once apply a rich herbal body lotion to seal in moisture.

508
Herbal bath for sore muscles

Rosemary, marjoram, and lavender will help ease sore muscles. Mix three tablespoons each of dried rosemary, marjoram, and lavender. Place the mixture in a double layer of cheesecloth, tie with a string, and toss into the bath as the tub is filling.

Aromatherapy Baths

In a warm bath, the vapors of essential oils are inhaled; the oils are absorbed through the skin. Choose fragrances that appeal to you, because scents can evoke vivid memories and emotions.

509
Uplifting bath

Together, grapefruit and lavender essential oils make a delightfully fragrant and uplifting blend. Whole milk or vodka will help prevent irritation of the skin.

4 drops grapefruit essential oil
5 drops lavender essential oil
1 tablespoon whole milk or vodka

Combine the essential oils with the milk or vodka. Add the mixture to a tub of warm water and stir into the water with your hand.

510
Sensuous bath

For a scented blend that lingers sensuously on the skin, follow the recipe for Uplifting bath (see No. 509), substituting four drops of sandalwood essential oil, two drops of rose essential oil, two drops of clary sage essential oil, and one drop of ylang ylang essential oil.

511
Calming bath

For a soothing and calming bath that helps you to balance your emotions, follow the recipe for Uplifting bath (see No. 509), substituting three drops of rose essential oil, three drops of

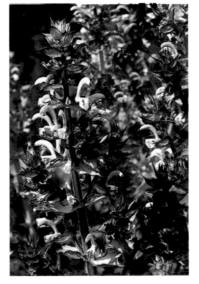

Clary sage has relaxing properties

neroli essential oil, and one drop of chamomile essential oil.

512
Relaxing bath

For a wonderfully relaxing, fragrant bath, follow the recipe for Uplifting bath (see No. 509), substituting four drops of lavender essential oil and two drops each of clary sage and sandalwood essential oils.

513
Energizing bath

For an energizing and refreshing bath, follow the recipe for Uplifting bath (see No. 509), substituting five drops

of lavender essential oil, two drops of rosemary essential oil, and two drops of peppermint essential oil.

514
Sweet dreams bath

For a deeply relaxing bath just before bed, follow the recipe for Uplifting bath (see No. 509), substituting four drops of vetiver essential oil and two drops each of clary sage and ylang ylang essential oil.

515
After-exercise bath

For a bath to ease muscle stiffness or soreness caused by overexertion, follow the recipe for Uplifting bath (see No. 509), using four drops each of eucalyptus, marjoram, and lavender essential oils.

516
Mind-clearing bath

For a bath to clear the mind after a long day at work, follow the recipe for Uplifting bath (see No. 509), substituting five drops of lavender essential oil and two drops each of spearmint and basil essential oil.

517
Meditative bath

For a bath that blends meditative calmness with feelings of love and compassion, follow the recipe for Uplifting bath (see No. 509), substituting four drops of sandalwood essential oil and two drops each of frankincense and rose oils.

Bath Salts

Adding earth and sea minerals to a bath replicates the healing waters found in natural mineral springs. Baths with mineral salts relax the mind and body, stimulate gentle purification, soothe tired and sore muscles, and soften the skin.

518

Earth-and-sea bath salts

Epsom salts and sea salt are purifying. Baking soda and borax leave your skin soft and smooth.

½ cup (60g) Epsom salts
½ cup (110g) sea salt
½ cup (60g) baking soda
½ cup (60g) borax

Combine the ingredients. Fill the tub with warm water and then add four to eight tablespoons of bath salts. Mix them into the water to dissolve.

519

Tension-relieving salts

This deeply relaxing bath eases tense and stiff muscles. The magnesium in Epsom salts helps relax the muscles and nervous system. Marjoram has sedative properties and eases muscle aches and stiffness. Lavender soothes both physical and emotional tension.

1 cup (125g) Epsom salts
1 cup (125g) baking soda
5 drops marjoram essential oil
5 drops lavender essential oil

Mix the ingredients together and add to the water just before entering the tub. Stir the water with your hand to dissolve the bath salts in the water. Soak for 20 to 30 minutes.

520

Relaxing bath salts

Sandalwood, lavender, and clary sage make a richly scented and relaxing bath blend.

1 cup (225g) sea salt
1 cup (125g) baking soda
30 drops sandalwood essential oil
10 drops lavender essential oil
10 drops clary sage essential oil

Combine the salt and baking soda. Add the oils, mix well, and store in a covered container. Dissolve four to eight tablespoons of the mixture in a tub is full of warm water.

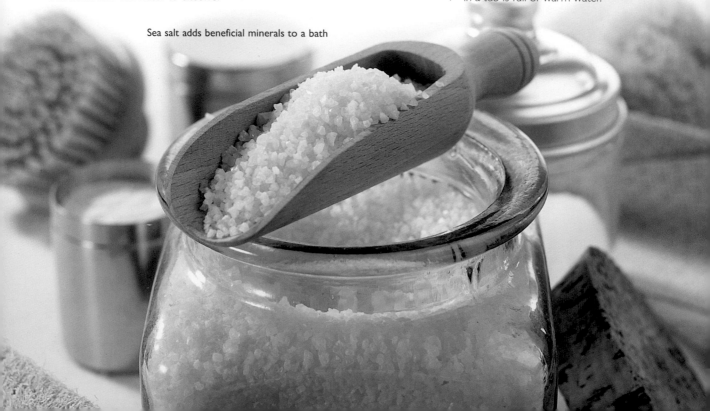

Sea salt adds beneficial minerals to a bath

521
Restorative bath salts

Follow the Relaxing bath salts recipe (see No. 520), substituting 30 drops of lavender, 10 drops of bergamot, and ten drops of geranium oils.

522
Invigorating bath salts

Follow the Relaxing bath salts recipe (see No. 520), substituting 25 drops of lavender, 10 drops of rosemary, 10 drops of petitgrain, and five drops of peppermint essential oils.

523
Uplifting bath salts

Follow the Relaxing bath salts recipe (see No. 520), substituting 25 drops of lavender, 15 drops of grapefruit, and 10 drops of bergamot oils.

524
Soothing bath salts

For a floral blend that soothes body, mind, and spirit, follow the Relaxing bath salts recipe (see No. 520), substituting 30 drops of lavender, 10 drops of clary sage, and five drops each of rose and chamomile oils.

525
Warming bath salts

For a warming bath on cold winter nights, follow the recipe for Relaxing bath salts (see No. 520), substituting 30 drops of sandalwood, 10 drops of sweet orange, five drops of ginger, and three drops of patchouli oils.

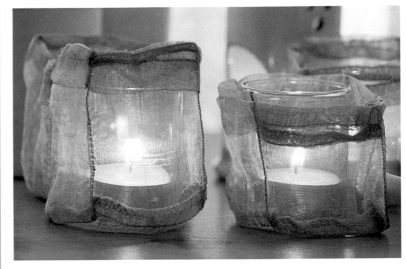

Candles help create the right atmosphere for a restorative bath

526
Meditative bath salts

For a bath that enhances a meditative state, follow the Relaxing bath salts recipe (see No. 520), substituting 25 drops of sandalwood, 20 drops of frankincense, and five drops of rose essential oils.

527
Sensuous bath salts

For an exotic, sensual bath blend with a lingering fragrance, follow the Relaxing bath salts recipe (see No. 520), substituting 30 drops of sandalwood, 10 drops of clary sage, five drops of rose, and two drops of ylang ylang essential oils.

528
Sweet dreams bath salts

For a deeply relaxing bath to enhance sleep and encourage dreams, follow the Relaxing bath salts recipe (see No. 520), replacing the sea salt with a cup (125g) of Epsom salts and substituting 30 drops of vetiver, 10 drops of clary sage, and five drops of ylang ylang essential oils.

529
Soothing bath salts for sore muscles

For a bath that stimulates circulation of the blood and eases sore or stiff muscles after overexerting yourself, follow the Relaxing bath salts recipe (see No. 520), substituting 20 drops of lavender and 10 drops each of eucalyptus, rosemary, and ginger essential oils.

530
Quick relaxer

For a mineral-rich bath that swiftly restores and relaxes you, add two cups (250g) of Epsom salts and one cup (125g) of baking soda as you fill a bath with warm water.

Oatmeal & Milk Baths

Oatmeal and milk baths are beneficial for all skin types and are especially healing for dry or irritated skin. Oats are anti-inflammatory and ease itching, while whole milk is rich in fats that nourish and smooth dry skin.

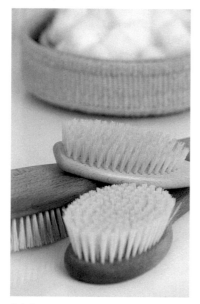

Soft brushes exfoliate dry skin

531
Remove dead skin cells

To prevent dry skin, avoid hot baths and use soap only where necessary because both strip away the skin's protective natural oils. Instead, use warm water and a soft body brush or bath sponge to slough off dead skin cells.

532
Soothing bath

For a bath that soothes both itchy skin or a rash, grind two cups (200g) of rolled oats into a fine powder in a blender, and add to a bathtub of warm water along with one cup (125g) of baking soda. Soak in the bath for 15 minutes.

533
Oatmeal bath

This is a simple and effective way to soothe rashes and dry, itchy skin.

2 cups (200g) rolled oats
10 drops lavender or chamomile
   essential oil

Grind the rolled oats in a blender and sprinkle the fine powder into a bathtub of warm water. Add the lavender or chamomile essential oil and stir the water with your hand to disperse the oats and oil. Soak for 20 minutes, then pat your skin dry without rinsing.

534
Herbal oatmeal bath

This bath softens your skin and helps condition it if it's dry.

2 cups (200g) rolled oats
2 tablespoons dried chamomile
2 tablespoons dried rose petals
2 tablespoons dried lavender

Grind the rolled oats into a coarse powder in a blender and mix with the chamomile, rose, and lavender.

Place half a cup (50g) of the mixture into the center of a double layer of cheesecloth. Tie the cloth with a piece of ribbon or string and toss it into the water as the tub fills.

535
Chamomile moisturizing milk bath

Chamomile, rolled oats, and whole milk can help moisturize dry skin and ease the itching that accompanies dryness.

4 tablespoons dried chamomile
2 cups (500ml) whole milk
1 cup (120g) finely ground rolled oats

Combine the chamomile and milk in a glass jar and steep overnight in the refrigerator. Strain, and add to a tubful of warm water. Grind the oats into a fine powder in a blender and add to the bath. Soak for 15 minutes. Gently pat your skin dry and immediately follow with a rich body lotion to seal in moisture.

536
Fragrant aromatherapy milk bath

Dry whole milk with lavender and ylang ylang oils creates a relaxing, fragrant, and skin-soothing bath.

½ cup (60g) powdered whole milk
7 drops lavender essential oil
2 drops ylang ylang essential oil

Add the powdered milk and the lavender and ylang ylang oils to a bathtub of warm water and stir them into the water with your hand. Soak for 15 to 20 minutes.

Natural Bath Oils

Adding oil to a bath creates a luxurious and moisturizing treatment that is excellent for dry skin. The oils float on top of the water and lightly cling to your skin after bathing.

537
Relaxing floral bath oil

Lavender, rose, and ylang ylang make a sweet, floral-scented, relaxing oil. Jojoba and almond oils moisturize and serve as a base for the bath oil.

2 tablespoons jojoba oil

2 tablespoons almond oil

25 drops lavender essential oil

10 drops rose essential oil

5 drops ylang ylang essential oil

Mix the oils in a tightly capped glass bottle. Add a teaspoon to a bathtub of warm water and stir the oil into the water with your hand. **Caution:** Bath oils make the tub slippery.

538
Uplifting citrus bath oil

For an uplifting, fragrant bath oil, follow the recipe for Relaxing floral bath oil (see No. 537), substituting 25 drops of lavender and 15 drops of grapefruit essential oils.

539
Energizing bath oil

For a bath that restores energy after a long day, follow the recipe for Relaxing floral bath oil (see No. 537), substituting 25 drops of lavender, 10 drops of rosemary, and five drops of peppermint essentail oils.

540
Calming bath oil

For a deeply relaxing and calming blend that has a wonderful lasting fragrance, follow the recipe for Relaxing floral bath oil (see No. 537), substituting 25 drops of sandalwood, 10 drops of lavender, and five drops of clary sage essential oils.

541
Sensual bath oil

For a sensual and exotic bath with a scent that lingers on your skin for hours, follow the recipe for Relaxing floral bath oil (see No. 537), substituting 25 drops of sandalwood, 10 drops of rose, and five drops of patchouli essential oils.

542
Moisturizing bath

Add one teaspoon of almond oil to the warm water in your tub for a simple moisturizing bath.

Bath Vinegars

Apple cider vinegar has mild deodorizing and cleansing properties and helps keep skin healthy by restoring its natural pH balance. Adding fresh or dried herbs infuses the vinegar with healing properties and gives it a pleasant scent.

543
Cooling bath vinegar

Fresh lemon, orange, and mint make a wonderfully scented, refreshing vinegar for a cooling summer bath.

¼ cup (6g) fresh mint

1 fresh, thinly sliced orange

1 fresh, thinly sliced lemon

2 cups (500ml) apple cider vinegar

Chop the mint coarsely. Place the orange, lemon, and mint in a glass canning jar along with the apple cider vinegar and cover with a lid. Allow the mixture to steep for two weeks. Strain into a bottle. Use a quarter of a cup (60ml) of the mixture per bath.

544
Bath vinegar for sensitive skin

A blend of lavender, rose petals, and chamomile makes a soothing bath vinegar for sensitive skin.

2 cups (500ml) apple cider vinegar

2 tablespoons dried lavender

2 tablespoons dried rose petals

2 tablespoons dried chamomile

Place the vinegar and herbs in a glass canning jar and cover with a lid. Allow the mixture to steep for two weeks. Strain into a bottle. Use a quarter of a cup (60ml) of the vinegar mixture per bath.

545
Lavender vinegar

For a simple scented bath vinegar, combine half a teaspoon of lavender essential oil with a cup (250ml) of apple cider vinegar in a bottle. Steep for one week before using. Shake the bottle once a day to disperse the oil in the vinegar. Use a quarter of a cup (60ml) of lavender vinegar per bath.

546
Rosemary invigorating bath vinegar

Rosemary, marjoram, and lavender help ease mental and physical fatigue. Fresh herbs are best in this vinegar, but you can use dried if necessary.

¼ cup (6g) fresh rosemary
    (or 2 tablespoons dried)
¼ cup (6g) fresh marjoram
    (or 2 tablespoons dried)
¼ cup (6g) fresh lavender
    (or 2 tablespoons dried)
2 cups (500ml) apple cider vinegar

Chop up the herbs coarsely and combine with apple cider vinegar in a covered glass canning jar. Allow the mixture to steep for two weeks. Strain into a bottle. Use a quarter of a cup (60ml) of the mixture per bath.

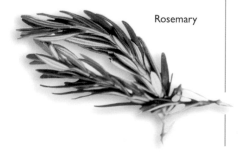
Rosemary

Aromatherapy Soaps

Adding essential oils to soap is one way to enjoy aromatherapy. But use soap sparingly, and only where you need it. To avoid overdrying your skin, wash in warm water instead of hot.

547
Uplifting soap

Lavender and grapefruit make an uplifting bath and shower soap.

25 drops lavender essential oil
15 drops grapefruit essential oil
4fl oz (125ml) liquid castile body soap

Add the oils to the soap and stir thoroughly. Store in a plastic squeeze-top bottle and shake before using.

548
Calming soap

Sandalwood, lavender, and clary sage make a calming soap.

25 drops sandalwood essential oil
10 drops lavender essential oil
5 drops clary sage essential oil
4fl oz (125ml) liquid castile body soap

Add the oils to the soap and stir thoroughly. Store in a plastic squeeze-top bottle and shake before using.

549
Energizing soap

Lavender, rosemary, and peppermint make an energizing soap.

20 drops lavender essential oil
10 drops rosemary essential oil
10 drops peppermint essential oil
4fl oz (125ml) liquid castile body soap

Add the oils to the soap and stir thoroughly. Store in a plastic squeeze-top bottle and shake before using.

550
Mood-boosting soap

Lavender, geranium, and bergamot together make a spicy-sweet bath and shower soap with mood-elevating properties.

20 drops lavender essential oil
10 drops geranium essential oil
10 drops bergamot essential oil
4fl oz (125ml) liquid castile body soap

Add the oils to the soap and stir thoroughly. Store in a plastic squeeze-top bottle and shake before using.

551
Sensual soap

Sandalwood, rose, and patchouli together make an exotic bath and shower soap, leaving you with a fragrant scent that lingers on your skin for hours.

25 drops sandalwood essential oil
10 drops rose essential oil
5 drops patchouli essential oil
4fl oz (125ml) liquid castile body soap

Add the oils to the soap and stir thoroughly. Store in a plastic squeeze-top bottle and shake before using.

Body Scrubs & Polishes

Body scrubs are wonderful allover exfoliating treatments. They slough off rough, dry skin and leave your entire body feeling smooth and silky. Use a gentle touch to avoid irritating delicate skin, and don't use body scrubs on sensitive areas such as the face and genitals.

552
Body scrub for dry, flaky skin

This moisturizing scrub removes flaky skin and soothes skin irritation.

¼ cup (45g) finely ground cornmeal

¼ cup (30g) finely ground rolled oats

¼ cup (30g) finely ground almonds

1 tablespoon almond oil

10 drops lavender essential oil

5 drops sandalwood essential oil

Mix the ingredients in a nonbreakable container. Wet your body in a warm shower, and apply the scrub to your legs, arms, and torso. Massage it into your skin with a circular motion. Rinse well, and pat your skin dry. **Caution:** Use a rubber tub mat to prevent falls.

553
Scrub for sensitive skin

This soothing scrub gently polishes, exfoliates, and moisturizes the skin.

½ cup (125ml) whole-milk yogurt

¼ cup (30g) finely ground rolled oats

¼ cup (15g) wheat bran

1 tablespoon honey

1 tablespoon almond oil

5 drops lavender essential oil

Mix the yogurt, oats, and wheat bran in a nonbreakable container. Mix the honey, almond oil, and lavender oil, and thoroughly combine the two mixtures. Wet your body in a warm shower. Apply the scrub to your legs, arms, and torso. Massage gently into your skin with a circular motion. Rinse well, and pat your skin dry. **Caution:** Use a rubber tub mat to prevent falls.

554
Strawberry exfoliating body scrub

Fresh strawberries make a fragrant body scrub that refreshes and gently exfoliates skin. Yogurt and honey moisturize, and bran polishes.

½ cup (125ml) whole-milk yogurt

½ cup (60g) fresh strawberries

1 tablespoon honey

½ cup (30g) wheat bran

Blend the yogurt, strawberries, and honey in a blender until smooth. Stir in the bran. Wet your body in a warm shower, and apply the scrub to your legs, arms, and torso. Massage it gently into your skin with a circular motion. Rinse, and pat your skin dry. **Caution:** Use a rubber tub mat to prevent falls.

555
Avocado moisturizing body scrub

Ripe avocados make a rich body scrub for moisturizing sensitive or dry skin. Cucumber soothes and cools irritated skin, and almond is a gentle exfoliant.

½ cup (110g) mashed ripe avocado

½ cup (110g) cucumber

¼ cup (40g) almonds

Purée the avocado and cucumber until smooth. Grind the almonds into a coarse meal in a blender and combine with avocado–cucumber purée. Wet your body in a warm shower, and apply the scrub to your legs, arms, and torso. Massage gently into your skin with a circular motion. Rinse well, and pat your skin dry. **Caution:** Use a rubber tub mat to prevent falls.

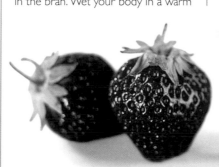
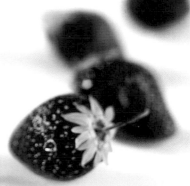

Strawberries

556
Sea salt body polishing scrub

For a simple body-smoothing scrub, mix half a cup (110g) sea salt with two tablespoons of almond oil. Take a quick, warm shower to dampen your skin. Standing in the bathtub, gently massage the mixture onto your skin, avoiding your face and genitals. Rub in a circular motion until your skin is rosy from the increased circulation. Rinse your body well with warm water, and towel yourself dry. **Caution:** Do not use this scrub on sensitive or irritated skin. Use a rubber tub mat to prevent falls.

557
Invigorating body scrub

Peppermint, rosemary, and lavender essential oils make an invigorating body scrub that leaves your skin tingling and refreshed. Almond oil is a mild exfoliant.

2 tablespoons almond oil
2 drops peppermint essential oil
3 drops rosemary essential oil
5 drops lavender essential oil
½ cup (110g) sea salt

Add the almond oil and the essential oils to the sea salt in a small plastic container and mix well. Dampen your skin in a warm shower, and gently massage the mixture onto your skin, avoiding your face and genitals. Rinse your body well with warm water and towel yourself dry. **Caution:** Do not use this scrub on delicate or broken skin. Use a rubber tub mat to prevent falls.

Body Splashes

Body splashes are refreshing toners for your entire body. Made from witch hazel, herbs, and fragrant essential oils, they cool and soothe your skin. Body splashes are especially welcome on hot summer days—spray your body liberally after showering and let your skin dry naturally. They are also great for traveling or after exercise.

558
Uplifting body splash

Lavender and grapefruit make an uplifting, fragrant body splash.

2 tablespoons dried lavender
½ cup (125ml) distilled witch hazel
10 drops grapefruit essential oil
5 drops lavender essential oil
½ cup (125ml) filtered or spring water

Steep the dried lavender in the witch hazel in a covered jar for one week. Strain, and pour into an 8fl oz (250ml) spray bottle. Add grapefruit and lavender essential oils and shake well. Add the water and shake again.

559
Invigorating body splash

A combination of rosemary, lavender, and peppermint makes a cooling and invigorating body splash.

2 tablespoons chopped fresh rosemary
2 tablespoons chopped fresh peppermint
½ cup (125ml) distilled witch hazel
10 drops lavender essential oil
½ cup (125ml) filtered or spring water

Steep the rosemary and peppermint in witch hazel in a covered jar for one week. Strain, and pour into an 8fl oz (250ml) spray bottle. Add lavender essential oil and shake well. Add the water and shake again.

560
Sensual body splash

A combination of sandalwood, rose, and clary sage makes a deliciously sensual body splash.

¼ cup (10g) dried rose petals
½ cup (125ml) distilled witch hazel
10 drops sandalwood essential oil
3 drops rose essential oil
2 drops clary sage essential oil
½ cup (125ml) filtered or spring water

Steep the rose petals in witch hazel in a covered jar for one week. Strain, and pour into an 8fl oz (250ml) spray bottle. Add sandalwood, rose, and clary sage essential oils and shake well. Add the water and shake again.

561
Soothing rose petal body splash

Rose essential oil and rose water make a gentle splash for delicate skin.

1 tablespoon distilled witch hazel
2 drops rose essential oil
1 cup (250ml) distilled rose water

Mix the witch hazel and the rose essential oil in an 8fl oz (250ml) spray bottle. Shake well. Add the rose water and shake again.

562
Cooling lavender water

To soothe skin irritation, spray your skin with cooling lavender water.

30 drops lavender essential oil
1 tablespoon distilled witch hazel

Mix the ingredients in an 8fl oz (250ml) spray bottle. Shake well, fill with filtered water, and shake again. Spray liberally onto irritated skin as often as desired. Refrigerate to enhance the cooling properties.

563
Lavender and aloe vera dry skin spritzer

You can ease the itching caused by dry skin with a mixture of lavender and sandalwood essential oils and aloe juice. Lavender and aloe calm itching as well as soothing and healing the skin. Sandalwood helps to moisturize dry skin.

4fl oz (125ml) aloe vera juice
10 drops lavender essential oil
10 drops sandalwood essential oil

Combine the aloe vera juice with the essential oils in a 4fl oz (125ml) spray bottle. Shake well, and spray itchy skin liberally several times a day.

564
Refreshing lime and mint body splash

Lime and peppermint make a wonderfully refreshing body splash.

¼ cup (10g) chopped fresh peppermint
1 fresh lime, sliced into thin rounds
½ cup (125ml) distilled witch hazel
½ cup (125ml) filtered or spring water

Steep the peppermint and the lime in the witch hazel in a covered jar for one week. Strain through a coffee filter, and pour into an 8fl oz (250ml) spray bottle. Add the water and shake again.

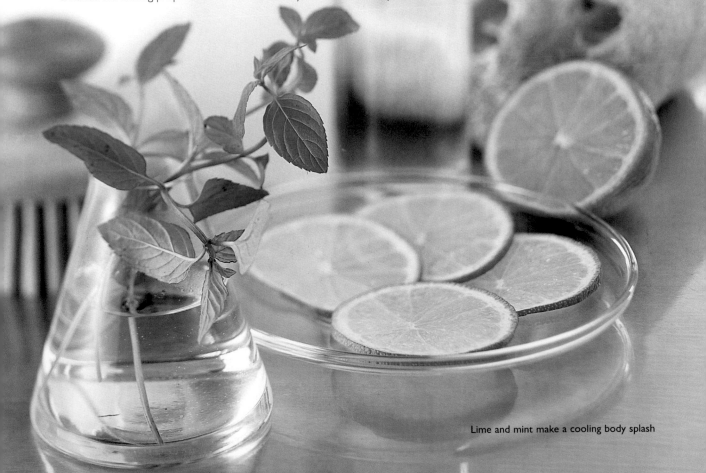

Lime and mint make a cooling body splash

Hydrotherapy Treatments

Hydrotherapy is a traditional way to purify and rejuvenate the body. It increases circulation of blood and lymph and helps the detox process by stimulating perspiration. Sipping herbal tea while soaking in a bath can further encourage detoxification. Purifying baths, saunas, and massages, combined with regular exercise and good nutrition, can also help eliminate cellulite.

565
Epsom salts purifying bath

A hot Epsom-salts soak with cypress, grapefruit, and ginger essential oils creates an effective purifying bath.

2 cups (250g) Epsom salts
3 drops cypress essential oil
3 drops grapefruit essential oil
3 drops ginger essential oil
1 tablespoon whole milk or vodka

Fill the bathtub with comfortably hot water, adding the Epsom salts while the water is running. Dilute the essential oils with milk or vodka and add to the bath after the tub has filled, thoroughly mixing the oils into the water with your hand. Soak in the tub for 15 to 30 minutes and follow with a cool rinse.

566
Hot and cold shower

For a simple daily hydrotherapy treatment, finish your hot morning shower with a blast of cold water. Alternating hot and cold water stimulates blood circulation and lymphatic flow. The key is to get really warm under the hot shower, so that the final cold rinse is a welcome treat.

567
Purifying parsley tea

Parsley is a natural diuretic and a gentle purifier. Sip a cup (250ml) of this tea while soaking in a detox bath.

2 cups (500ml) boiling water
4 tablespoons chopped fresh parsley

Pour the water over the parsley and cover. Steep for 15 minutes, strain, and add lemon and honey if desired.

568
Body brushing

While running your bath, gently brush your skin with a dry loofah sponge or a brush with natural bristles. This massage stimulates circulation and sloughs off dry skin. Using gentle strokes, begin with the soles of your feet; move up your legs, hips, and abdomen, then up your arms from fingertips to shoulders, across your torso and back. Finish with your neck. Follow with a bath of your choice.

569
Herbal purifying tea

To enhance the detoxifying effects of a bath, sip a cup (250ml) of cleansing herbal tea while you are soaking in the water. This tea, which contains burdock root, dandelion root, licorice root, nettle, peppermint, and red clover, gently detoxifies and purifies the body by stimulating the waste disposal functions of the skin, liver, kidneys, and intestines.

1 teaspoon burdock root
1 teaspoon dandelion root
1 teaspoon licorice root
3½ cups (875ml) water
1 teaspoon nettle
1 teaspoon peppermint
1 teaspoon red clover

Combine the burdock root, dandelion root, and licorice root with water in a covered pot. Bring to a boil, and simmer gently for about 15 minutes. Remove from the heat; add the nettle, peppermint, and red clover. Cover, steep for 10 minutes, and strain. Drink up to three cups (750ml) a day for up to three weeks.

570
Seaweed detox bath

Mineral-rich seaweed and Epsom salts create a powerful detoxifying bath. Sea salt is purifying while the baking soda leaves your skin soft and smooth.

½ cup (60g) Epsom salts
½ cup (110g) sea salt
½ cup (25g) dried kelp or dulse
1 cup (125g) baking soda

Combine the Epsom salts, sea salt, and kelp in a blender and grind into a fine powder. Add the mixture to a tub of hot water along with the baking soda. Soak for 20 minutes, and rinse with lukewarm water.

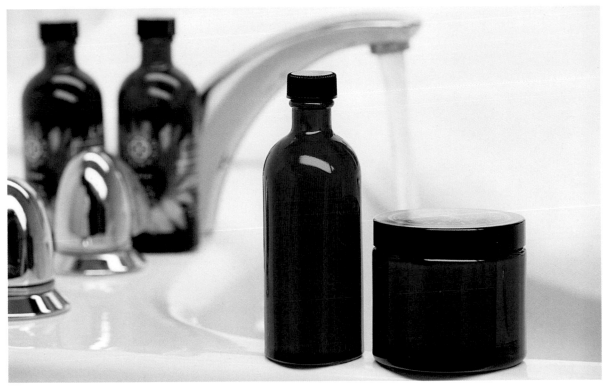

Essential oils, when used in a bath, stimulate detox

571
Simple aromatherapy detox bath

Make a quick and easy bath for detoxifying yourself with juniper and grapefruit essential oils. Adding the whole milk or the vodka to the mixture helps prevent irritation of the skin.

4 drops juniper essential oil
4 drops grapefruit essential oil
1 tablespoon whole milk or vodka

Thoroughly mix the ingredients together and add them to a bathtub of hot water, stirring with your hand to evenly disperse the oils. Soak in the bath for 20 to 30 minutes and then rinse with lukewarm water.

572
Scented sauna

Essential oils can greatly enhance the experience of a sauna. To fill a sauna with scented steam, add a few drops of eucalyptus, spruce, or frankincense essential oil to water that is poured onto the hot sauna rocks.

573
Salt scrub for cellulite

Used frequently, this scrub stimulates the circulation and enhances the flow of lymph, which helps reduce cellulite. Wet your body in a warm shower. Massage a handful of sea salt on your buttocks and thighs for two minutes. Rinse well with warm and then cold water. Your skin will tingle as your circulation increases. Use this massage daily if desired. **Caution:** Do not use this scrub on broken or inflamed skin.

574
Self-massage for cellulite

While soaking in a purifying bath, self-massage areas affected by cellulite. For soft cellulite, firmly grip the tissue, lifting it away from the muscle below. Using a twisting and kneading motion, work deeply to bring the circulation back. For firm cellulite that is hard to lift away, vigorously rub the area with the knuckles of your fists. Cellulite massage may feel slightly painful. Take care to avoid bruising yourself, but don't be afraid to massage firmly.

Natural Massage Oils

Massage not only feels great, it's good for you as well. Massage relaxes tight muscles, stimulates circulation of blood and lymph, encourages the elimination of toxins from tissues, and calms the nervous system. Treat yourself at least once a month to a full-body massage. It's easy to create your own oils from pure vegetable oils and fragrant essential oils. **Caution:** Don't use essential oils during pregnancy without professional advice.

Fragrant essential oils add healing power to massage oils

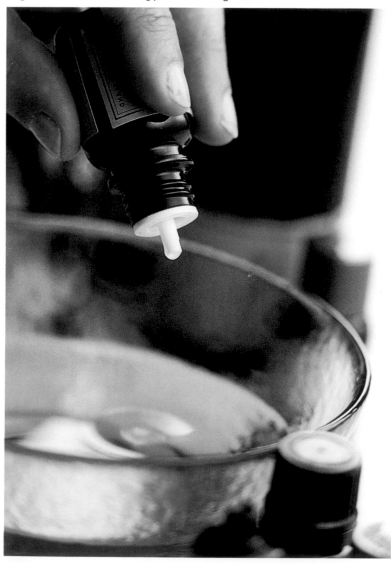

575
Choose your own oil

To make your own massage oil, add 10 drops of your favorite essential oil to one fluid ounce (30ml) of base oil, such as almond, grape-seed, or jojoba.

576
Energizing massage oil

This massage oil is wonderful for restoring energy after a long day. Rosemary and peppermint are stimulating, and lavender helps bring balance to a tired body and mind.

6 tablespoons almond oil
2 tablespoons jojoba oil
25 drops lavender essential oil
10 drops rosemary essential oil
5 drops peppermint essential oil

Mix the oils in a tightly capped bottle and shake well before using.

577
Sensual massage oil

For a sensual, exotic oil with a scent that lingers on your body, follow the Energizing massage oil recipe (see No. 576), substituting 25 drops of sandalwood, 10 drops of rose, and five drops of patchouli essential oils.

578
Relaxing massage oil

For a deeply relaxing blend with a lasting scent, follow the Energizing massage oil recipe (see No. 576), substituting 20 drops of sandalwood, 15 drops of lavender, and five drops of clary sage essential oils.

579
Warming massage oil

For a warm and spicy massage oil, follow the Energizing massage oil recipe (see No. 576), substituting 20 drops of sandalwood and 10 drops each of frankincense and ginger essential oils.

580
Calming massage oil

For a spicy-sweet massage oil which has calming and antidepressive properties, follow the Energizing massage oil recipe (see No. 576), substituting 20 drops of lavender and 10 drops each of geranium and bergamot essential oils.

581
Mood-uplifting massage oil

For a delightfully fragrant massage oil that lifts your mood and raises your spirits when you are feeling down, follow the Energizing massage oil recipe (see No. 576), substituting 20 drops of lavender and 20 drops of grapefruit essential oils.

Relaxation

Relaxation is a great beauty enhancer. If you practice just a few minutes of relaxation at intervals throughout the day you can make an enormous difference in your physical and emotional well-being. Consciously practicing relaxation improves your circulation and digestion, reduces the production of harmful stress hormones, and helps rejuvenate your body.

582
Centering breath

Practice this exercise anywhere and anytime to center yourself and calm your mind and body. Sit with your spine comfortably erect and your feet flat on the floor. Gently focus your attention on your breathing. Relax, and inhale through your nose to a count of five, counting at a pace that is comfortable for you. Pause, holding your inhalation for a count of five. Exhale through your slightly opened mouth to a count of 10, keeping the exhalation smooth and controlled. Repeat for five complete cycles.

583
Chest expander

This yoga exercise loosens your tight back muscles and expands your breathing capacity. Stand with your spine comfortably straight and your feet hip-width apart. Interlock your fingers behind your back, resting your hands on your buttocks. Inhale, and raise your arms behind you and as high as you comfortably can, keeping your fingers interlocked and your shoulders relaxed. Exhale, and lower your arms, again resting your hands on your buttocks. Repeat the sequence several times.

584
Alternate nostril breathing

This breathing exercise is immensely calming, and helps relax the body and clear the mind of worries. Sit in a comfortable position with your spine straight and shoulders relaxed. Gently press your right nostril closed with your right thumb and inhale slowly and deeply through your left nostril. Gently press your left nostril closed with the ring finger of the right hand. Retain the breath for a few seconds, then release your thumb, exhaling slowly and completely through your right nostril. Immediately inhale through your right nostril with a slow and steady breath. Close your right nostril with your right thumb and retain the breath for a few seconds. Release your ring finger, and exhale slowly and steadily through your left nostril. Repeat the exercise at least 10 times, keeping your breath even and controlled.

585
Relaxing yoga exercise

Practice this restorative yoga pose daily. Lie flat on your back with your legs a comfortable distance apart. Place your arms next to your body with your palms facing up. Close your eyes and scan your body for any areas of tension. Relax those areas. Use your breath to help you relax. Each time you exhale, imagine you are breathing out tension. Visualize your worries and problems ebbing away. Remain in this yoga pose for at least 10 minutes.

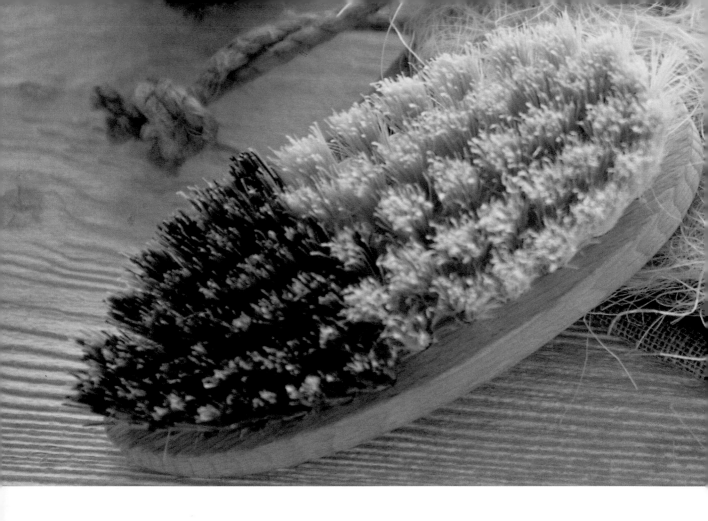

NATURAL
HOUSE &
GARDEN

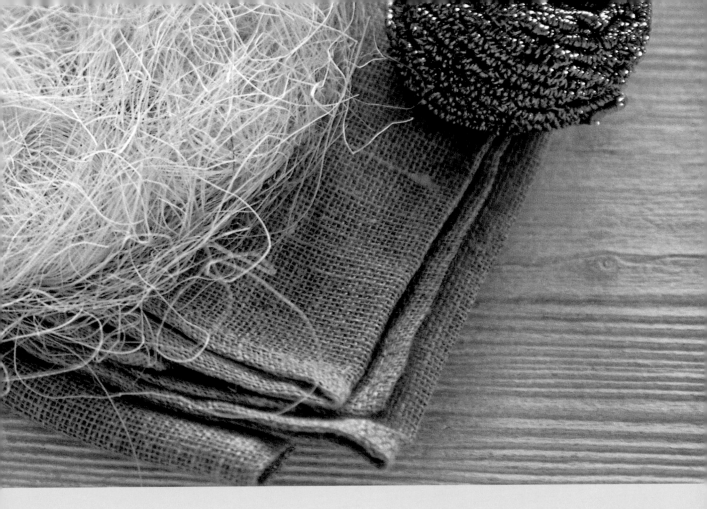

Homes today are often tightly sealed to make them more energy efficient, but in the process, natural ventilation is hindered, allowing pollutants and toxins to accumulate. To prevent this, I've always relied on natural products for cleaning, and fragrant essential oils rank at the top of my favorite household cleaning supplies. Many essential oils have antimicrobial properties, which make them excellent for killing the germs that cause colds, flus, and other infections. But they don't contribute to the problem of chemical-resistant microbes. There is a marvelous side benefit to cleaning with essential oils—my friends always remark on how wonderful my home smells!

Gardening is one of the great pleasures in my life. I don't have acres of land—in fact, my property is small even by city standards. Yet I grow a wide variety of herbs, vegetables, fruits, and flowers. By creating a haven for wildlife and plants, I have created a special place right outside my back door that revives my body, nourishes my spirit, and produces wonderful harvests.

For more than a quarter of a century, I have been committed to a natural organic approach to caring for my home and garden. You will discover much of this wisdom in the pages that follow. It takes a bit of effort, but creating a nontoxic home environment is essential for both the health of my family and the well-being of the earth.

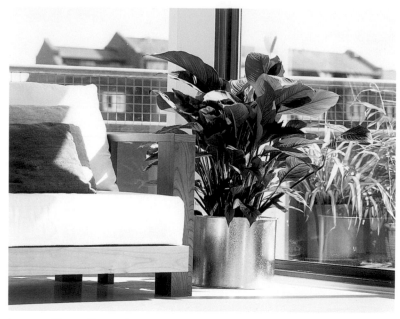

Let peace lilies purify your home

Creating a Natural Home

While you might not have much control over outdoor pollutants that you are exposed to, you do have a great deal of control over the toxins and pollutants in your home. The following guidelines will reduce unwanted chemicals in your indoor environment and help create a healthful and natural home.

586
Bring in fresh air

To reduce the pollutants accumulating within your home, open the windows to let fresh air circulate: 15 minutes in the morning and evening is sufficient. Do this during the winter months. If you live with a person who smokes or if your home is in a heavily polluted area, consider buying an air purifier. Air filters can be installed in the ventilation system of your home, or portable air filters can be used in individual rooms.

587
Reduce formaldehyde

Formaldehyde is a volatile, toxic, and carcinogenic gas found in products such as plywood, particle board, paneling, wood finishes, carpeting, furniture, permanent press fabrics, and household cleaners. To minimize outgassing of formaldehyde, keep the indoor temperature around 65–70°F (18–21°C) and the humidity between 35 and 50 percent. Install humidity and temperature gauges and read them regularly.

588
Purify your home with plants

Common houseplants such as aloe vera, philodendron, spider plant, ficus, English ivy, peace lily, and schefflera are a pleasing way to purify the air. They remove a variety of pollutants, including benzene, carbon monoxide, and formaldehyde, from the air.

589
Prevent mold and mildew contamination

Keeping humidity levels low helps control mold, mildew, and dust mites. Proper ventilation helps remove excess moisture—install exhaust fans in the bathroom and a range hood exhaust fan in the kitchen that vents to the outside. Dehumidifiers and air conditioners also help remove surplus moisture from the air.

590
Remove shoes indoors

Start a new policy: remove your shoes as soon as you enter your house; ask visitors to do so as well. This helps prevent outdoor contaminants found in dirt (such as pesticides) from coming indoors.

591
Abstain from dry-cleaning

Avoid dry-cleaning your clothing and other fabrics. Many dry-cleaners use perchloroethylene, a solvent that stays in your clothes and has a link to cancer. If you do dry-clean your clothes, make sure you air them out (preferably outside of your house) for several days before you hang them in a closet.

592
Inspect heating and cooling systems

You can keep the air in your home cleaner by making sure combustion-based systems are inspected annually. These include furnaces, chimneys, and other systems associated with central air. If these systems use filters, change them every month or two during periods of use. If you have a fireplace, have it cleaned regularly and burn only aged or cured wood.

593
Prevent carbon monoxide poisoning

Fuel-burning appliances that are not operating properly are potential sources of carbon monoxide. This is an odorless gas that causes flulike symptoms at low concentrations and, at higher concentrations, death. Install a carbon monoxide detector and alarm to warn you of its presence.

594
Use gas-burning appliances properly

Read the manuals for your appliances to make sure that you are using and maintaining them properly, and then check them to see if they work correctly. For gas appliances, the flame should burn with a blue color.

A flame which has a persistent yellow tip generally indicates increased pollutant emissions and the need for adjustment. Call your gas company to have the appliance fixed.

595
Install nontoxic flooring

Carpets are notorious air polluters. Not only is the formaldehyde (typically used to produce and install them) a problem, but they also trap fumes, dust, and other air pollutants and then later release them. If you can, replace carpets with hardwood floors and use a water-based sealant as a finish. Vinyl floors are another potential problem because they emit chemicals called plasticizers. Consider replacing vinyl floors with ceramic tiles, hardwood, or natural linoleum.

596
Use air filters for pure air

To remove dust, pollen, smoke, pet dander, and mold spores from the air in your house, buy a high efficiency particulate air (HEPA) filter. You might also want to buy a HEPA vacuum cleaner, which captures airborne dust mites along with particles of dirt and dust.

597
Avoid lead-based paints

When you paint your house, choose water-based products. Have your home thoroughly checked for the presence of lead paint, which could have been used in any home built before 1980. Ingesting or inhaling large amounts of lead over time

Choose water-based paints for your home

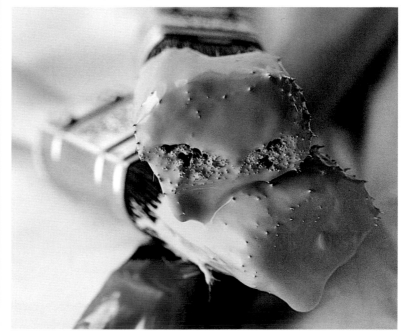

can cause permanent neurological damage, and children are the primary victims. If lead paint removal is necessary, hire professional help.

598
Check for radon and asbestos

Check your home for radon, a radioactive gas that occurs naturally in certain soils and rocks. It can accumulate in houses to dangerous levels, and long-term exposure has been linked to lung cancer. You can buy a test kit at a hardware store. If you find your home contains high levels of radon, call a professional to fix the problem. If your house was built before 1980, have it checked for the presence of asbestos, too. Asbestos was often used as insulation and is sometimes also found in ducts, vinyl floor tiles, and exterior shingles. Breathing asbestos fibers is directly related to lung cancer, but risks only exist when the fibers are released into the air.

599
Reduce chlorine exposure

Chlorine is suspected of damaging the immune system and contributing to degenerative diseases. It is also known to combine with other contaminants in water to form powerful cancer-causing substances. Install a water purifier to remove chlorine and other contaminants from your drinking and cooking water. In addition, install a filter for your shower that removes chlorine.

600
Avoid toxic furnishings

Use natural materials and furnishings in your home instead of synthetics whenever possible. Buy solid wood furniture instead of particle board or plastic, and upholster furniture with natural fabrics. Choose metal or wood blinds and natural fabric window drapes. For the bedroom, buy pure cotton sheets. Avoid permanent press sheets, which are treated with formaldehyde, a highly toxic chemical. Choose pillows, comforters, and blankets that are made of down, wool, or cotton.

601
Keep electrical pollution out of your bedroom

Get rid of any unnecessary electrical products in your bedroom. These include electric blankets, alarm clocks, personal computers, and televisions. The electromagnetic fields (EMFs) emitted from these appliances can disturb your sleep patterns and interfere with your health. They may even contribute to cancer. Instead of an electrical alarm clock, use one that's battery-powered or wind-up, and use a hot-water bottle in place of an electric blanket.

The Natural Kitchen

Making meals from natural foods begins with creating a healthy kitchen environment. Make sure your kitchen is clean and hygienic, has good air circulation, and is equipped with nontoxic cookware. There are a number of ways of preparing and safely storing natural foods so that they retain their freshness and their taste.

602
Cleaning berries and leafy greens

To clean soft or difficult to scrub fruits and vegetables such as grapes, broccoli, berries, or leafy greens, fill a basin with water and half a teaspoon of dishwashing liquid. Soak the produce for several minutes. Rinse thoroughly in several changes of water to remove all the soap. Before soaking leafy greens such as lettuce and cabbage, remove the outer leaves as they contain more chemical residues than the inner ones.

603
Washing greens

Dark leafy greens such as collards, kale, and spinach are some of the richest sources of health-protective antioxidants. Cleaning them can be difficult, however, because the crinkly leaves hold onto sand and grit. The only truly effective way to wash leafy greens is to immerse them in a large pot or sink of water. The leaves will float on the surface, but the sand and grit will sink to the bottom. Gently swish the greens in the water, and remove them. Repeat with a fresh

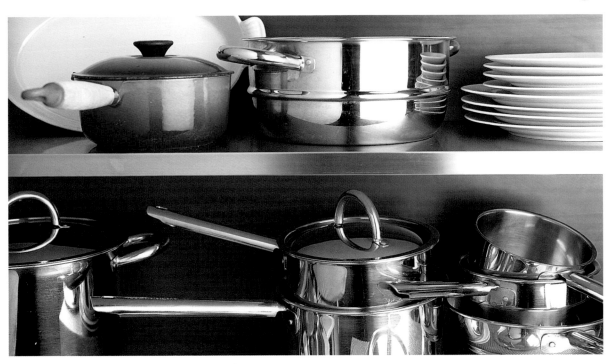

Use only stainless steel, enameled, or cast-iron cookware

pot of water as many times as necessary until there is no sand at the bottom of the pot or sink.

604
Natural vegetable wash

Wash vegetables with a small amount of a mild, natural dishwashing liquid based on vegetable oil. Scrub with a bristled scrub brush and warm water. Rinse well. This will safely remove dirt, waxes, and some pesticides, herbicides, and fungicides commonly applied to conventional produce.

605
Cellulose sponges

To keep your vegetables fresh and crisp, place a couple of natural cellulose sponges in the vegetable

bins in your refrigerator. These will keep the air-dry by absorbing excess moisture caused by condensation.

606
Safe cookware

Cookware made from aluminum or synthetic nonstick surfaces can leach toxins into your foods. Instead, use stainless steel, glass, porcelain, enamel-coated cast iron, natural clay, or cast-iron cookware. Cast-iron cookware must be well seasoned to be effective. To season a cast-iron pan, rub it with a generous amount of olive oil and place in an oven set on low for one hour. Let the pan cool and wipe off the excess oil. After using the pan, wash it with hot water, but no soap, and thoroughly dry it by heating it on a burner over low heat.

607
The right temperature

Temperature is most important for food storage. Any warmer than 40°F (4.5°C) and the bacteria that can make you sick multiply rapidly. Store perishable foods right away, or leave them out at room temperature for no more than two hours.

608
Storing fresh food

The sooner you eat fresh food, the better. The longer you store it, the less appetizing it tastes and the more vitamins are lost. Most vegetables and fruits store best in the refrigerator in plastic bags. Potatoes and onions stay fresh at room temperature in a cool, dark area.

609
Transfer canned goods

Refrigerating foods in the original can after opening probably won't put your health in jeopardy, but they will look better and taste better if you store them in glass containers. Foods with acidic contents such as tomatoes or pineapple can corrode the metal lining of cans, producing an off-flavor or discoloration.

610
Protect bulk items

Take nonperishable items such as beans and grains out of their plastic bags and put them in sealed glass or plastic containers in a cool, dark cupboard to keep them fresh and free of pests. Store nuts and whole grain flours in the refrigerator or freezer, because processing makes their oils prone to rancidity.

611
Don't wait to eat fish

Fresh fish is usually about a week old when you buy it, which means you should cook or freeze it within one or two days. Oily fish such as salmon keeps for two months in the freezer, while other varieties keep up to four months. Wrap the fish tightly when freezing to prevent freezer burn.

612
Chill dairy products

If milk has been properly bottled and transported, it can last between seven and 10 days after the sell-by date. To ensure milk stays fresh, check that the temperature of your refrigerator is maintained at 40°F (4.5°C) or below, and store dairy products on the top shelf in the back. Do not put either milk or eggs in the door because this is the warmest place in the refrigerator. Properly stored eggs will keep for three weeks.

613
Use meat quickly

Cook or freeze ground meat and poultry within one to two days of purchase. Fresh cuts last three to five days in the refrigerator. Ground meats can be stored in the freezer for up to four months; whole cuts of meat and poultry can be frozen for up to one year.

614
Rewrap cheese and meat

Some supermarkets wrap hand-cut cheese and meats in plastic film made from PVC (polyvinyl chloride), which can leach a carcinogenic chemical into fatty foods. If you're uncertain about whether or not your grocery store uses PVC, remove the original wrap and rewrap your cheese and meat in waxed paper or a safer film such as polyethylene.

615
Repel weevils

Place a couple of bay leaves in your grain and bean storage containers to repel weevils.

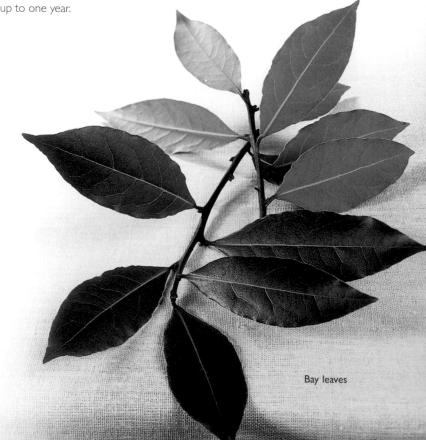

Bay leaves

Natural Pest Control

There's no need to use toxic chemicals to control pests such as ants, cockroaches, flies, and mice. To keep these unwanted visitors from setting up house, make your home an unappealing destination for them with the following tips. If a few of the creatures do find their way into your home, natural deterrents and traps will quickly take care of the problem without danger to you or to the environment.

616
Tips for controlling pests

You can control pests in various ways. Cut off their food supply by cleaning up the kitchen immediately after meals (or at least, rinse the dishes to remove food residues). Sweep up crumbs, wipe the counters, and wash out jars, bottles, and cans destined for recycling. Store your food in tightly covered containers, and empty garbage cans and kitchen compost bins daily. Insects are attracted to sources of water; repair leaking faucets and check for leaking pipes under sinks. To eliminate hiding places, get rid of stacks of newspapers, paper bags, and cardboard boxes. Use caulk to seal cracks in windows and walls where insects can enter.

617
Plant herbs to keep ants away

Planting herbs such as lavender, peppermint, and tansy around your house will help keep ants away. Plant them in the ground or in pots around doorways and place small pots of mint in your windowsills.

618
Natural ant control

Dried peppermint, cayenne, and borax help deter ants.

¼ cup (7.5g) dried peppermint leaves
¼ cup (35g) powdered cayenne
¼ cup (30g) borax

Mix the ingredients together, and sprinkle the mixture liberally around the area where ants are entering your home.

619
Repel ants with oils

Peppermint, spearmint, and citronella essential oils help deter ants. Place a few drops of one oil on a cotton ball and put in areas where you have seen ants. Renew the oil every two days to keep the scent strong.

620
Homemade ant trap

Make a simple ant trap by mixing the following in a screw-top jar.

3 cups (750ml) water
1 cup (225g) sugar
4 teaspoons boric acid

Poke holes in the lid, and place the jar near ant trails but out of reach of pets and children.

621
Eliminate cockroaches

A combination of borax, cocoa, and flour lures and kills cockroaches.

2 tablespoons flour
2 tablespoons powdered cocoa
4 tablespoons borax

Combine the ingredients and place the mixture in some small shallow containers in cabinets, under sinks, and other areas where you know cockroaches congregate.

622
Trap cockroaches

Place half an overripe banana and half a bottle of beer in a quart (1.25 liter) glass canning jar. Rub a thick margin of petroleum jelly on the inside lip of the jar. Lean a one-inch (25mm) wide strip of heavy cardboard at an angle against the outside of the jar to provide the roaches with easy access. Once inside the jar, the roaches won't be able to get out.

623
Repel cockroaches with essential oils

Cockroaches don't like the scent of eucalyptus or rosemary essential oils. Place a few drops of essential oil on cotton balls and put in areas where you have seen roaches. Renew the essential oil every couple of days to keep the scent strong.

624
Keep flies away

Keep your garbage containers tightly covered. Install screen doors that open outward so flies are not pulled into the house each time the door is used. Window fans that blow air outward help keep flies from entering through windows. Keep fly swatters handy—aim one and a half inches (4cm) from the fly's back because flies jump up and backward when they take off.

625
Repel flies with herbs

To keep flies away, put out bowls of fresh orange and lemon peels mixed with dried cloves. Planting rue and tansy near doorways also helps prevent the pests entering the house.

626
Control flies with oils

Flies don't like the scent of lavender, eucalyptus, or cedar. Use one or a combination of these essential oils in an aromatherapy diffuser or on cotton balls placed around the room. Add a few drops of an oil to small bowls of hot water to help disperse the scent throughout the room.

627
Homemade fly paper

Create your own flypaper by spreading molasses onto strips or squares of bright yellow posterboard. Hang the strips in doorways or lay squares of flypaper on the kitchen counters and other places where flies are a problem.

628
Banish mice

Seal all potential entryways and stuff steel wool into the openings around plumbing where mice might enter. Live traps work well, but make sure you release the captured mice at least a mile (1.6km) away from your home so they do not return. You can also try a sonic repellent (available at some hardware stores). This device emits high-frequency sound waves to scare away rodents.

Orange, lemon, and cloves repel flies

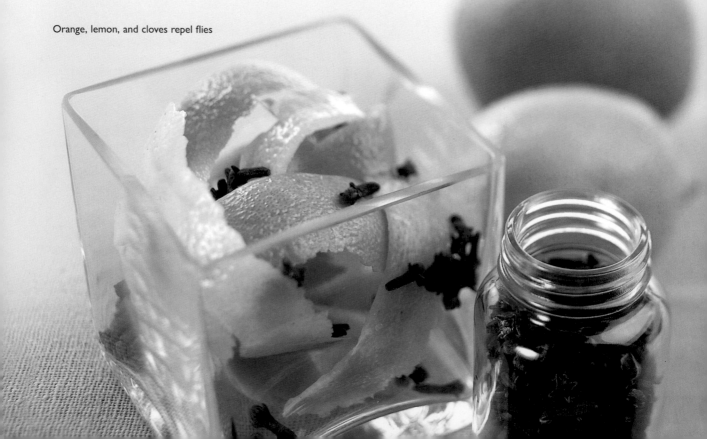

Natural Air Fresheners

A pleasant, clean fragrance is an essential part of an inviting home. Most conventional air fresheners simply mask unpleasant odors with strong chemical fragrances. Instead, use pure essential oils and herbs and, most importantly, open your windows for at least a few minutes every day—even in winter.

629
Lavender and citrus air freshener

Lavender and grapefruit essential oils make a light, refreshing air freshener.

1 teaspoon vodka
15 drops lavender essential oil
10 drops grapefruit essential oil
2 cups (500ml) water

Mix together the vodka and essential oils in a 16fl oz (500ml) spray bottle and shake well. Add water and shake again. Spray a fine mist into the air. Avoid spraying directly on fabrics or wood surfaces.

630
Pine forest air freshener

A blend of sandalwood, pine, and juniper essential oils create an earthy, forest-scented room deodorizer.

1 teaspoon vodka
10 drops sandalwood essential oil
10 drops pine essential oil
10 drops juniper essential oil
2 cups (500ml) water

Mix the vodka and oils in a 16fl oz (500ml) spray bottle and shake well. Add water, shake again, and spray a fine mist into the air. Avoid spraying directly on fabrics or wood surfaces.

631
Air freshening spray

Mix 25 drops of an essential oil of your choice with a teaspoon of vodka in a 16fl oz (500ml) spray bottle and shake well. Fill the bottle with water and shake again. Spray into the air but avoid fabrics or wood surfaces to prevent possible staining.

632
Antiseptic air freshener

Use this extra-strength room spray when someone in the house has a cold or the flu. Juniper, eucalyptus, and lavender essential oils all have antimicrobial properties.

1 teaspoon vodka
20 drops juniper essential oil
20 drops eucalyptus essential oil
20 drops lavender essential oil
2 cups (500ml) water

Mix the vodka and oils in a 16fl oz (500ml) spray bottle and shake well. Add water, shake again, and spray a fine mist into the air. Avoid spraying directly on fabrics or wood surfaces.

Lavender is an excellent air freshener

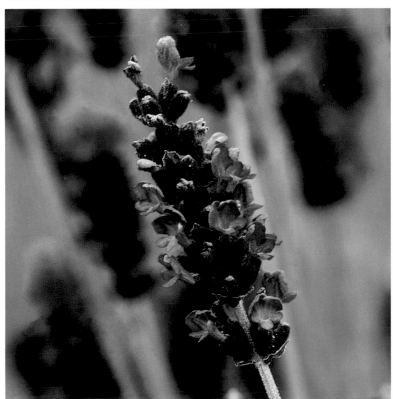

633
Scented fire logs

If you have a fireplace or a hearth, you can scent a room around it by placing a drop or two of essential oil onto each log that you add to the fire. Try cedarwood, juniper, pine, or cinnamon essential oils.

634
Fresh herbal bouquets

Freshly cut herbs make natural fragrant bouquets for scenting a room. Lavender, rosemary, lemon balm, bergamot, sage, thyme, and mint are all good choices and will last up to a week in a vase with water.

635
Fragrant humidifier

Place a bowl of water with two drops of essential oil on top of a wood stove or radiator to create humidity and at the same time add fragrance to a room.

636
Neutralize cooking odors

Cooking odors, especially from fish and strong-smelling vegetables such as broccoli, tend to linger in the kitchen. To freshen the air after cooking, throw a few slices of lemon or orange into a pot along with three cups of water and simmer, uncovered, over low heat for 30 minutes. If you like a spicy fragrance, add a couple of cinnamon sticks or a few cloves.

637
Herbal hearth

Add sprigs of fresh rosemary, sage, or lavender to the logs and coals of a burning fire to scent a room.

638
Vanilla freshener

For a simple room freshener, place a few drops of pure vanilla extract on a cotton ball in a shallow saucer. Replace when the scent dissipates.

Vanilla extract makes a fragrant air freshener

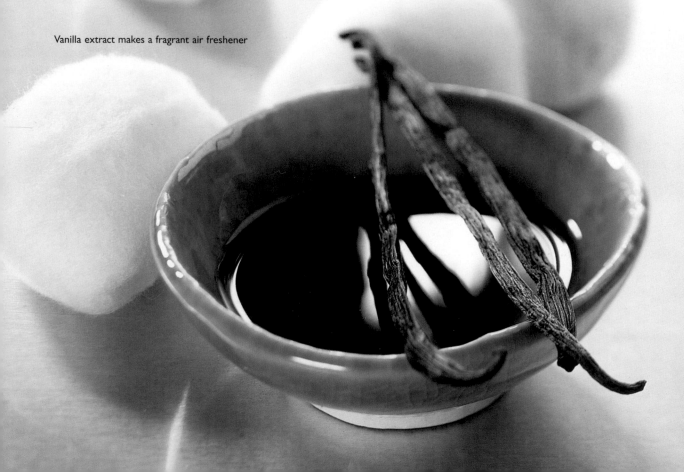

Cleaning Surfaces

Most surfaces around your home can be easily cleaned with kitchen ingredients that you probably have on hand, such as vinegar and liquid dishwashing soap. Essential oils add a pleasant fragrance and, in addition, many have antimicrobial properties, which make them excellent for killing the germs that cause colds, flus, and other infections. The following natural cleaners are nontoxic, inexpensive, and easy to make, and are good for removing dirt, grease, and grime.

639
Antiseptic hand soap

Essential oils such as lavender, eucalyptus, and lemon are natural antimicrobials.

- 8fl oz (250ml) liquid natural hand and body soap
- 30 drops lavender essential oil
- 20 drops eucalyptus essential oil
- 10 drops lemon essential oil

Combine the ingredients together in a plastic bottle or soap dispenser and mix well.

640
All-purpose spray

Borax, vinegar, and soap will dissolve dirt and greasy residues on surfaces around the home. Lavender and rosemary essential oils have natural antiseptic properties.

- 1 teaspoon borax
- 2 cups (500ml) warm water
- 2 tablespoons distilled white vinegar
- ½ teaspoon natural liquid dishwashing soap
- 10 drops lavender essential oil
- 5 drops rosemary essential oil

Combine the borax and water in a spray bottle and shake well. Add the vinegar, soap, and essential oils and shake again. Spray on surfaces such as countertops, walls, and woodwork and wipe clean with a sponge.

641
Soapy spray cleanser

Grimy, greasy surfaces need the added power of orange essential oil.

- 1 teaspoon borax
- 1 cup (250ml) warm water
- ¼ cup (60ml) distilled white vinegar
- ¼ cup (60ml) natural liquid dishwashing soap
- 10 drops orange essential oil

Combine the borax and water in a spray bottle and shake well. Add vinegar, soap, and orange essential oil and shake again. Spray on surfaces and wipe clean with a sponge. Rinse well with water.

642
Vinegar glass cleaner

A combination of white vinegar and water makes an inexpensive yet effective window and glass cleaner.

Adding lemon essential oil gives a pleasing fragrance.

- ⅔ cup (170ml) water
- ⅓ cup (80ml) distilled white vinegar
- 2 drops lemon essential oil

Mix the ingredients in a spray bottle and shake well. Spray onto surfaces and wipe with a clean, lint-free towel.

643
Heavy-duty glass cleaner

Windows sometimes need a stronger cleanser—adding a bit of soap helps remove grease and grime.

- 1 cup (250ml) distilled white vinegar
- ¼ teaspoon natural liquid dishwashing soap
- 1 cup (250ml) warm water

Mix the ingredients in a spray bottle and shake well. Spray onto surfaces and wipe with a clean, lint-free towel.

644
Remedy for streaky windows

Streaky windows might be caused by a buildup of wax from previous commercial cleaners. Use this formula to remedy the problem, then switch to a simple water and vinegar window cleaner (see No. 642).

- ½ cup (125ml) isopropyl alcohol
- ½ cup (125ml) warm water
- ¼ teaspoon natural liquid dishwashing soap

Mix the ingredients in a spray bottle. Shake well. Spray onto windows and wipe dry with a clean, lint-free towel.

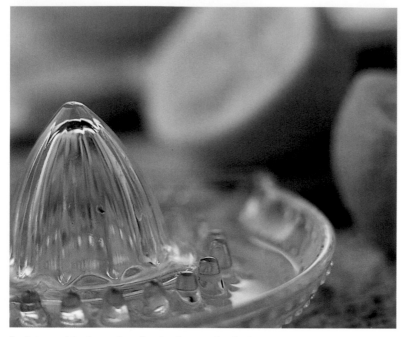

Fresh lemon juice is excellent for cleaning wooden furniture

Furniture Care

Wood, leather, bamboo, and upholstered furniture last longer and look better with regular cleaning; with just a few simple ingredients you can make excellent furniture polishes and cleaners. You'll find furniture first-aid remedies for spills, burns, stains, and scratches in this section, too.

645
Lemon furniture polish

Extra-virgin olive oil helps protect the wood in the furniture. Lemon essential oil cleans the wood and provides a refreshing scent.

½ cup (125ml) extra-virgin olive oil
¼ teaspoon lemon essential oil

Mix the ingredients in a glass bottle, shake, and store. Rub a small amount onto wood furniture with a soft cotton cloth.

646
Raw walnut rub

To remove white, hazy water rings from wood surfaces, rub the mark with half a raw walnut.

647
First aid for heat marks

Hot cookware can mar wooden surfaces with white discoloration. To repair the damage, rub a candle on to the mark (choose a light or dark colored candle, depending on the color of the wood surface). Cover with a double thickness of paper towels, and press the area with a warm iron. Buff with a soft cloth and repeat if necessary.

648
Wood furniture cleaner

A mixture of extra-virgin olive oil and fresh lemon juice is excellent for cleaning wood furniture.

2 tablespoons extra-virgin olive oil
2 tablespoons fresh lemon juice

Combine the ingredients in a small glass jar. Shake well. Apply to furniture with a soft cotton cloth.

649
Remove water stains from wood

To remove hazy water spots from wooden surfaces, mix baking soda and mayonnaise to the consistency of a thick paste. Gently rub a small amount of the paste into the wood and leave it for five minutes. Buff the surface with a clean, soft cloth.

650
Spilled candle wax

To clean the drips and puddles of wax that collect around candles, first let the wax cool thoroughly and then carefully scrape it from the wooden surface with a dull knife. Wash off the remainder of the wax residue with hot soapy water, rinse, and dry. When the surface is completely dry, apply an oil polish.

651
Repair wood scratches

Superficial scratches may disappear when rubbed with an oil-based furniture polish. To repair deeper scratches, melt a few drops of a wax crayon that matches the color of the wood and fill the scratch. (Heat a dull kitchen knife over a flame and hold the knife blade against the crayon to cause it to melt.) Smooth the wax even with the surface of the wood and let it cool. Scrape away excess wax with a dull knife and buff the surface with an oil furniture polish.

652
Remove sticky labels

Vegetable oil safely removes gummed and sticky labels from wood finishes and surfaces. Apply a liberal amount of oil to the label, leave overnight, and then rub it off with a soft cloth.

653
Caring for bamboo, rattan, and wicker

Bamboo, rattan, and wicker furniture benefit from regular vacuuming and dusting. A large, soft brush cleans woven furniture thoroughly. To prevent drying and splitting, take the furniture outside and hose it down once a year with a fine spray from the garden hose to restore moisture to the canes. Alternatively, spritz woven furniture with a plant mister every couple of months.

654
Clean upholstery

Regularly vacuum your upholstered furniture to prevent dust from accumulating. To freshen and clean upholstery, apply a simple homemade foam cleanser, which helps remove the dirt without soaking the fabric with water. Lavender essential oil provides a fresh scent.

¼ cup (60ml) hot water
1 teaspoon borax
2 tablespoons natural liquid dishwashing soap
3 drops lavender essential oil
(**To make and use, see below**)

655
Clean leather upholstery

Vinegar, olive oil, and lemon essential oil will clean and condition leather.

2 tablespoons distilled white vinegar
2 tablespoons extra-virgin olive oil
2 drops lemon essential oil

Mix the ingredients in a small jar and shake well. Test it on an inconspicuous area to check for color changes to the leather. Then apply it sparingly—rub it in thoroughly, and buff with a soft cloth to remove excess oil.

MAKING AND USING A FOAM CLEANSER FOR UPHOLSTERY

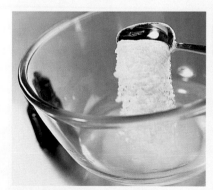

1 Pour the hot water into a medium-sized bowl and add the borax, stirring thoroughly to dissolve it. Allow the mixture to cool to room temperature.

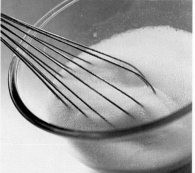

2 Add the natural dishwashing soap and the drops of lavender essential oil to the mixture. Beat with a wire whisk or egg beater to create foam.

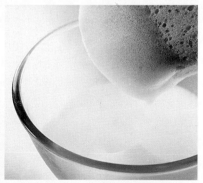

3 Working on a small section at a time, rub the foam onto upholstery with a damp sponge. Immediately remove with a damp cloth. Let it dry.

Cleaning Floors & Carpets

A household policy that bans street shoes indoors helps keep floors and carpets clean. Using essential oils while vacuuming carpets or mopping wood floors gives the entire house a fresh, clean scent. You'll find remedies for carpet stains in this section, and a tip for cleaning garage floors, too.

656
Refreshing wood floor cleaner

A combination of vinegar, water, and soap with lavender and orange essential oils cleans floors and leaves a sweet, refreshing scent.

½ cup (125ml) distilled white vinegar
2 tablespoons natural liquid dishwashing soap
2 gallons (10 liters) warm water
10 drops lavender essential oil
5 drops orange essential oil

Mix all the ingredients together in a large bucket and stir well. Wash your wooden floors with either a mop or rag as desired. Afterward, rinse each floor with clean water.

657
No-rinse wood floor cleaner

If your floor is not really dirty but just needs damp mopping, a bit of vinegar and lavender essential oil in a bucket of water does the trick.

2 gallons (10 liters) warm water
¼ cup (60ml) distilled white vinegar
15 drops lavender essential oil

Mix the ingredients in a large bucket and mop the floor.

658
Natural carpet freshener

Baking soda helps absorb odors and lavender essential oil adds a pleasant, fresh scent.

20 drops lavender essential oil
2 cups (250g) baking soda

Mix the oil thoroughly into the baking soda with a wire whisk. Sprinkle a fine layer of the mixture onto your carpet and leave for at least a couple of hours. Vacuum thoroughly.

659
Remove stains from carpeting

Stains are easiest to remove from carpeting if you act immediately. Blot—do not rub—the stain with paper towels or a soft, clean cloth to soak up as much as possible of the substance. Then, depending what has caused the stain, apply a cleaner (see No. 660). Avoid saturating the carpet with liquid; instead, apply a small amount, blot the stain, and repeat if necessary. Then blot the area with a clean damp sponge or cloth. Make sure you repeat this several times to remove all traces of the stain cleaner. Dry the area thoroughly by covering it with a clean, dry towel and applying pressure with a heavy object. Replace the towel with a dry one as soon as it becomes saturated.

Baking soda and lavender freshen carpets

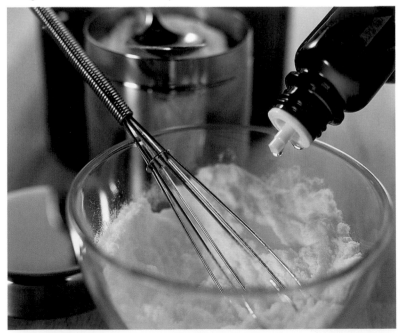

660
All-purpose carpet stain remover

A combination of liquid dishwashing detergent and vinegar removes many types of stain.

1 teaspoon natural liquid dishwashing soap
¼ cup (60ml) distilled white vinegar
1 cup (250ml) warm water

Thoroughly mix the ingredients together in a spray bottle. Shake well, and spray onto the stain. Blot the carpet with a clean, damp sponge.

661
Foam carpet cleaner

Use this gentle foam cleaner to spot clean carpets. Lavender essential oil adds a fresh, pleasant scent.

¼ cup (60ml) natural liquid dishwashing soap
½ cup (125ml) warm water
6 drops lavender essential oil

Mix the ingredients together in a large bowl and beat into a stiff foam with an electric mixer. Apply the cleaner with a damp sponge to the soiled areas, and remove with a damp cloth. Repeat if necessary. Let the carpet dry and then vacuum.

662
Filter bag freshener

To neutralize the musty smell of a vacuum cleaner, place a couple of drops of a fragrant essential oil of your choice on the filter bag just before vacuuming.

663
Alcohol stains

Blot the carpet with a damp sponge soaked in club soda until as much as possible of the stain is removed. If you need, follow with All-purpose carpet stain remover (see No. 660).

664
Chocolate stains

Gently rub a mixture of equal parts of vegetable glycerin and warm water into the carpet stain. Rinse with lukewarm water. Repeat if necessary.

665
Coffee and tea stains

Sponge with cold club soda until the carpet is clean. If necessary, sponge it with a solution of one teaspoon borax diluted in one cup (250ml) of water. Rinse with clean water.

666
Grease stains

Sprinkle baking soda onto the stain and gently rub it in. Leave overnight, and vacuum. Follow with All-purpose carpet stain remover (see No. 660).

667
Pet stains

Treat pet stains quickly to prevent damage to the carpet.

½ cup (125ml) distilled white vinegar
½ cup (125ml) water
1 teaspoon natural liquid dishwashing soap

Mix the ingredients in a spray bottle and shake well. First mop the stain with paper towels and then spray the formula onto the stain. Blot with a damp sponge, and rinse with water.

668
Cleaning mud

Let the mud dry thoroughly and then vacuum the carpet. Follow with All-purpose carpet stain remover (see No. 660).

669
Removing chewing gum

Rub the gum with an ice cube until it hardens, and then scrape it from the fibers of the carpet with a dull knife.

670
Removing wax

With a dull knife, carefully scrape off as much excess wax as possible from the carpet. Place a brown paper bag over the remaining wax, and press with a warm iron. The wax will melt and transfer onto the paper bag. Place a fresh section of the paper bag over the spot, and continue pressing until all the wax has been removed.

671
Garage floor cleanup

Sprinkle a thick layer of clean cat litter over an oil leak or antifreeze spill. Let it sit for several hours. Sweep up the litter and throw it away. Follow by cleaning with a citrus-based natural cleaning product to remove any remaining oil or grease.

Cleaning Metal

Cleaning metal surfaces such as copper, brass, and silver is easy with common ingredients such as vinegar, salt, baking soda, and lemon juice. For best results, clean metal surfaces regularly, before a heavy layer of tarnish builds up and makes the object difficult to clean.

672
Polishing copper with vinegar and salt

Fill a spray bottle with distilled white vinegar and spray liberally onto the tarnished copper surface. Sprinkle salt over the vinegar and rub with a soft cloth. Rinse with warm water. Heavily oxidized copper may need more than one treatment.

673
Cleaning brass

Mix lemon juice with baking soda to the consistency of toothpaste. Rub the mixture onto the metal surface and let sit for five minutes. Rinse well with warm water.

674
Brightening brass

To keep brass brighter after polishing, rub a bit of olive oil onto it with a soft cloth.

675
Removing tarnish from silver

Place a large sheet of aluminum foil in a sink of very hot water. Add half a cup (110g) of salt and stir to dissolve.

Place the sterling silver cutlery or serving pieces in the sink and allow them to soak for five minutes. Rinse the silver items thoroughly with clean water and dry. Tarnish is easiest to remove if the silver is cleaned regularly in this way.

676
Simple silver polish

Light tarnish can be cleaned from silver using the mild abrasive action of baking soda. Dampen a clean sponge and sprinkle it with baking soda. Rub the silver cutlery or serving pieces until they are clean. Rinse them thoroughly with clean water, and dry. For stubborn tarnish, make a paste of baking soda and water, and apply to the silver. Let the silver items dry, and then rinse them with warm water. An old toothbrush will help to clean intricate pieces of silver.

Clearing Drains

Drains become clogged when hair, grease, and soap residues accumulate over a period of time. Most of the commercial drain cleaners rely on lye, a highly corrosive chemical, to dissolve the clog or blockage. Instead, try these nontoxic alternatives for keeping your drains clear.

677
Unclogging drains with a plunger

The best way to unclog a blocked drain is to use a rubber plunger (available from any hardware store). First remove the strainer if you have one, and make sure the drain is completely covered with the plunger as you need to create sufficient pressure to break through the clogging substance. To prevent drains from becoming blocked in the first place, always use a strainer in your bathroom sink and tub drains to trap loose hair, and never pour grease down your kitchen sink.

678
Natural drain cleaner

Use the following formula once a week to keep your kitchen sink drain clean and free of soap and grease residues that can accumulate and cause blockages.

$^1/_2$ cup (60g) baking soda
$^1/_2$ cup (110g) salt
$^1/_2$ cup (125ml) distilled white vinegar

Pour the baking soda, salt, and white vinegar through the plughole and into the drain. Wait 15 minutes, and pour a teakettle of boiling water down the drain, taking care not to burn yourself with the steam.

Cleaning the Kitchen

Washing dishes, scrubbing pots and pans, and cleaning appliances can all be accomplished with simple ingredients such as baking soda, natural liquid dishwashing soap, and essential oils. You'll find quick fixes here for everything from deodorizing sink disposals to cleaning coffeemakers.

679
Citrus dishwashing liquid

Lemon and orange essential oils are antibacterial and help cut grease.

4fl oz (125ml) unscented natural liquid
    dishwashing soap
10 drops lemon essential oil
10 drops orange essential oil

Mix the ingredients, shake well, and use as usual for washing dishes.

680
Citrus vinegar rinse

This scented vinegar makes your glassware sparkle and smell clean.

8fl oz (250ml) apple cider vinegar
20 drops lemon essential oil
20 drops orange essential oil

Shake the ingredients and add two tablespoons to the rinse water when dishwashing by hand.

681
Cleaning stainless steel

To clean and polish stainless steel cookware, rub a thin paste of baking soda and vinegar onto the metal surface, rinse well with water, and dry.

682
Tackling baked-on food

Sprinkle baking soda over baked-on or burned foods and add enough hot water to moisten. Let it sit overnight; the food should be easy to remove. Alternatively, half-fill a pot or pan with hot water and a squirt of natural dishwashing soap. Bring to a boil, cover, and simmer for 15 minutes.

683
Dishwasher formula

Before using this formula, rinse the food off the dishes.

3 tablespoons baking soda
1 tablespoon borax
2 drops lemon essential oil

Mix the ingredients together and use the mixture in your dishwasher.

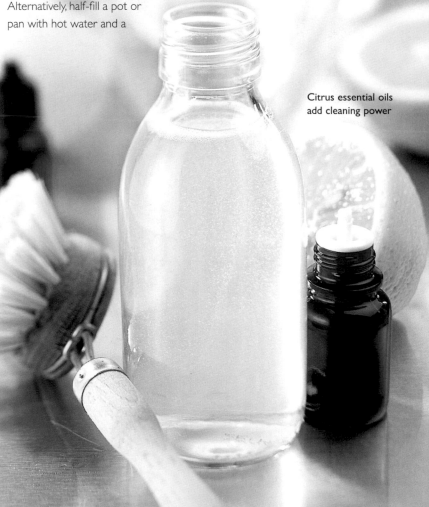

Citrus essential oils add cleaning power

684
Kitchen cleaning spray

This light spray is great for cleaning kitchen countertops and other surfaces. Vinegar helps remove the oily film that collects in kitchens, and lavender and lemon essential oils are natural antimicrobials.

1/2 cup (125ml) distilled white vinegar
1/4 teaspoon natural liquid dishwashing soap
1/2 cup (125ml) water
1/4 teaspoon lavender essential oil
1/4 teaspoon lemon essential oil

Combine all the ingredients together in a spray bottle. Shake well before using on kitchen surfaces.

685
Grease-cutting cleanser

This heavy-duty cleanser removes the greasy buildup that can accumulate on kitchen walls and cabinets.

1/4 cup (30g) baking soda
1/2 cup (125ml) distilled white vinegar
1 teaspoon natural liquid dishwashing soap
1 gallon (5 liters) hot water
5 drops lemon essential oil

Mix all the ingredients together in a bucket and use on a sponge to clean walls and cabinets.

686
Kitchen floor cleaner

Baking soda helps neutralize kitchen odors while soap and vinegar cut the greasy film that accumulates on kitchen floors. Eucalyptus and orange essential oils add a refreshing scent and help kill germs.

1/4 cup (30g) baking soda
1/2 cup (125ml) distilled white vinegar
2 tablespoons natural liquid dishwashing soap
2 gallons (10 liters) hot water
10 drops eucalyptus essential oil
5 drops orange essential oil

Combine the baking soda, vinegar, soap, and water in a bucket and stir thoroughly. Add the oils and stir again. Wash the floor with a sponge, rag, or mop. Rinse with clean water.

687
Cleaning the disposal

A kitchen sink disposal can harbor food residues, unpleasant odors, and bacteria. This mixture will help to clean and disinfect it.

1/4 cup (30g) borax
1/4 cup (30g) baking soda
1/2 lemon rind

Combine the ingredients and pour the mixture down the disposal. Turn it on, using plenty of hot water.

688
Oven degreaser

This formula works well with steel-wool soap pads.

1 tablespoon natural liquid dishwashing soap
1/2 cup (125ml) distilled white vinegar
1/2 cup (125ml) warm water

Mix the ingredients in a spray bottle. Spray liberally onto the oven interior and rinse with warm water.

689
Cleaning your oven the nontoxic way

To clean without toxic ingredients, spray the oven with warm water and sprinkle a thin layer of baking soda on to the bottom of the oven. Spray again with water, and let the mixture sit overnight. In the morning, scrub the oven with steel-wool soap pads and rinse well with water.

690
Cleaning automatic coffeemakers

Lime and other minerals in water can build up as sediment in coffeemakers and cause clogging. Pour one cup (125ml) of distilled white vinegar into the coffeemaker as though you were making coffee. Follow with two full pots of water to thoroughly flush the vinegar from the coffeemaker.

691
Removing sediment from teakettles

Vinegar and salt remove the mineral sediments that accumulate at the bottom of teakettles.

1 1/2 cups (375ml) distilled white vinegar
1 1/2 cups (375ml) water
3 tablespoons salt

Combine the ingredients in the teakettle, bring to a boil, and simmer for 15 minutes. Leave the mixture in the teakettle overnight. In the morning rinse thoroughly with several changes of water.

692
Remove cutting board odors

Apply a paste of baking soda and warm water to a cutting board after you have chopped garlic and onions. Let it stand for 15 minutes, and rinse.

693
Baking soda deodorizer

Every month, cut off the top of a box of baking soda and place it in your refrigerator to keep it smelling fresh.

694
Refrigerator deodorizing cleanser

Baking soda and lemon juice will clean and deodorize the refrigerator.

$1/2$ cup (125ml) freshly squeezed lemon juice

2 cups (500ml) hot water

1 tablespoon baking soda

Mix the ingredients, dip a sponge in the solution, and thoroughly wash the interior of the refrigerator. Finish by wiping with a clean, damp cloth.

Cleaning the Bathroom

Bathrooms are warm, moist environments and so become prime targets for mold, mildew, and bacterial growth. The following natural antimicrobial cleaning treatments will help you keep your bathroom fresh and clean.

695
All-purpose spray

Lavender, eucalyptus, and lemon essential oils make an all-purpose spray that leaves your bathroom clean and pleasantly scented.

1 teaspoon borax

2 cups (500ml) hot water

$1/2$ teaspoon natural liquid dishwashing soap

3 tablespoons distilled white vinegar

15 drops lavender essential oil

10 drops eucalyptus essential oil

5 drops lemon essential oil

Mix the borax and hot water and let it cool to room temperature. Pour into a spray bottle and add remaining ingredients. Shake well.

696
Mold and mildew spray cleaner

This spray cleaner makes use of the antimicrobial properties of lavender and eucalyptus essential oils, and will help you prevent mold and mildew from growing in your bathroom.

$1 3/4$ cups (450ml) hot water

2 tablespoons borax

$1/4$ cup (60ml) distilled white vinegar

$1/2$ teaspoon eucalyptus essential oil

$1/2$ teaspoon lavender essential oil

Dissolve the borax in the hot water. Let it cool to room temperature, and pour into a 16fl oz (500ml) spray bottle. Add the vinegar and essential oils and shake well.

697
Preventing mold and mildew

Mold and mildew are far easier to prevent than to remove. Both thrive in a dark, moist environment, so make sure your bathroom is well-ventilated. Open the window after you bathe or shower and, if you have one, use the exhaust fan. Regular cleaning (at least once a week) also keeps fungi from gaining a foothold. Scrub the tiles and grout with a soft bristle brush and use an old toothbrush to clean smaller areas, such as the caulking around the tub or sink.

698
Heavy-duty mold and mildew cleaner

A strong solution of borax and tea tree oil helps eliminate heavy concentrations of mold or mildew.

1 cup (120g) borax

2 cups (500ml) hot water

$1/2$ teaspoon tea tree essential oil

Dissolve the borax in hot water, let it cool to lukewarm, and add the tea tree oil. Apply to the mildewed area with a sponge or brush. Let it sit for a few hours, and rinse well with water.

699
Grout cleaner

The grout between ceramic tiles is a favorite target for mildew and grime.

$1/2$ cup (60g) baking soda

$1/2$ cup (60g) borax

$1/3$ cup (80ml) distilled white vinegar

Mix the ingredients into a smooth paste. Scrub into the grout with a toothbrush and rinse well.

700
Gentle bathroom cleaner

This cleanser helps disinfect surfaces and stop mildew growing.

1 tablespoon borax
2 cups (500ml) hot water
1/2 cup (125ml) natural liquid dishwashing soap
20 drops juniper essential oil
20 drops eucalyptus essential oil

Dissolve the borax in the hot water and let it cool to room temperature. Combine the solution with the soap and oils in a plastic squeeze bottle and shake well. Dampen the sink or tub and apply the cleaner with a sponge or rag. Rinse with clean water.

701
Sink and tub cleanser

A gentle polishing with baking soda, borax, and liquid soap cleans enamel, porcelain, and fiberglass surfaces

without damaging the finish. Lavender and eucalyptus essential oils help disinfect and add a fresh scent.

1/3 cup (40g) baking soda
1/3 cup (40g) borax
1 teaspoon natural liquid dishwashing soap
5 drops lavender essential oil
5 drops eucalyptus essential oil

Mix the ingredients together in a small plastic container. Dampen the sink or tub and apply the scrub with a sponge or rag. Rinse well.

702
Natural bleaching cleanser

Hydrogen peroxide helps bleach out stains that affect porcelain and fiberglass fixtures.

1/2 cup (60g) baking soda
1/2 teaspoon natural liquid dishwashing soap
1 teaspoon hydrogen peroxide

Mix the ingredients in a small plastic container. Dampen the sink or tub and apply the scrub with a sponge or rag. Rinse well with clean water.

703
Floor disinfectant

Dissolve a quarter of a cup (30g) borax in one gallon (5 liters) of hot water. Add five drops of patchouli essential oil and stir well. Use a mop, sponge, or rag to clean the floors.

704
Shower head cleaner

When a shower nozzle becomes clogged with mineral deposits, soak the shower head in a mixture of equal parts of distilled white vinegar and hot water. Leave for one hour, and then scrub with a toothbrush.

705
Removing rust stains

Rub a paste of cream of tartar and lemon juice into the rust stains on porcelain sinks and bathtubs and leave for 30 minutes. Rinse well. Repeat if necessary.

706
Cleaning toilet bowls

Borax and lemon juice clean and deodorize toilet bowls and help remove mineral deposits. Pour a cup (120g) of borax and a quarter of a cup (60ml) of lemon juice into the bowl. Let it sit overnight. Scrub with a toilet brush, and flush to rinse. If the bowl is stained from mineral deposits, scoop water out of the toilet to lower the water level. Make a borax and lemon juice paste and rub it onto the inside of the bowl. Let it stand overnight, then scrub and rinse.

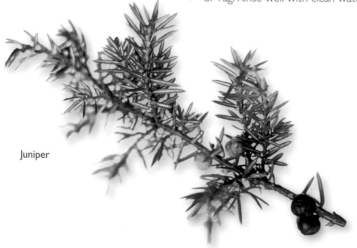

Juniper

707
Removing stubborn toilet rings

Mineral deposits that aren't removed with borax and lemon juice can be buffed off with a pumice stick or fine steel wool. Scoop water out of the toilet to lower the water level and expose the stains. Dampen the porcelain, and buff gently with the pumice stick or steel wool.

708
Polishing chrome fixtures

Remove water spots from chrome bathroom fixtures with a mixture of equal parts baking soda and distilled white vinegar. Apply to the fixtures, let dry, and polish with a soft cloth.

709
Shower curtain cleaner

Mix half a cup (60g) of borax, half a cup (125ml) of distilled white vinegar, and three drops of eucalyptus essential oil. With a soft-bristled scrub brush, scrub the mixture on to vinyl shower curtains and shower curtain liners once a month. Rinse well with warm water.

710
Cleaning fabric shower curtains

Wash your fabric shower curtains with a mixture of half a cup (60g) of borax, half a cup (125ml) of distilled white vinegar, a mild natural laundry detergent, and warm water.

Natural Clothing Care

Laundering clothing with natural cleaning agents such as vinegar, baking soda, and gentle detergents is easier on your clothing, skin, and the environment than strong chemical detergents. In this section, you'll also find tips for removing a variety of stains, as well as for cleaning accessories such as jewelry, shoes, and handbags.

711
Freshening clothing

Many times, clothing is not really dirty, but simply needs to be rinsed and freshened. To remove perspiration and odors from fabrics, try adding a quarter of a cup (30g) of baking soda and a quarter of a cup (30g) of borax as your washing machine is filling and put it on a rinse cycle.

712
Holding the colors

To help keep colors from fading in the wash, add one tablespoon of distilled white vinegar to each load of your laundry.

713
Eliminating detergent residue

Residues from detergents can irritate sensitive skin and cause itching and dryness. Use half the recommended amount of detergent for a load of laundry, and add one cup (250ml) of distilled white vinegar to the final rinse water to remove the residues. **Caution:** Avoid vinegar if you are using chlorine bleach because the combination produces toxic gases.

714
Natural oxygen bleach

Oxygen bleaches rely on hydrogen peroxide, not chlorine, to whiten clothing. They are gentler on fabrics and better for the environment. They work best if you presoak your white clothing for two hours in the bleach solution. Follow by laundering in the hottest water recommended for your fabric. To prevent dinginess and discoloration, always wash white laundry separately from other colors.

715
Clothes softener

To soften and deodorize clothing, add half a cup (60g) of baking soda to your laundry during the rinse cycle.

716
Alternatives to dry-cleaning

To minimize trips to the dry-cleaner, keep clothing clean by brushing regularly with a lint brush. Hanging clothing outdoors on a sunny day helps remove stale odors and keeps clothing fresh. If you do have clothing dry-cleaned, hang it in a well-ventilated place (outdoors is best—weather permitting) for a week before wearing it to allow the dry-cleaning solvent to evaporate.

717
Natural laundry soap

Castile soap, baking soda, and borax provide extra cleaning action for dirty clothing. Grapefruit and lavender essential oils add a fresh, clean scent.

10 drops grapefruit essential oil

10 drops lavender essential oil

1 cup (125g) baking soda

1 cup (120g) borax

1 cup (120g) powdered castile soap

Add the essential oils to the baking soda drop by drop, mixing thoroughly with a hand sifter. Combine this with the borax and soap, and mix again. Store in a tightly covered container. To use the soap, add one-half cup (60g) to each load of laundry.

Clean laundry the natural way

718
Laundry starch

If you like the look of crisply ironed cotton and linen, treat your fabrics with this spray. Mix half a tablespoon of cornstarch and one cup (250ml) of water in a spray bottle. Shake well. Spray lightly onto fabrics as you iron.

719
Natural all-purpose stain remover

This removes many types of stain, especially if you treat them quickly.

1 tablespoon vegetable glycerin

1 tablespoon natural liquid dishwashing soap

1/2 cup (125ml) water

Mix the ingredients, shake well, and store in a plastic squeeze bottle. Rub into the stain and launder as usual.

720
Berry stains

Stretch the item over a large bowl and sprinkle with cream of tartar. Pour boiling water onto the stain and continue until you have removed as much as possible. Rub in a little vegetable glycerin and launder.

721
Blood stains

Sponge with hydrogen peroxide and then rub in liquid dishwashing soap and soak in cold water overnight. Launder as usual.

722
Grass stains

Dampen the fabric with cold water and rub cream of tartar into the stain. Follow this by rubbing with

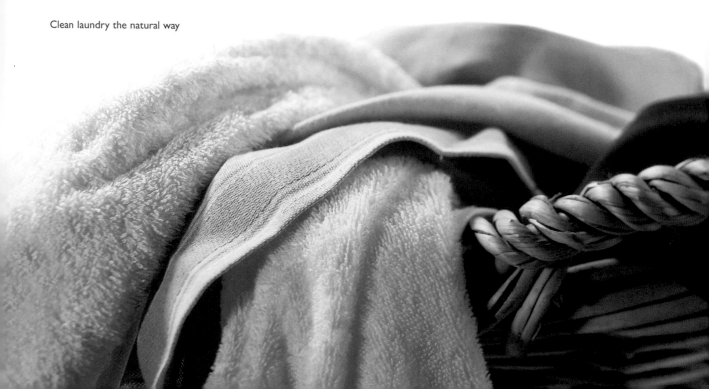

a mixture of equal parts vegetable glycerin and liquid dishwashing soap. Rinse, and launder as usual.

723
Chocolate stains

Sponge the clothing with hydrogen peroxide to remove as much of the stain as possible. Mix a paste of borax and water and apply to the stain. Launder as usual.

724
Coffee and tea stains

Rinse the coffee or tea stain with cold water or club soda. If the stain is still evident, sponge it with a solution of one teaspoon of borax diluted in one cup (250ml) of water. Rinse thoroughly with clean water and launder as usual.

725
Grease stains

Cover the stain with cornstarch and rub in gently. Allow to sit for 15 minutes and brush to remove. Rub liquid dishwashing soap into the stain and launder in the hottest water appropriate for the fabric.

726
Ink stains

Rub a small amount of vegetable glycerin into the ink stain and then apply a paste of cream of tartar and lemon juice. Leave the paste on for several minutes, then rinse off with warm water, and repeat if necessary. Launder as usual.

727
Mildew stains

Rub with a paste of buttermilk and salt and then launder in hot water. If the item is white or light-colored, hang it outdoors to take advantage of the sun's natural bleaching action.

728
Perspiration stains

Combine a tablespoon of salt and a tablespoon of baking soda. Add enough water to make a paste and rub into the stain. Let it sit for an hour and then launder.

729
Protein stains

For milk or egg stains, soak the item in cold water. Follow by rubbing liquid dishwashing soap into the stain and launder as usual.

730
Red wine stains

Using an absorbent towel, blot up as much of the wine as possible. Apply a thick layer of salt; leave on until the salt has absorbed the wine, and then rinse. Alternatively, try soaking the stain with club soda.

731
Collar stains

To remove the ground-in dirt and oils that stain collars, make a paste of liquid dishwashing soap and baking soda. Rub the mixture into the stain, let it sit for one hour, and launder.

732
Removing chewing gum

Rub the gum with an ice cube until it freezes; you should then be able to pull the gum off of the fabric. Follow by rubbing distilled white vinegar into any remaining sticky areas.

733
Removing wax

With a dull knife, carefully scrape off as much excess wax from the fabric as possible. Place a brown paper bag over the remaining wax, and press with a warm iron. The wax will melt and transfer onto the paper bag. Place a fresh part of the paper bag over the spot, and continue ironing until you have removed all the wax from the fabric.

734
Preventing clothes moths

Although clothes moths can be extremely destructive, they are also easily destroyed by laundering, fresh air, and sunlight. Moths are attracted to wool, mohair, angora, and other animal hair fibers, and also to food stains and perspiration. Make sure your clothing is clean before storing it. A simple way to kill moth larvae is to hang clothing outdoors in the fresh air and sunshine. For added protection against moths, add a few drops of cedar or eucalyptus essential oil to the final rinse water when washing sweaters or other clothing and allow to soak for about 30 minutes.

735
Herbal moth repellents

Herbs that work well to repel moths include eucalyptus, lavender, and peppermint. Place a handful of dried herbs in the center of a cotton handkerchief and tie with a ribbon. Use bags of herbs generously: the stronger the fragrance, the more protection herbal repellents provide. To protect clothing and linens from moths, place cotton balls sprinkled with a few drops of patchouli essential oil in closets and drawers. Replenish the essential oil when the scent begins to diminish.

736
Repel moths with cedar

Cedar is excellent for repelling moths. Either buy cedar shavings in pet stores for sachets, or use solid blocks of cedar, which are commonly available as natural moth repellents. Cedar blocks should be sanded every few months to renew their fragrance or treated with a few drops of cedar essential oil.

737
Freshening hairbrushes and combs

To remove residues of hair-styling products and to keep hairbrushes and combs clean and fresh, soak them weekly in a basin of warm, soapy water to which you have added a quarter of a cup (30g) of baking soda. Soak for 30 minutes, and scrub if necessary with a nailbrush. Rinse thoroughly with warm water.

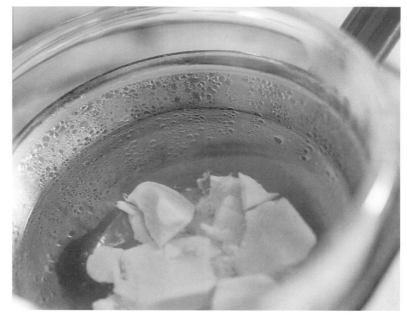
Renew leather with olive oil and beeswax

738
Jewelry cleaning tips

Most precious gems, except pearls, can be cleaned in lukewarm, soapy water with a soft toothbrush. Rinse thoroughly with clear water and dry. To enhance the luster of pearls, rub them with a few drops of vegetable glycerin and buff with a soft cloth.

739
Clean gold and silver

Items of jewelry containing silver or gold can be cleaned with this paste.

$^{1}/_{4}$ teaspoon natural liquid dishwashing soap
2 tablespoons baking soda

Mix the ingredients into a paste. Apply with a soft toothbrush and buff gently. Rinse in warm water, and dry.

740
Caring for leather

Clean dirty leather with a sponge and a solution of mild soapy water. Rinse thoroughly, and dry with a soft cloth.

$^{1}/_{4}$ cup (60ml) olive oil
2 teaspoons grated beeswax

Heat the ingredients in a saucepan until the beeswax has melted. Pour into a small jar and let cool. Apply a small amount of polish to leather at least every three months to keep it from drying and cracking. Rub it in well, and buff to remove excess.

741
Remove stains from leather

Beat an egg white until stiff and rub into the leather with a soft cloth. Repeat until the stain has gone.

Soil, Compost, & Mulches

Healthy soil is the foundation of a pest free, disease resistant, and abundant garden. Instead of chemical fertilizers, use natural soil enrichments such as manure and compost. Buy a soil-testing kit and discover the pH and nutrient content of your soil; this knowledge will help you bring the best out of your garden.

742
Loosening the clay soil in your garden

Clay soil is heavy and sticky and can suffocate plant roots, but it does retain abundant moisture and is often rich in nutrients. To improve the drainage of clay soil, work it with a garden fork and add horticultural sand or gravel to the depth of at least 12in (30cm). Avoid working in clay soil when the ground is wet; standing on or digging in wet soil will cause it to compact even more.

743
Improving sandy soil

Sandy soil drains quickly but does not retain nutrients or moisture well. Add soil improvers such as compost or leaf mold and dig it in to a depth of at least 12in (30cm). To make the job easier, simply spread a layer of organic matter over the surface of garden beds in the fall. By spring, most of the compost or leaf mold will have been broken down and worked into the soil by earthworms and other beneficial soil organisms.

Clean garden tools in a bucket of sand and oil

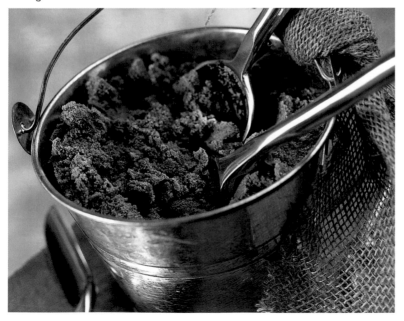

744
Creating new beds in your garden

Clearing an area of grass and weeds is a lot of hard work. You can make it easier by killing the grass and weeds first. In the summer or fall, cover the area you want cleared with large flattened cardboard cartons. Place leaves, grass clippings, or straw over the cardboard, making at least a 6in-(15cm-) thick layer of mulch. Remove the cardboard and mulch the following spring, and your ground will be ready to prepare for planting.

745
Keep fingernails clean

To keep fingernails clean when gardening, scratch your nails over a bar of soap before heading out to the garden. The soap beneath your fingernails will prevent dirt from accumulating and makes cleaning up much easier.

746
Keeping your garden tools clean

If you keep your garden tools clean you help keep them sharp, prevent rust, and lengthen their life span. Wipe your tools clean with a piece of rough burlap after every use, and apply a small amount of mineral oil to prevent rust. For an easy way to clean up small tools, fill a large bucket with sand and add mineral oil to dampen the sand. Stick the metal end of trowels and other hand tools in the sand until their next use.

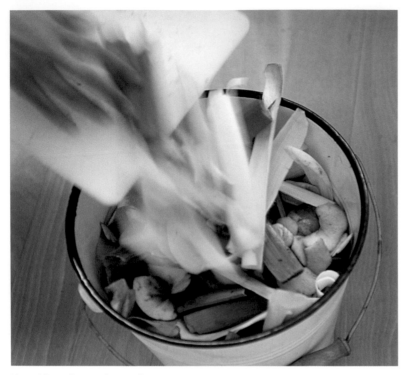

Vegetable peelings make excellent compost

747
Compost for soil health

One of the most effective ways of improving your soil is to use compost from grass clippings, yard prunings, leaves, and kitchen wastes such as fruit and vegetable peelings, eggshells, coffee grounds, and tea leaves. To avoid attracting animals and pests, do not use meats or fatty foods and do not include diseased plants or weeds that have gone to seed.

748
Green and brown composting materials

Good healthy compost needs approximately equal amounts of green and brown materials.

Brown materials:
Dried leaves, dried garden flowers and plants, straw, and shredded newspaper.

Green materials:
Grass clippings, fresh plant and flower clippings, vegetable and fruit peelings, and manure.

749
Making a simple compost pile

A wire or wood slat bin that is about 3ft (1m) in diameter makes a good compost bin. Begin your compost pile by spreading a layer of brown material (such as dried leaves) about 6in (15cm) thick. Follow this with a layer of green material (such as grass clippings) about 6in (15cm) thick.

Cover this with about one inch (25mm) of garden soil. Then add another layer of brown material and moisten the compost pile with water. Continue layering the pile with approximately equal amounts of brown and green materials mixed with a little soil, and keep the pile about as moist as a damp sponge. Turn the pile every two weeks with a garden fork. When the compost pile is about 3ft (1m) tall, start another pile. In approximately two months to one year, the compost will be dark brown, soft, crumbly, and ready to use in your garden.

750
Speed up composting

To speed up the composting process, cut up all the materials you want to use into small pieces before adding them to your compost pile.

751
Making leaf mold

Leaf mold is an excellent, nutrient-rich compost to add to your garden. An easy way to make leaf mold is to fill heavy plastic lawn bags with leaves raked from your lawn or a neighbor's lawn. Wet the leaves down by spraying with a hose, and poke a couple of dozen holes in the bag with a garden fork. Fold the top of the bag to close it and place a heavy brick on top of the bag. Let it sit for six months or longer in a sunny location, until the leaves have decomposed into a rich compost. A hot, humid climate will break down the leaves more quickly than a cold, dry climate.

752
Using compost in your garden

All soils can be improved by the regular addition of compost. To add nutrients and improve soil texture, spread 2in (5cm) of aged compost on to vegetable and annual beds in the spring. Turn the compost into the soil, and then seed or put in transplants. During the growing season, add compost as a mulch to vegetable gardens to further enrich the soil.

753
Making potting soil

Compost makes a potting soil of excellent quality. Before using, first filter the compost through a coarse mesh screen to remove large chunks of organic material.

2 cups (360g) good garden soil
1 cup (160g) compost or leaf mold
1 cup (120g) vermiculite
1 tablespoon bone meal

Mix the ingredients together and use the mixture for your houseplants or for starting seeds.

754
Feed the soil

To ensure that your plants remain healthy, it is more important to feed the soil in which they grow than it is to add fertilizer to the plants. Create a soil rich in nutrients by adding large amounts of organic materials such as compost and leaf mold to your soil throughout the year.

755
Nourish your plants with compost tea

Plants flourish when fed with a tea made from aged compost. Compost tea can be used as a root fertilizer, and sprayed on leaves to nourish the plant through the foliage. It provides a rich source of nutrients for all types of plants and also helps control pests and diseases when used as a spray. To make compost tea, fill a cloth bag with aged compost and tie the top closed. Submerge the bag in a clean trashcan, add water to cover the bag by 6in (15cm), and cover. Let steep for a couple of weeks. During this time, the compost tea will ferment and create a population of beneficial bacteria. To use, pour the desired amount into a watering can or garden sprayer and dilute with three parts water. Use weekly to keep plants healthy.

756
Mulching your garden

Mulching plants is one of the biggest time-saving practices in your garden. Adding mulch to a garden conserves soil moisture, inhibits weed growth, and helps maintain a consistent soil temperature to protect plant roots from excessive heat or cold. Bark chips, shredded bark, cocoa shells, and pine needles are attractive mulches and are best suited to flower beds and for mulching around shrubs and trees. Compost, leaf mold, shredded leaves, grass clippings, and straw are excellent mulches for vegetable gardens. They decompose fairly quickly and can be turned in to the soil at the end of the season, helping improve soil texture and adding nutrients. In general, apply layer of mulch at least 3in (7.5cm) thick to beds and plants.

757
Using mulch correctly

Mulching plants keeps soil moist and prevents plants from drying out, but it can harbor plant pests. To avoid these, occasionally rake the mulch to keep pests from setting up house. It is best to keep mulch an inch (2.5cm) away from the base of plants; this improves air circulation and prevents potential problems with excess dampness.

758
Soaker hoses

To conserve water and deliver it directly to the roots of plants, lay soaker hoses (available at garden supply stores) under the mulch.

759
Acid-loving plants

Pine needles are an excellent mulch for acid-loving plants such as azaleas and rhododendrons.

A Word About Plants

When you have chosen the most suitable plants for your garden, make sure they get off to a good start by planting them correctly in the soil. This discourages diseases and pests, and ensures the best possible harvest.

760
Figuring plant spacing

A common mistake when planting is to underestimate the size that a plant or shrub will be when it is full grown. Planting too close together means crowded roots, increased potential for disease, and a lot of extra work created by the necessity to move plants. A good general rule is to space a plant one-half the distance of its mature size from neighboring plants—for example, if a plant will be 2ft (60cm) wide, plant it 12in (30cm) away from other plants. If you are uncertain about a plant's mature size, consult a gardening book or ask an expert at a nursery or garden center.

761
Beneficial planting

Plant closely enough so that, at their mature size, plants will touch and slightly overlap their leaves. This will create a beneficial environment for most plants, conserving moisture and helping shade out weeds.

762
Rotate crops

Crop rotation plays an important role in preventing pests and diseases from overtaking your garden. By not planting the same crop repeatedly in the same spot in your garden, you keep the particular pests and diseases that attack specific plants from gaining a stronghold. Ideally, avoid planting the same crop in a garden bed more than once every three years.

763
Avoid compacting soil

When you are planting, stand on a board at least 12in (30cm) wide so that you are distributing your weight over a larger area. This will help you avoid compacting the soil.

764
Align rows north–south

Lay out your vegetable garden rows running north to south so that both sides of the row will receive an equal amount of sunlight during the day.

765
How to plant straight rows

If you want to grow vegetables in straight rows, lay a narrow board on top of the soil and either plant along the edge of the board or make a furrow the length of the board and plant the seeds in the furrow. Another simple way of ensuring straight rows is to place stakes at the ends of where you want the rows to be; tie a string between the stakes and plant beneath the string.

766
Preparing seeds for planting

Seeds often carry disease-causing pathogens and should be treated before they are planted or stored. To lessen the possibility of disease, use this sterilizing bath.

1 tablespoon apple cider vinegar
1 quart (1.25 liters) water

Combine the vinegar and water in a bowl. Place the seeds into the center of a piece of clean cheesecloth, gather the ends together, and secure with a rubber band. Dip the bag of seeds into the vinegar solution a few times. Remove the seeds from the bag and place them on several thicknesses of paper towels to dry. Make sure the seeds are thoroughly dry before storing.

767
Eggshell planting pots

To make simple individual planting pots for seedlings, cut the top off of an egg carton. After you've eaten the eggs, save the shell halves, and poke a small drainage hole in the bottom of each. Place the eggshell into the egg carton, fill with planting soil mix, and plant the seeds. When the seedlings reach transplant size, plant them in your garden in the eggshell, crushing the shell as you do so.

768
Freeing rootbound plants

Transplants destined for the flower or vegetable garden often become rootbound in small pots. To help the roots spread out and to keep them from continuing to grow in a tight mass, use a dinner fork to pull the roots apart. If roots are really tightly bound, make a light cut with a utility knife vertically down each of the four sides of the root mass.

769
Water thoroughly before planting out

The best way to ensure that the plant will be adequately watered when transplanted is to soak the plant thoroughly while it is in the container. In addition, after digging a hole for the plant, fill the hole with water and let it drain before putting in the new plant. After placing the plant and filling in the hole with soil, water again thoroughly.

770
Individual greenhouses from plastic bottles

A plastic bottle makes an excellent greenhouse for protecting young vegetable plants from a late frost. Cut off the bottom of the bottle, about 3 pints (1.8 liters) in size, and place it over the plant, pushing it 2in (5cm) down into the soil. Leave the top off the bottle to prevent temperatures from getting too hot during the day.

771
Guard plants from frost damage

An unseasonably cold spring or fall night can wreak havoc with tender plants. To protect your garden from frost damage, cover plants with a couple of layers of newspaper held down by rocks when the weather forecast predicts some freezing temperatures. This simple solution raises the temperature around the plant by at least 10°F (4°C).

772
Keep container plants from freezing

Protect your container plants and their pots from unexpected freezing temperatures. Wrap each pot in several layers of newspaper, followed by a layer of burlap on top. Tie the layers in place with string. To protect the plant, cover it with a brown paper grocery bag.

773
Prevent scorching

Avoid watering your plants during the heat of the day to prevent the leaves and flowers from being scorched by the sun's rays.

774
Blanching cauliflower

If you want to grow pure white heads of cauliflower, most varieties must be blanched while they are growing. Without blanching, the heads turn an unappetizing yellowish brown.

Choose a sunny day when the plant is completely dry and the cauliflower head is about the size of a golf ball. Tie the leaves of the plant up over the head and secure with a rubber band. Water only the roots of the plant, and unwrap the cauliflower every few days to check for pests.

775
Grow straight carrots

Carrots need loose, rock-free soil to grow properly. Prepare a garden bed by thoroughly digging and loosening the soil to at least 12in (30cm) deep, and make sure you remove all the rocks and roots, and break up the clumps of soil. This will allow the carrots to grow straight down. Spread 2in (5cm) of compost on top of the garden bed and dig it in to loosen the soil. If the soil is really heavy, add an additional 2in (5cm) of coarse builder's sand and thoroughly dig it in. When the carrot tops are 2in (5cm) tall, thin the seedlings to one inch (25mm) apart. Thin them again about two weeks later to 3in (7.5cm) apart. Failing to thin the seedlings properly results in misshapen carrots.

776
Encourage a bigger broccoli harvest

Many varieties of broccoli produce not only a central head, but also smaller side shoots that are just as tasty as the head. Try to encourage the production of these side shoots to receive a bigger harvest from your plants. When you remove the central head, cut it by taking just 2in (5cm)

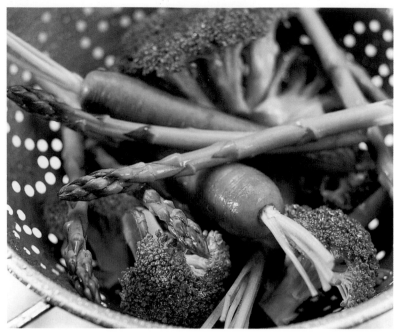

Grow better vegetables with natural methods

780
Produce more apples

To improve the yield of an apple tree, spray the foliage with seaweed extract, available at garden centers, three times—when the buds fill out, after the petals drop, and once again when the fruits are half an inch (12mm) in diameter. To increase the size and flavor of apples, thin fruit on trees by removing the smaller apples in each cluster of fruit before they reach one inch (25mm) in diameter. Remove all but one apple in each cluster on small trees; you can leave two apples per bunch on larger trees.

781
Shade lettuce naturally

Plant leafy greens and cool-loving plants such as lettuce and spinach beneath tall flowering plants, such as nicotiana or sunflowers, or beneath trellises of cucumbers or squash.

782
Pollinate plants by hand

The flowers of vine crops such as squash, zucchini, and pumpkin need to be pollinated to produce fruit. Ideally, beneficial insects do this, but plants sometimes need assistance. If the tiny fruit on a vine is dying, it has not been pollinated. To hand-pollinate flowers, take a small soft artist's paintbrush and touch it to the pollen-bearing stamens in the male flowers and then brush the pollen gently on the tip of the pistil in the female flower (those with a tiny fruit at the base of the flower).

of the stem. At the same time, apply additional fertilizer to the plant by scratching in a quarter of a cup (30g) of balanced organic fertilizer per broccoli plant. If you want to produce tender heads of broccoli, make sure you mulch the plants heavily and water them regularly.

777
Produce more and better asparagus

To improve the productivity and health of your asparagus bed, add pickling salt to the soil at the rate of 2.5lb (1.5kg) for each 100ft (30m) of row. Sodium chloride rock salt improves the growth of asparagus and increases resistance to disease. Don't use salt on asparagus beds that are less than one year old, and don't use iodized table salt.

778
Produce more beans

Dust the seeds of beans and peas with a bacterial inoculant just before planting. This helps beans gather nitrogen, improving growth and increasing harvest. Pick beans when they are tender and about the diameter of a pencil. Harvesting daily also encourages bean production.

779
Grow better cucumbers

To save space and produce healthier cucumbers, train the vines on a trellis instead of letting them sprawl on the ground. Cucumbers need plenty of water while growing to prevent deformed or bitter fruits. To keep the vines producing, pick cucumbers frequently, while they are still young.

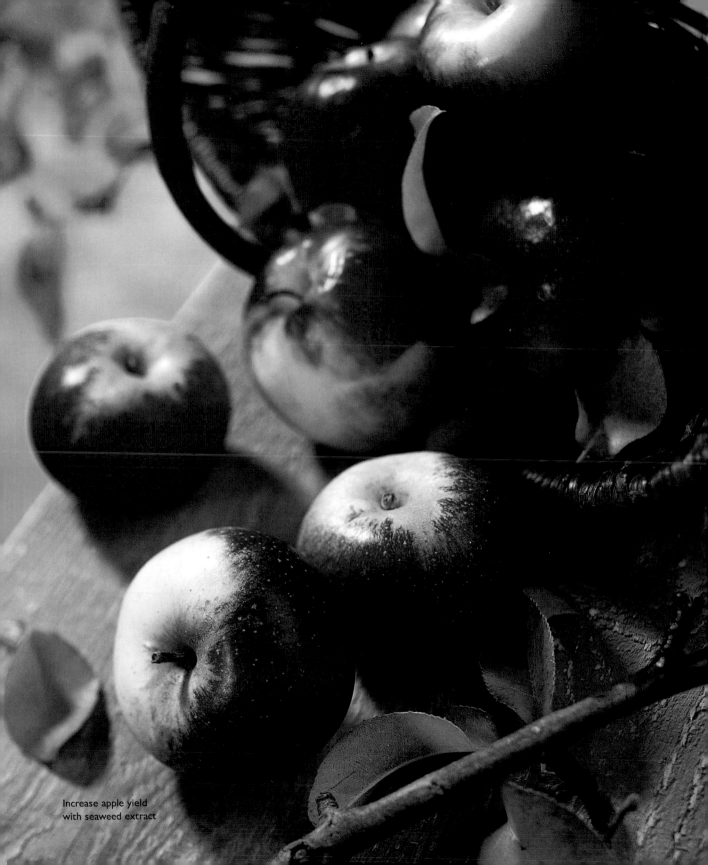

Increase apple yield
with seaweed extract

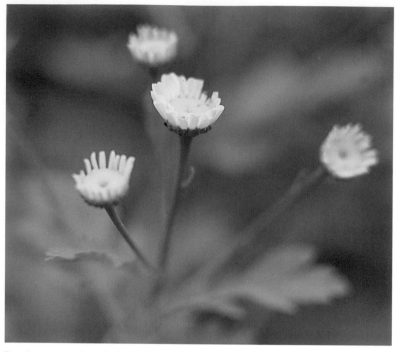

Feverfew attracts beneficial insects

Beneficial Animals & Plants

Many insects including ladybugs, green lacewings, and parasitic wasps are beneficial visitors to your garden, as are spiders and many birds. They prey on destructive pests such as aphids and cabbage worms, and prevent damage to your vegetable crops and flowers. Certain plants, such as dill and garlic, are also beneficial because they can protect crops and flowers, such as roses.

783
Plants that attract beneficial insects

You can encourage beneficial insects to visit your garden by providing their favored habitats and food sources, such as anise hyssop, borage, catmint, comfrey, cornflower, echinacea, feverfew, fennel, garlic chives, golden marguerite, lavender, lupine, mint, sweet alyssum, and yarrow.

784
Provide water for helpful insects

Beneficial insects need water to drink, and providing a convenient source will help attract them to your garden. To provide dry areas for the insects to land, fill a shallow container with rocks and add water, leaving some of the rocks exposed.

785
Let some of your vegetables bloom

To attract beneficial insects to your garden, let a few of your vegetables bloom, such as salad greens or broccoli, bok choy, kale, and other members of the brassica family.

786
Protect your brassicas with dill

Plant dill among your broccoli, cauliflowers, cabbages, and other brassicas. The ferny, delicate leaves of the herb attract beneficial parasitic wasps, which keep pests, such as cabbage worms, under control.

787
Guard your cucumbers with nasturtiums

Plant colorful nasturtiums among your cucumbers to repel cucumber beetles. The broad nasturtium leaves weave among the cucumber vines and also provide a sheltered habitat for beneficial spiders that trap and eat destructive pests.

788
Protect your roses with garlic

Plant garlic beneath your rosebushes to help ward off the pests that prey on roses. The tall purple pom-pom flowers make an attractive addition to your garden. Other allium family members, such as garlic chives, are equally effective.

789
Protect your tomatoes with basil

Planting basil with your tomato plants helps control tomato hornworms. The leaves of the herb also provide tasty garnishes for tomato dishes.

790
Safeguard your corn with pole beans

Corn and pole beans make excellent garden companions. Tall corn stalks act as natural supports for climbing pole beans, and the pole beans repay the favor by attracting beneficial insects that protect corn from pests.

791
Repel pests with marigolds

Common marigolds will help repel many insect pests from your vegetable garden. The stronger the scent of the marigold, the more vigorous are the repellent properties. French marigolds also help repel nematodes in nearby plants. For best results, plant patches of marigolds throughout your garden.

792
Guard your cabbages with thyme

Plant thyme among your cabbage plants to help deter cabbage pests, including cabbage-white butterflies, cabbage maggots, and imported cabbageworms.

793
Entice birds to your garden

Birds are wonderful in helping keep destructive garden pests under control. Provide additional food and water to entice them. A mixture of millet and black sunflower seeds will draw many common insect-eating birds such as wrens, robins, and jays. Set up a birdbath or a shallow dish with water; a birdhouse with the appropriate size entry for the type of bird you want to attract will help keep residents close to your home.

794
Attract pollinating insects

Fruit trees and fruiting vegetables, such as cucumbers and squashes, need the help of pollinating insects to produce their crops. You can attract these beneficial insects into your garden with a spray of sweet sugar water.

¹/₄ cup (55g) sugar
1 cup (250ml) water
2 quarts (2.5 liters) water

Boil the sugar with the cup of water until it dissolves. Allow the solution to cool to room temperature. Pour it into a pump-type garden sprayer, add the remaining water, and spray onto your garden.

795
Attract ladybugs with zinnias

Common garden zinnias attract ladybugs, which feast on aphids. Plant zinnias liberally in vegetable gardens to protect broccoli, cauliflower, and leafy greens.

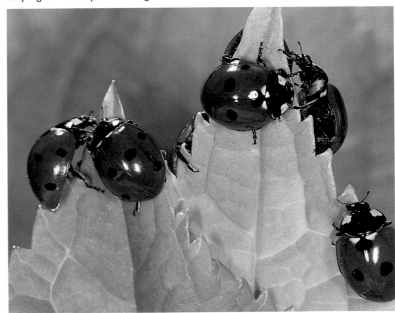

Ladybugs feast on aphids in the garden

Nontoxic Pest Control

Preventing insect damage is easiest if you keep a close eye on your garden. Check your plants at least once a week for pests. You can remove slugs, snails, and other large pests by picking them off plants; wash aphids off with a strong spray of water from the hose. To keep down populations of pests, keep your garden beds clean and free of weeds and other debris.

796
Tips for using garden sprays

Natural insecticidal sprays can be effective controls for garden pests, but they can also cause damage by burning leaves or harming tender plants. To be on the safe side, first test a few plants (or a few leaves if you are treating one large plant) for sensitivity before spraying an entire bed. Check for damage after a couple of days. Apply an insecticide spray in the evening, and soak the plant thoroughly with the spray, including the undersides of leaves.

797
Simple soap spray

This spray kills a wide variety of soft-bodied insects, including spider mites, mealybugs, aphids, and whiteflies.

- 1 tablespoon natural liquid dishwashing soap
- 2 quarts (2.5 liters) water

Mix the ingredients together in a pump-type garden sprayer and shake well. Apply the spray liberally to your plants each week and after every rain until you have the pest problem under control.

798
Avoid spraying plants in the sun

To prevent the sun's rays from damaging a plant's leaves, use soap and other insecticide sprays in the evening or on a cloudy day.

799
Simple garlic spray

Garlic fends off many leaf-eating garden pests.

- 1 head chopped garlic
- 1 quart (1.25 liters) warm water

Mix the ingredients and steep for four hours. Strain through a coffee filter, pour into a spray bottle, and spray affected plants every other day for two weeks.

800
Garlic and pepper spray

A garlic and hot pepper spray keeps insects from eating plants.

- 1 head garlic
- 8 hot jalapeño peppers
- 1 quart (1.25 liters) water
- ½ teaspoon natural liquid dishwashing soap

Wearing rubber gloves, chop up the garlic and peppers and blend with water in a blender. Steep overnight. Strain through a coffee filter into a pump-type garden sprayer. Add the soap and shake well. Spray your plants liberally once a week and after each rain until the pests are under control. Store the spray in your refrigerator for up to a month.

801
Herbal repellent spray

A spray made from rue, feverfew, and chives helps repel destructive leaf-eating garden insects.

- 1 quart (1.25 liters) boiling water
- 1 cup (40g) chopped fresh feverfew leaves
- ½ cup (20g) chopped fresh rue
- ½ cup (20g) chopped fresh chives
- ½ teaspoon natural liquid dishwashing soap

Pour the boiling water over the herbs, cover, and steep until cool. Strain and pour into a pump-type garden sprayer. Add the soap, shake well, and spray your plants.

802
Tansy spray for cabbage worms

Tansy tea, sprayed onto cauliflower, broccoli, and other members of the brassica family, helps repel imported cabbageworms.

- 1 quart (1.25 liters) boiling water
- 2 cups (80g) chopped fresh tansy leaves
- ½ teaspoon natural liquid dishwashing soap

Pour the water over the tansy, cover, and steep until cool. Strain through a coffee filter and pour into a pump-type garden sprayer. Add the soap, shake well, and spray your plants.

803
Wormwood spray for aphids

A strong tea of wormwood helps to keep aphids away from plants.

1 quart (1.25 liters) boiling water
2 cups (80g) chopped fresh wormwood
 leaves
1/2 teaspoon natural liquid dishwashing
 soap

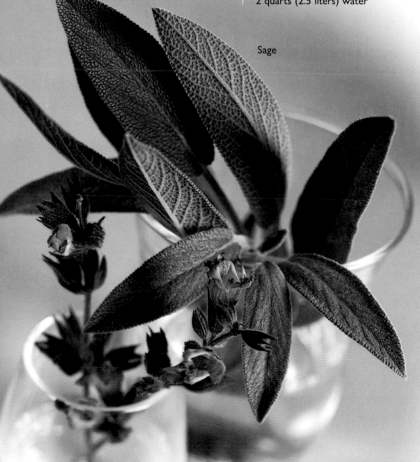

Sage

Pour the boiling water over the wormwood, cover, and steep until cool. Strain through a coffee filter and pour into a pump-type garden sprayer. Add the dishwashing soap, shake well, and spray your plants.

804
Essential oil repellent spray

Thyme, sage, and lavender essential oils help control a variety of destructive garden insects.

3 drops thyme essential oil
3 drops sage essential oil
5 drops lavender essential oil
1 teaspoon vodka or rubbing alcohol
2 quarts (2.5 liters) water

Mix the essential oils with the vodka to help them disperse evenly in the water. Combine with the water in a pump-type garden sprayer and thoroughly spray your plants.

805
Tobacco spray

Nicotine is toxic to various pests, especially aphids, leafhoppers, thrips, and leafminers. It's toxic to beneficial insects, too, so use as a last resort.

1/2 cup (15g) dried crushed tobacco
 leaves
2 quarts (2.5 liters) warm water
1 teaspoon natural liquid dishwashing
 soap

Soak the tobacco in water for half an hour and strain. Add the dishwashing soap and shake well. Using a pump-type garden sprayer, spray the leaves thoroughly with the solution. Store in a cool place in a tightly covered container for up to two weeks.

806
Tomato leaf spray

Tomato leaves are rich in alkaloids that are highly toxic to insects. A tomato leaf spray can help control aphids and corn earworms.

2 cups (80g) chopped tomato leaves
1 quart (1.25 liters) water
1 teaspoon natural liquid dishwashing
 soap

Soak the tomato leaves in water overnight. Strain through cheesecloth, pour into a pump-type garden sprayer, and add the soap. Shake well, and spray your plants liberally.

807
Hot pepper dust to combat ants

A combination of powdered cayenne pepper, garlic, and dill helps keep ants away from plants.

½ cup (65g) powdered cayenne pepper
½ cup (60g) powdered garlic
½ cup (60g) powdered dill

Buy powdered herbs or grind dried herbs into a powder in a coffee grinder. Mix them together, and sprinkle liberally around affected plants in a wide margin.

808
Potato flour spray for suffocating pests

A spray made from potato flour is nontoxic, but kills by suffocating pests. It helps control aphids, thrips, whiteflies, and spider mites.

¼ cup (30g) potato flour
1 quart (1.25 liters) warm water
1 teaspoon natural liquid dishwashing soap

Mix the potato flour with the water until it is thoroughly dissolved. Pour into a pump-type garden sprayer and add the dishwashing soap. Shake well and spray your plants liberally.

809
Defeat cabbage root flies with paper

Cabbage root flies deposit their eggs around the base of cabbage, broccoli, cauliflower, and other brassicas. The eggs hatch into maggots, which tunnel into roots and kill plants. To foil cabbage root flies, place a 6in (15cm) square of heavy paper around the base of each young plant. Cut a slit in the paper large enough to slide the plant stem through before planting.

810
Control aphids

One of the most common garden pests, aphids multiply rapidly and blanket tender new growth of roses, vegetables, and perennials. Aphids weaken plants by sucking out the sap. This spray helps control them.

1 teaspoon natural liquid dishwashing soap
2 teaspoons light cooking oil
2 quarts water (2.5 liters)

Combine the soap, oil, and a cup (250ml) of water and mix together thoroughly. Pour the mixture into a pump-type garden sprayer. Shake well, add the remaining water, and then shake again. Liberally spray each and every aphid-infested plant with the solution once a week, and after each shower of rain until the aphids are under control.

811
Eggshell barrier to combat slugs and snails

To discourage slugs and snails from gaining access to your plants, place a generous barrier of coarsely crushed eggshells in a circle around the base of each plant.

Crushed eggshells deter slugs and snails

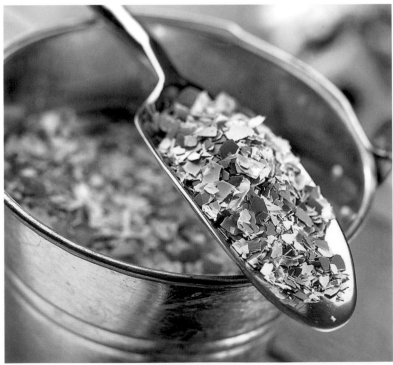

812
Banish slugs and snails

Slugs and snails come out at night, and eat large, ragged holes in leaves and chew off tender new growth. Handpick them at night; sprinkle salt on slugs to dehydrate them. During the day, they hide in cool, moist places. Set out large plastic flower pots turned upside down with one edge lifted slightly for the pests to crawl under. Each morning, dispose of the slugs and snails you find there.

813
Protect plants from slugs and snails

To prevent both slugs and snails from chewing on your plants, place a ring of diatomaceous earth around the perimeter of the garden or around the specific plants you wish to protect. Diatomaceous earth is a fine powder made from the microscopic skeletons of marine algae and can be purchased at garden supply centers. Their razorlike structure cuts into snails and slugs and dehydrates them. To be effective, diatomaceous earth must be reapplied after every rain.

814
Lure snails and slugs with beer

Snails and slugs are attracted to traps of stale beer. Bury a shallow pan so the top is level with the soil and fill it halfway with beer. Place pans where you have seen evidence of snail and slug activity. In attempting to drink the beer, the pests fall in and drown.

815
Copper barriers

Copper strips, available at garden centers, make an effective slug and snail barrier. Slugs and snails generally will not cross copper; they receive a mild electric shock when their slimy bodies touch the metal. To protect garden beds, bury a 4in (10cm) wide strip of copper one inch into the ground, and bend the top half inch (12mm) of the metal outward to create a lip.

816
Remove cabbage loopers

These small green inchworms love cabbage family plants, but also eat large holes in the leaves of lettuce, spinach, tomatoes, and peas. They are easy to spot and can be picked off by hand. Garlic spray (*see No. 799*) also deters them. Crops can be treated with *Bacillus thuringiensis* (BT), a naturally occurring bacteria which kills caterpillars and is not toxic to humans or other mammals. Use BT specifically on plants that are infested with pest caterpillars to avoid killing the larvae of other butterflies.

817
Cover plants with fabric

To protect your plants from pests, cover them with sheer fabrics, such as cheesecloth or nylon mesh, tacked onto simple bamboo or wood frames. Buy special lightweight floating row covers at garden centers, which allow your plants plenty of sun but protect them from insect damage.

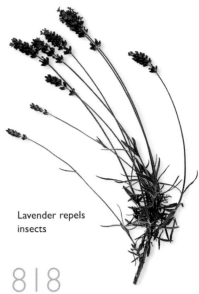

Lavender repels insects

818
Natural insect repellent

Citronella, lavender, and eucalyptus oils help keep mosquitoes and other biting insects at bay without the toxic side effects of chemical repellents.

1¹/₂ teaspoons citronella essential oil
1¹/₂ teaspoons lavender essential oil
³/₄ teaspoon eucalyptus essential oil
1 teaspoon jojoba oil
8fl oz (250ml) distilled witch hazel

Mix the essential oils and jojoba oil in a glass spray bottle. Shake well. Add the witch hazel and shake again. Spray on your body and clothing, avoiding your eyes and mucous membranes.

819
Thwart cutworms

Cutworms are rarely seen in daylight hours, but at night, these fat gray or brown caterpillars cause serious damage in the vegetable garden. They devour small seedlings and transplants, and sever young plant stems at soil level. Protecting plants from cutworms is the most effective approach. Save cardboard rolls from paper towels and toilet paper; cut to 6in (15cm) high, and place around the plant to create a physical barrier, sinking the tube one inch (25mm) below the soil level.

820
Enlist birds to eliminate cutworms

Birds love cutworm larvae and, if given a chance, will quickly eliminate a significant number of the pests from your garden. To expose the larvae, dig over your soil several times over a period of a couple of days before planting—you'll find that birds will quickly descend on your garden for a cutworm feast.

821
Trap wireworms

Wireworms are the larvae of click beetles; they burrow into root vegetables such as carrots and potatoes as well as flower bulbs. To trap them, cut chunks of potatoes and thread one or two pieces onto a bamboo skewer. Bury the chunks near root vegetable crops, using the skewer as a marker. Check the traps after a couple of days and dispose of the larvae infested potatoes.

822
Eradicate root-knot nematodes

These nematodes are microscopic soil-dwelling worms that infest the roots of many garden vegetables, especially lettuce, tomatoes, and carrots. Nematodes weaken plants and cause wilting, pale or yellowed leaves, and stunted flowers and fruit. If you pull up a plant, the root will be swollen and knotted. To treat a nematode infestation, remove the plants from the bed and plant a thick cover crop of strongly scented marigolds. Turn the marigolds into the bed in the fall.

823
Get rid of earwigs with oil and molasses

Earwigs are small brown insects with telltale pincers protruding from their backsides. They like to feed on soft plants such as lettuces and flowers. They hide during the day and come out at night to feed. To make a trap for earwigs, fill an unwashed 6oz (175g) tuna can with half an inch (12mm) of vegetable oil and half a teaspoon of molasses. Place several cans of this mixture around your garden near susceptible plants. Replace weekly or as needed.

824
Foil earwigs with newspaper traps

Earwigs search out dark, moist spots during the hours of daylight. Rolled-up newspapers secured with a rubber band and moistened with water provide just the kind of place they like to hide. Place a few of these newspaper traps around your garden; in the morning dispose of the pests.

Preventing Plant Diseases

Keeping diseases from gaining a foothold is an important part of making sure your garden remains healthy. Keep a close eye on your garden and take immediate action at the first sign of disease. To prevent problems, choose disease-resistant varieties of plants whenever possible.

825
The correct way to water plants

To discourage fungal diseases such as powdery mildew, water the plants in your garden early in the day so that the foliage is completely dry by nightfall. The best time to water is in the early morning. Avoid watering during the heat of the day because plants can easily be scorched when the water droplets on the leaves magnify the sun's rays.

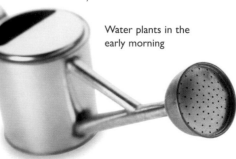

Water plants in the early morning

826
Tips for healthy plants

Keep your soil healthy and nourished by adding compost and other organic nutrients during the year. Provide plants with sufficient water to keep them strong, feeding them as needed with organic fertilizers. Keep your garden clean; regularly pick up leaves, fruits, and berries from the ground.

827
Enlist the sun to kill soilborne pests

If you are struggling with soilborne, disease-causing, or tenacious pests such as nematodes, try solarizing your soil. This raises soil temperature high enough to eradicate diseases and pests. Because it also kills beneficial insects and soil organisms, solarization should only be used as a last resort. To solarize soil, remove all plants and weeds, cultivate the soil, rake it smooth, and thoroughly water it. Dig a trench 6in (15cm) deep around the perimeter of the bed and stretch a sheet of medium-weight plastic over the bed, pressing it down so that it touches the soil. Tuck the plastic into the trench, fill it with soil, and leave the plastic in place for two months. When you remove it, add compost to help restore the beneficial microorganisms to the soil.

828
Treat powdery mildew

Powdery mildew looks like a white or gray coating on foliage. It spreads quickly and causes leaves to shrivel, and deforms new growth. This fungus affects many vegetables and flowering plants, and is most troublesome in the fall. Wash the leaves weekly to keep the spores from germinating or spreading, then spray on this formula.

1 teaspoon light vegetable oil
10 drops tea tree essential oil
1 teaspoon baking soda
1 gallon (5 liters) water

Mix the oils together and add to the baking soda and water. Shake well, and spray liberally onto affected plants once a week.

829
Prevent blossom end rot

Tomatoes, peppers, cucumbers, squashes, and melons can all suffer from blossom end rot, a disease that causes a dark, sunken area at the blossom end, which enlarges and can cover up to half the fruit. It's often caused by a calcium deficiency or by uneven watering. To prevent blossom end rot, add composted manure or bone meal to supply calcium when preparing garden beds prior to planting. Make sure that plants are getting approximately one inch (25mm) of water per week from either rain or irrigation, and mulch plants to keep the soil moist.

830
Prevent damping-off

Damping-off is caused by soilborne fungi that make seedling stems rot and collapse at the soil level. The fungi can also decay seeds before they sprout. To prevent this, avoid planting seeds too deep and keep the soil moist, but not soggy. Make sure plants have good air circulation if you're planting them indoors. Planting in a sterilized planting mix eliminates the possibility of fungi in the soil. If you are re-using containers that have been previously used to grow plants, clean them thoroughly to destroy damping-off fungi. Wash them in hot soapy water, rinse well, and let them dry in the sun for a couple of days.

831
Prevent black spot

Black spot is a common fungal disease that affects many roses. The disease appears as round black spots surrounded by yellow rings on the leaves; it can seriously weaken plants. To prevent black spot, avoid overhead watering and apply fresh mulch each spring. To treat it, remove and dispose of infected leaves and spray with the following formula.

1 tablespoon baking soda
1 teaspoon natural liquid dishwashing soap
1 gallon (5 liters) lukewarm water

Mix the ingredients together in a pump-type garden sprayer and spray on your plants once a week.

832
Epsom salts boost

To improve calcium uptake and prevent diseases such as blossom end rot, add two tablespoons of Epsom salts to the hole in which you are planting tomatoes, peppers, cucumbers, squashes, or melons.

Lawns, Weeds, & Blooms

Organic gardening techniques work just as well for lawns and flower gardens as they do for vegetable gardens. There's no need for toxic chemicals and synthetic fertilizers when you follow the principles of healthy gardening.

833
Feeding your lawn

Once every year in the fall, feed your lawn by spreading a quarter to half an inch (6–12mm) of compost over the grass or use an organic fertilizer specifically for lawns. Do not overfeed your lawn—excessive fertilizer makes the grass grow too fast and makes it more susceptible to disease.

834
Mowing your lawn

Mow your lawn often, and leave grass at least 2in (5cm) high to help it develop strong roots. To reduce the lawn's need for fertilizer, allow grass clippings to remain after mowing to provide nutrients as they decompose.

835
Watering your lawn

Frequent watering of a lawn causes the grass to develop a shallow root system. Instead, water thoroughly once a week, or twice if really necessary. To calculate how much water you have given your lawn, place a straight-sided glass jar near a sprinkler. When one inch (25mm) has collected, it's time to move the sprinkler to another area.

836
Combat pet urine

If you catch a dog or cat urinating on your lawn, soak the area with water at once to prevent the grass from scorching and turning brown.

837
Natural weed control

Weeds are easy to restrain without chemical herbicides if you establish a consistent weed-prevention and control program. To prevent weeds from gaining a foothold, don't leave patches of bare ground available. Mulch garden beds heavily, and scatter grass seed on thin spots in your lawn as soon as they appear. Mow your lawn often, but do not cut it too short. Leaving grass 2–3in (5–7cm) tall promotes stronger growth and helps crowd out weeds. Mowing frequently also cuts down on weeds by removing the flowering heads that spread seeds.

838
Weeding in drought

When soil is extremely dry, don't pull weeds as it disturbs the soil and causes additional moisture loss. Instead, remove weeds at the surface of the soil with an oscillating hoe.

839
Eat your weeds

Many common weeds, such as lamb's quarter, dandelion, and purslane, add taste and health to spring salads. Use tender leaves, not the roots.

840
Tulip and daffodil care

Cut tulip and daffodil flower stalks to the ground after they bloom. But let the leaves remain for at least eight weeks to help the bulbs generate energy for next year's spring flowers. For neatness, bundle the leaves together and secure them with a rubber band to keep them tidy.

841
Everblooming biennials

Biennial plants, such as foxglove, forget-me-nots, and clary sage, bloom only in the second year of their life cycles and then die. They are excellent self-sowers, though, and a new crop of plants will appear each spring. To create a yearly show of blooms, plant biennials two years in a row, and allow a few flowers to go to seed each year. Shake the dried flower heads over the area where you want new plants to grow before removing the dead plants.

842
Stimulate flower bloom

To keep your annuals blooming for as long as possible, regularly remove withered blossoms to keep the plant from going to seed and to stimulate reblooming. To encourage the growth of full, bushy plants, pinch off the tips of new growth with your fingers.

843
Rejuvenate perennials

Most perennials need to be divided every few years to prune out weak or dead sections and rejuvenate the plant. The best time to do this is on a cool day in the spring or fall, when it is least traumatic for the plant. Dig up the plant, including as much root as possible. Divide it with a sharp spade by cutting through the center of the root mass; divide again into the size of plants you want. Throw away unhealthy or damaged parts. Replant the divided sections immediately.

844
Keep roses blooming

Remove spent flowers regularly before they create a seed pod. This encourages a rose to produce more flowers instead of putting energy into making seeds. To stimulate the best blooms, remove the flower by cutting the stem at an angle just above the third set of leaves.

845
Boost rose blooms and color with Epsom salts

The magnesium in Epsom salts helps roses absorb nutrients more readily, stimulating more blooms and better color. Sprinkle a teaspoon per 12in (30cm) of plant height and scratch into the soil in the spring. Repeat after the roses have bloomed.

Houseplant Care

Houseplants come from various habitats of the world. Some find it easy to adapt to indoor environments, but others need special care to cope with less than optimal conditions, such as excessive heat, poor light, and lack of humidity.

846
Watering houseplants

The water needs of your houseplants depend on their species and will vary according to the indoor environment in your home, especially its room temperature, humidity, and light exposure. As a general rule, water houseplants when their soil dries out and not according to a schedule. Soak thoroughly, and let the soil dry out between waterings.

847
Use lukewarm water

Always water your houseplants with lukewarm water as cold water can shock the plant and damage the roots.

Grass-type houseplant

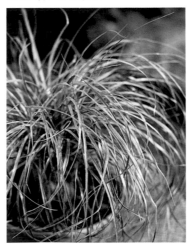

848
Mist plants for health

Most homes are very dry because of air conditioning and heating. If the tips of your houseplants turn brown, it's a sure sign that the plant needs more humidity. To keep houseplants healthy, mist them at least a couple of times a week using a plant mister.

849
High-nutrient plant spray

Comfrey tea provides beneficial minerals and encourages growth.

2 cups (500ml) boiling water
2 tablespoons dried comfrey leaf

Pour the water over the comfrey, cool to room temperature, and strain. Spray plants liberally once a week. Comfrey tea can stain so avoid contact with fabrics. Refrigerate leftover tea for up to one week.

850
Sugar water for longer-lasting flowers

Cut flowers last longer if you feed them with lukewarm sugar water. Dissolve one teaspoon of sugar in two cups (500ml) of water. Change the water in the vase every couple of days.

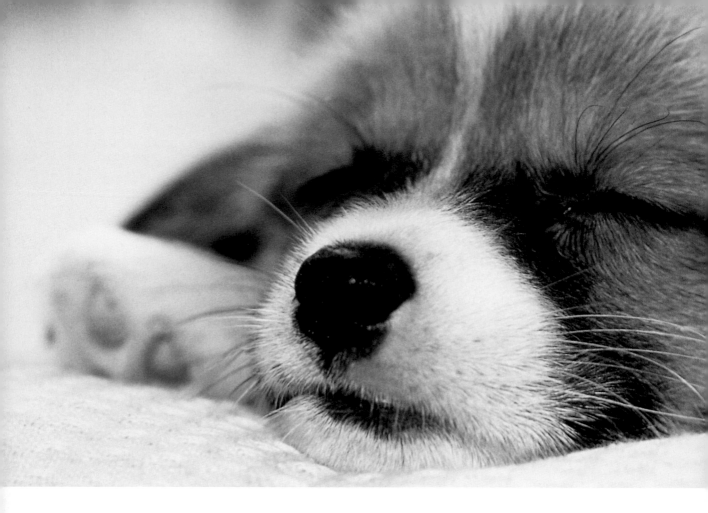

NATURAL
PET CARE

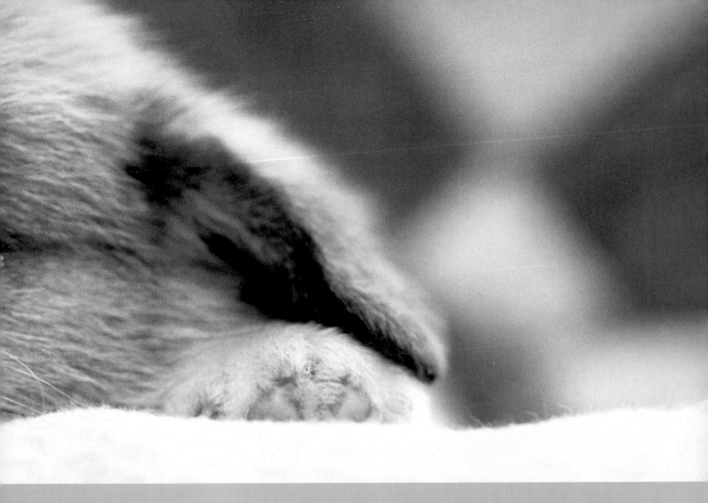

For many of us, our pets are valued family members. They provide companionship, joy, and unconditional love, and, in return, they depend on us for a well-balanced diet, a safe and comfortable home, opportunities for play and exercise, and regular veterinary care. Moreover, they instinctively create pleasure in their lives and can be wonderful teachers for us; both cats and dogs spend most of their time each day playing and relaxing.

Natural remedies are often a safe and easy way to treat many minor health problems that your pet may encounter. Herbs, vitamins, aromatherapy, homeopathy, and hydrotherapy are just as effective for your pet as they are for humans, and are much safer than many pharmaceutical drugs. But not every remedy that is appropriate for humans is appropriate for a pet. When in doubt, always check with a vet or an herbalist.

In the first part of this chapter, you will find suggestions for creating a healthful lifestyle for your dog or cat. In the second part, Caring for Your Sick Pet, you will find remedies for treating common health problems that affect both dogs and cats. Many individual remedies provide special instructions for treating dogs and cats. Check with your vet for any symptoms that do not resolve within a couple of days of home care, such as prolonged vomiting or diarrhea.

Your Dog's Healthy Home

Dogs need a space to call their own, and most have definite preferences about that space. Some like to be outside, others prefer to be indoors, some like soft bedding, and others would rather sleep on a cool kitchen floor or on the grass. Paying attention to your dog's habits will make life easier for both you and your pet. Wherever your dog is most comfortable, make sure that it is a healthy and safe place.

851
A comfortable dog bed

Most dogs like a soft, comfortable bed for sleeping. A soft padded dog bed with a washable cotton or flannel cover or blanket is a good choice. Avoid wicker dog beds—many dogs find them irresistible for chewing and the splinters can be dangerous if they are swallowed. Regularly wash the bedding in a mild, unscented natural laundry detergent and rinse well to prevent skin irritation.

852
Prevent heat exhaustion

In hot weather, make sure that your dog has a covered shelter such as a porch or doghouse that provides respite from the sun. In addition, always make sure that your dog has plenty of fresh, cool water available both outdoors and indoors.

853
Avoid exposure to toxic materials

Make sure that your dog has a safe environment by checking your home, garage, and yard for such harmful substances as household and garden chemicals, insecticides, paints, and solvents. Avoid using toxic chemical fertilizers and pesticides on your lawn or garden. Instead, choose from one of the many natural nonchemical alternatives, which are available at most garden centers. Be especially careful to clean up antifreeze spills, which dogs will drink if they find it.

Caution: Antifreeze is toxic and causes severe kidney damage; if you suspect that your dog has been drinking antifreeze, seek immediate veterinary attention.

854
Avoid self-feeders

Self-feeders are a convenient device for pet owners, but there are a few significant health drawbacks to their use. First, bacteria can quickly contaminate food (often within a matter of hours). Second, roaches, flies, and other vermin can infest the food. Finally, many dogs will overfeed themselves and become overweight. It's better when possible to feed your pet a rationed amount of fresh food once or twice daily.

Your Dog's Healthy Diet

A dog's health is directly related to what it eats, and it is dependent on you to provide it with optimal nutrition. Signs of a nutrient-deficient diet include a dull coat, dry or itchy skin, gas, low energy, unpleasant body odor, diarrhea, vomiting, and behavioral problems. Changing to a health-supportive diet usually yields positive results within a few weeks.

855
What to feed your dog

Many commercial dog foods are of poor quality and will not support optimal health for your pet. The best pet foods are those made from high-quality meat products. Do not use soy-based foods as these are difficult for a dog's digestive system to process. Avoid any brands that contain preservatives, chemical additives, and artificial flavors and colorings. Canned foods are the favorite of most dogs and are high in necessary dietary fats. Dry food offers more concentrated protein and helps keep teeth clean and healthy. The best option for feeding your dog may be to mix canned and dry food in equal proportions, and to supplement this with other healthful foods such as vegetables, eggs, and cottage cheese.

856
Healthful treats for dogs

Give your dog various treats such as beef jerky, lean meat, raw knuckle bones, cheese, cottage cheese, vegetables, dried and fresh fruit, whole grain dog biscuits, and yogurt.

857
Supplement your dog's diet with raw foods

A diet of canned or dry food, no matter how high the quality, is not sufficient for optimal health for your pet. Dogs need fresh, raw food daily to provide the nutrients and enzymes not found in processed foods. Some of the nutritious raw foods that dogs enjoy include carrots, apples, dark green lettuces, and broccoli. Grate or chop these and add a couple of tablespoons per 10lb (4.5kg) of body weight to your dog's regular food. Start with small amounts to give your dog's digestive system time to adjust since too much raw food can cause diarrhea.

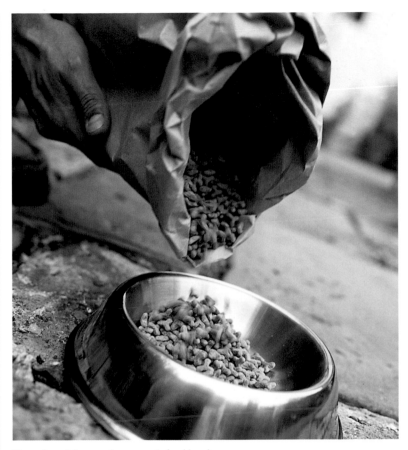

Use only stainless steel or ceramic food bowls

858
Add a bit of raw meat

Adding a bit of raw meat to your dog's diet helps approximate the natural diet of its ancestors. Most dogs love a bit of raw beef or organ meat a couple of times a week. Choose organic meat to avoid the hormones and other chemicals found in conventionally produced meats. Start with small amounts to avoid digestive upsets and to give the dog's system time to adjust. In general, feed your dog approximately 2oz (60g) of raw meat per 10lb (4.5kg) of body weight per meal.

859
Establish a regular feeding schedule

Your dog will be healthiest if you feed him regular meals—twice daily, once in the morning and again in the early evening. Serve the food at room temperature instead of straight out of the refrigerator—it will be more appealing to your dog, and easier on the digestive system. Stainless steel or ceramic bowls are best for food and water; avoid plastics, because they can leach toxic plastic molecules into food and water.

860
Raw eggs for a lustrous coat

Raw eggs are rich in protein and minerals that create a thick, healthy coat. Add the yolk of one raw egg to your dog's food ration every day if desired. However, do not feed your dog raw egg whites more than once a week because raw egg whites eaten too frequently can interfere with protein balance.

861
Garlic for immune health

Dogs benefit from eating raw fresh garlic daily because it fights harmful bacteria, viruses, and parasites and strengthens the cardiovascular and immune systems. Add a quarter of a clove of finely minced garlic per 10lb (4.5kg) of body weight to your dog's daily food. **Caution:** Speak to your vet before feeding garlic to your dog as it may cause health problems in some dogs.

862
Yogurt for digestion

Adding a small amount of plain natural yogurt to your dog's daily diet will help keep the digestive system functioning optimally. Natural yogurt contains beneficial bacteria, such as *Lactobacillus acidophilus*, which maintain a healthy environment in your dog's intestinal tract. Choose yogurt that is labeled as containing live microorganisms, and add one tablespoon per 10lb (4.5kg) of body weight to your dog's food each day.

863
Fiber for digestion

Adding a small amount of fiber in the form of wheat bran to your dog's diet every day will help keep the digestive system functioning optimally. Wheat bran acts like a natural broom, cleaning the intestinal tract and helping prevent constipation. Add a quarter of a teaspoon of wheat bran for each 10lb (4.5kg) of body weight to your dog's food once every day.

864
Cooking meals for your dog

To prepare homemade food for your dog, base the meal on cooked whole grains, such as oatmeal, brown rice, millet, or bulgur wheat. Feed about three-quarters of a cup (130g) of grain for a 10lb (4.5kg) dog. Add the following ingredients to the grain: a third of a cup (75g) of protein in the form of cooked chicken, turkey, or beef; two tablespoons of fresh, raw, grated vegetables; half a teaspoon of extra-virgin olive oil; a quarter of a clove of raw garlic; a tablespoon of yogurt; and a powdered supplement of both vitamins and minerals. Adjust the proportions of these additional ingredients according to your dog's weight, metabolism, and activity level.

Caution: Speak to your vet before feeding garlic to your dog as it may cause health problems in some dogs.

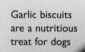

Garlic biscuits are a nutritious treat for dogs

865
Garlic biscuits

Dogs like the flavor of garlic, and these biscuits provide a nutritious homemade treat.

2 cups (260g) whole wheat flour
2/3 cup (115g) stone-ground cornmeal
1/2 cup (100g) sesame seeds
3 eggs
1/4 cup (60ml) milk
1/2 cup (125ml) chicken broth
2 tablespoons olive oil
2 cloves minced garlic
(**To make, see below right**)

Caution: Speak to your vet before feeding garlic to your dog as it may cause health problems in some dogs.

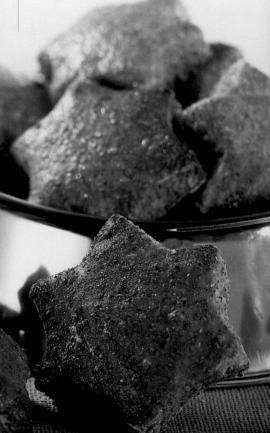

866
Raw bone treats

A juicy raw meat bone is a treat for most dogs. But buy only large bones: round knuckle bones, which your dogs can safely chew onto their hearts' content, are best. Smaller bones can be dangerous because your dog may attempt to swallow them. Never feed your dog cooked bones of any variety: they can splinter and pierce the throat or intestines.

867
Nutritional supplement formula

For optimal health, feed your dog a nutritional supplement made from a combination of concentrated whole foods. Nutritional yeast is a good source of B-complex vitamins and wheat germ is rich in vitamin E. Barley grass is an excellent source of chlorophyll, which helps in the detox process, and kelp is rich in both iron and minerals.

1 cup (120g) nutritional yeast
¼ cup (30g) raw wheat germ
2 tablespoons powdered green barley grass
2 tablespoons powdered dried kelp

Mix the ingredients together and add half a teaspoon per 10lb (4.5kg) of body weight to your dog's daily food ration.

868
Other special treats for your dog

Dogs love treats. If chosen carefully, they can be healthful additions to the daily diet. Many commercial treats are loaded with harmful fats, sugars, and chemicals, but dogs just as readily like hard biscuits, small bits of meat, and

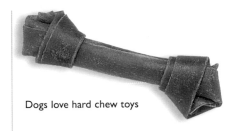

Dogs love hard chew toys

even fruits and vegetables. Give small amounts of treat foods to avoid upsetting your dog's digestive tract, and don't allow treats to take the place of regular balanced meals.

869
Give your dog plenty of water

Make sure you provide your dog with plenty of fresh water at all times to prevent dehydration. Keep a bowl filled both indoors and out, and make water available throughout the day, not just at mealtimes.

MAKING GARLIC BISCUITS FOR YOUR DOG

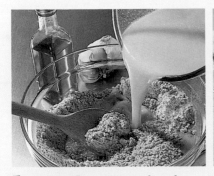

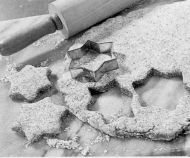

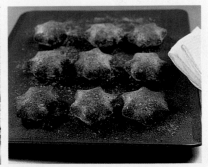

1 Mix the flour, cornmeal, and sesame seeds in a large bowl. Beat two eggs with the milk and add the chicken broth, olive oil, and garlic. Stir the wet ingredients into the dry and mix well into a firm dough. Leave for 15 minutes.

2 Place the dough on a lightly floured surface. Roll out the dough to a thickness of a quarter of an inch (6mm) and cut it into whatever shapes you want. Beat the remaining egg and brush the biscuits with the egg.

3 Place the biscuits onto a lightly greased cookie sheet and bake them in a 350°F (180°C) oven for 25 to 35 minutes, or until they turn a golden color. Remove the biscuits from the baking sheet and then leave them to cool.

The Importance of Exercise

Daily exercise prevents obesity, strengthens the cardiovascular system, encourages healthy digestion, and keeps muscles and bones strong. A daily walk is a wonderful opportunity to exercise with your dog and share companionship.

870
Exercising tips

Most dogs love to go for a walk. Be aware of their need for water, and don't let them become overheated. Look for signs of overexertion: heavy panting, fatigue, and an awkward gait are signs that your dog needs to slow down and rest. If the exercise is more energetic, such as running beside you, ask your vet to make sure it won't be harmful; some breeds suffer problems that stressful exercise makes worse.

871
Preventing injuries

After walking or running with your dog, check its feet for pebbles, bits of glass, or other debris that may be embedded in its footpads. In addition, inspect the footpads for cuts; if you find any, wash them with lukewarm soapy water and rinse with an herbal antiseptic made by combining equal parts of water and echinacea extract. Then apply calendula gel to speed healing.

873
Protect the ears

When bathing your dog, gently place a cotton ball into each ear opening to prevent water from entering the ear canal. Water in the ear is not only uncomfortable but can also lead to ear infections.

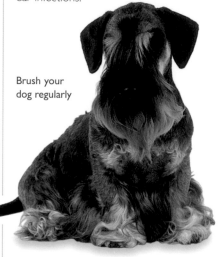

Brush your dog regularly

Grooming Your Dog

Dogs have different grooming requirements, depending on the length and thickness of their hair and whether they are indoor or outdoor dogs. Many grooming tasks such as bathing, brushing, and cleaning ears and eyes are easy to perform at home and will keep your pet healthy and looking its best.

872
Bathing your dog

Many dogs resist baths, even those that love to play in water. How often you bathe your dog depends on how dirty it gets and how strong its natural odor is. At most, bathe your dog once a week. More frequent bathing removes protective oils from the coat and can cause dryness and irritation of the skin. Before giving your dog a bath, brush its coat thoroughly to untangle any knots in the hair. To make bathtime less traumatic for your dog, use lukewarm water and a mild castile shampoo diluted half with water. Be gentle and give your dog a lot of praise while bathing it. To prevent chills and stress, thoroughly dry your dog after the bath, either by rubbing it briskly with a towel or by using a blow-dryer set on warm.

874
Brushing your dog

Dogs with long hair need to be groomed daily to prevent tangling and knots, but all dogs benefit from frequent brushing. Brushing helps clean and condition the dog's skin and coat and removes shedding hair. Choose your grooming tools according to the amount and type of hair your dog has. Thick hair requires a wide-toothed comb; fine hair needs a comb with closely spaced teeth. To prevent scratching your dog's skin, make sure the comb has rounded teeth. Comb the coat thoroughly to remove tangles and loose hair, and then finish by brushing to distribute oils throughout the coat.

875
Removing tar, paint, and other substances

Sticky substances such as tar, paint, glue, and gum are difficult to remove from the hairs on a dog's coat. Do not use solvents such as turpentine on your dog as they can burn its skin and are toxic if ingested. Rub petroleum jelly into tar to help dissolve it; ice will help harden gum and makes it easier to remove. In general, most sticky substances will need to be trimmed out of the hair.

876
Cleaning your dog's ears

Cleaning your dog's ears should be part of its regular grooming routine. Once a month, clean the exterior ear opening and the outer folds of the inner ear with a cotton swab dipped in pure vegetable oil. Gently remove excess wax, but be careful to not push wax into the ear canal. Most dogs will learn to tolerate this if you are patient, gentle, and persistent. Some dogs, especially those with long, floppy ears, have excessive hair in the ears. Have a groomer trim this hair to prevent infection.

877
Removing tear stains

Some dogs are prone to dark tear stains on the facial hair at the inner corners of the eyes. Remove them with a solution of hydrogen peroxide.

1 teaspoon hydrogen peroxide

3 tablespoons water

Mix the hydrogen peroxide with the water. Dip a cotton swab into the mixture and gently swab the stained hair until the stain is removed. **Caution:** Take extra care to prevent the peroxide solution from getting in your dog's eyes.

878
Trimming the nails

If your dog regularly walks outdoors on hard surfaces, its nails probably need to be trimmed only rarely. But dogs that spend most of their time indoors or running around on grassy backyards require regular nail trimming to prevent injury—long nails can snag on carpeting or hinder the way a dog walks. To make the job easier, buy a pair of special nail clippers at a pet store. Make sure when you trim the nails to make the cut where the nail curves downward, just below the pink area of the nail to avoid cutting into the blood vessels. Most dogs balk at toenail trimming— you will have the best results if you train your dog as a puppy to be calm while its nails are trimmed. If you find nail trimming difficult, have a groomer do it for you.

879
Cleaning your dog's teeth

Keeping your dog's teeth clean will help alleviate bad breath and protect your dog's health. Just like humans, dogs can suffer from tooth decay and periodontal disease. Some dogs do not mind having their teeth cleaned, especially if they have been trained

from puppyhood. Gently scrub your pet's teeth with a clean cloth or a dog toothbrush and water at least once a week. If your dog resists, have its teeth checked and cleaned by your vet.

880
Baking soda toothpaste

To whiten and clean your dog's teeth, mix up a paste of baking soda and water and use a small amount as a toothpaste. Baking soda polishes the teeth and helps neutralize bad breath. Avoid human toothpaste— dogs don't like the taste.

881
A daily biscuit

To keep your dog's teeth and gums strong and healthy, give it hard dog biscuits daily. The rough surfaces scrape plaque off of the teeth and help keep teeth sharp.

Dog biscuits

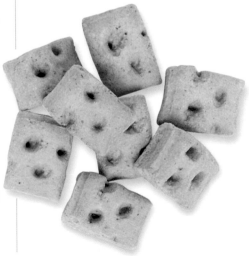

Your Cat's Healthy Home

Cats are naturally curious and independent creatures, which is part of their appeal. Most cats have a mind of their own, and prefer to choose where to sleep, when and what to eat, and when they want to socialize. Regardless of how independent your cat is, though, it still depends on you to provide it with a healthy and safe home.

882
Adjusting to a new home

To help your cat or kitten adjust to a new home, make the space as reassuring as you can by leaving a light on and playing soothing music in the room where your cat will be sleeping. Let your pet adjust to its surroundings at its own pace; it may hide or eat very little while it is getting comfortable with its new home, but will usually become an active member of the family within a couple of days. Remove breakable objects and keep electrical cords out of reach until your new cat or kitten is well-trained.

883
A cozy cat bed

Although your cat will undoubtably select its own favorite places to curl up and nap, it will also appreciate having its own bed. Cats love soft, warm, and comfortable places. A washable pillow and cozy cotton blanket are good choices. Wash the bedding every couple of weeks in a mild, natural laundry detergent (available at natural food stores) and rinse well to prevent skin irritation.

884
Provide a scratching post

Scratching objects is a normal and necessary behavior for your cat because it helps strengthen muscles, and sharpen and trim the claws. To save wear and tear on your furniture and to prevent unnecessary tension between you and your pet, provide your cat with a scratching post. The best type is a tall, upright post with a coarse, rough covering. To encourage your cat to make use of the scratching post, sprinkle some catnip on it.

885
Avoiding exposure to toxic materials

Follow the advice for dogs (see No. 853). In addition, if your home or yard contain poisonous plants, such as philodendron, dieffenbachia, and Easter lily, which could harm your cat if ingested, then remove them.

Your Cat's Healthy Diet

Your cat's health is directly related to what it eats, and it is dependent on you to provide it with optimal nutrition. Signs of a nutrient-deficient diet include a dull coat, dry or itchy skin, gas, low energy, unpleasant body odor, diarrhea, vomiting, and behavioral problems. Changing to a health-supportive diet usually yields positive results within a few weeks.

886
What to feed your cat

Cats are notoriously finicky eaters. To keep your cat happy and healthy, provide it with a varied diet of nutritious foods and treats. Add a tablespoon of dry food to some high-quality canned food, and supplement with table scraps and healthful whole foods. Avoid brands containing meat by-products, chemical additives, preservatives, and artificial flavors and colorings.

887
Tasty leftovers and table scraps

Most cats love to eat table scraps. A teaspoonful or two of appropriate leftovers (see No. 888) will provide interesting variety as well as a tasty and beneficial addition to your pet's meals. High-protein foods, such as fish, meat, eggs, and cheese, are good choices. So, too, are cooked or steamed vegetables such as corn, yams, and broccoli.

888
Healthful treats for cats

Give your cat various treats such as baked yams or winter squash, cheese, cooked corn, cooked chicken liver, raw vertebrae bones, sardines, soft-boiled egg, nutritional yeast tablets, steamed vegetables, and yogurt.

889
Dangerous bones

Never feed your cat cooked poultry bones, which can splinter and damage the intestinal tract. Poultry neck vertebrae are an exception, because they crumble instead of splintering.

890
Feed regularly

Your cat will be healthiest if you feed it twice daily, in the morning and in the evening. Avoid self-feeders if you can (see No. 854). Leave food for 30 minutes and then remove it. Serve it at room temperature, not out of the refrigerator. Ceramic or heavy stainless steel bowls are best for food and water; avoid plastics, because they can leach toxic plastic molecules into food and water.

891
Raw food supplement

Cats need a certain amount of raw fresh food each day to provide the nutrients and enzymes not found in processed foods. Some of the raw food cats enjoy include beef, fish, poultry, egg yolks, and finely grated carrots and zucchini. Start with half a teaspoon of raw food mixed in with canned food to give your cat time to adjust to a new, healthier diet. You can also give a nutritional supplement (see No. 867): mix into the food half a teaspoon per 10lbs (4.5kgs) body weight once daily.

892
Raw eggs for a lustrous coat

Raw eggs are rich in protein and minerals that create a thick, healthy coat. Add a raw egg yolk to your cat's food ration several times a week if desired. Do not feed your cat raw egg whites, however, because they can interfere with protein balance and create a nutrient deficiency.

893
Fiber for a healthy digestion

Adding a small amount of fiber in the form of wheat bran to your cat's daily diet will help keep the digestive system functioning optimally. Wheat bran acts as a natural broom for the intestinal tract and helps prevent constipation. Add half a teaspoon of bran to your cat's food once daily.

894
Cooking for your cat

If you want to prepare homemade food for your cat, base the meal on proteins such as raw ground beef, raw chicken, raw egg yolks, and cooked poultry or beef. About 60 percent of the meal should be protein, with the remaining 40 percent divided equally between cooked grains and vegetables. Appropriate grains include brown rice, millet, oats, and sweet corn; healthful vegetables include steamed broccoli, dark leafy greens, carrots, baked sweet potatoes, and winter squash. Supplement the diet with a natural powdered vitamin and mineral supplement for cats to ensure your pet gets all the nutrients it needs for optimal health.

895
Yeast treat

Offer your cat a couple of nutritional yeast tablets as a crunchy between-meal treat. Nutritional yeast is rich in B-complex vitamins, and most cats love the flavor.

Sardines

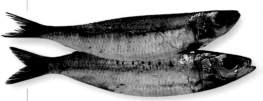

896
Special treats

Cats adore special treats. Use them in moderation to reward desired behavior. Commercial cat foods are loaded with sugars, salt, and artificial flavors to which many cats become addicted. Wean your cat to a more healthful natural diet by adding small amounts of treats to its diet. These include sardines, cooked chicken livers, and jarred natural baby foods.

The Importance of Play

Cats need to play for both their emotional and physical well-being. Daily play offers them an outlet for energy that can otherwise be destructive. In addition, a good session of active play is a great opportunity for healthful exercise.

897
Toys for your cat

Cats naturally love to play, and will try to get you involved by batting at your feet or ambushing you as you enter a room. Toys such as a catnip mouse or a ball with a ribbon will encourage a playful nature and stop teeth and claws from injuring you.

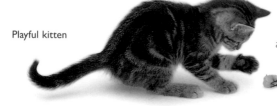

Playful kitten

898
Prevent injuries

String or yarn can be swallowed and cause strangulation or life-threatening intestinal obstruction. Instead, use a scarf or a wide piece of ribbon for playtime. Avoid buying toys that can easily fall apart, or those with glued-on parts. Safe, inexpensive toys include brown paper bags, ping-pong balls, and cardboard tubes from toilet paper rolls.

Grooming Your Cat

Cats spend a great deal of time grooming themselves, but they also benefit from regular grooming by their owners. Cats have different grooming requirements, depending on the length and thickness of their coat. Many grooming tasks such as brushing, and cleaning ears and eyes are easy to perform at home and will keep your pet healthy and looking its best.

899
Bathing your cat

Cats generally dislike baths, and most will rarely, if ever, need to be bathed. However, your pet may need a bath if it becomes very dirty or is infested with parasites. To make bathtime less traumatic, use lukewarm water and a mild castile shampoo diluted half with warm water. Be gentle and give it praise and encouragement. Do not spray it with water, submerge its head in water, or get water into its eyes. To prevent chills and stress, thoroughly dry your cat by patting it with a towel. Keep it in a warm room until it is completely dry, then brush its coat to redistribute the natural protective oils through its fur.

900
Prevent tangled hair

Always groom your cat thoroughly before bathing it. This prevents tangled hair from forming into matted knots that can be difficult to remove.

901
Brushing and combing

Cats with long hair need grooming at least once a week to prevent tangling and knots, but all cats benefit from frequent brushing. Grooming helps clean and condition the cat's skin and coat and removes shedding hair. Choose your grooming tools according to the amount and type of hair your cat has. Thick hair requires a wide-toothed comb, fine hair needs a comb with more closely spaced teeth, and a short-haired cat needs a slicker brush. To prevent scratching your cat's skin, make sure the teeth of the comb have rounded ends. Untangle knots carefully with your fingers; if this is not possible, carefully cut the knots out or take your cat to a professional groomer to have the knots removed.

902
Removing the shampoo

An after-bath rinse of apple cider vinegar and warm water removes all traces of shampoo from your cat's coat and helps balance the natural acidity of the skin. Mix one tablespoon of apple cider vinegar in two cups (500ml) of lukewarm water and pour over your cat's fur. Rinse well with warm water.

903
Give the coat a shine

An after-bath rinse of rosemary and lavender makes your cat's coat shiny and sweet smelling. Pour one cup (250ml) of boiling water over one teaspoon each of dried rosemary and lavender; cover and steep until cool. Strain and dilute with an equal amount of lukewarm water.

904
Removing tar, paint, and other substances

Sticky substances such as tar, paint, glue, and gum are difficult to remove from a cat's fur. Do not use solvents such as turpentine on your cat because they can burn its skin and are toxic if ingested. Rub petroleum jelly into tar to help dissolve it; ice will help harden gum and make it easier to remove. In general, most sticky substances will need to be trimmed carefully out of the hair.

905
Cleaning your cat's ears

Once a week, check your cat's ears for excess ear wax or dirt. If necessary, clean the exterior ear opening and the outer folds of the inner ear with a cotton swab dipped in pure vegetable oil. Gently remove all the excess wax, but be careful to not push wax into the ear canal. Most cats will learn to tolerate this cleaning process if you are patient, gentle, and persistent.

Regularly check your cat's ears for wax

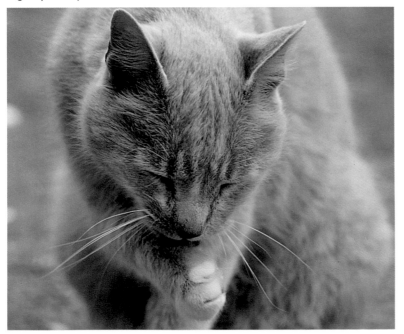

906
Cleaning your cat's eyes

Some cats, particularly Persians, are susceptible to narrowed tear ducts that cause tears to build up, leaving brown stains on the fur around the eyes. The tears should be wiped off at least twice a day with a soft tissue. Your vet may prescribe eyedrops to help with this condition, or you can make these saline eyedrops.

$1/8$ teaspoon of sea salt
$1/2$ cup (125ml) boiling water

Make a gentle saline solution by dissolving the sea salt in the boiling water. Cool and refrigerate for up to one week in a covered glass jar. Heat the solution to a comfortably warm temperature before using by placing the jar in a bowl of hot water. Place a couple of drops in the inside corner of each eye twice daily.

907
Remove dark tear stains

Dark tear stains can be removed with diluted hydrogen peroxide. Mix one teaspoon of hydrogen peroxide with three tablespoons of water. Dip a cotton swab into the mixture and gently swab the stained hair, taking care to not get the peroxide solution into the cat's eyes.

908
Strong and healthy teeth

To keep your cat's teeth and gums strong and healthy, give it a small amount of dry food daily, and provide her with the neck vertebrae from a raw chicken to gnaw on a couple of times a week.

909
Cleaning your cat's teeth

Keeping your cat's teeth clean will help alleviate bad breath and protect it from getting periodontal disease. The following solution will help.

$^1/_2$ teaspoon sea salt

$^1/_2$ teaspoon baking soda

$^1/_2$ cup (125ml) lukewarm water

Mix the ingredients into a solution and use it to wet a clean cloth. If your cat lets you, wipe its teeth and gums once a week. If it resists, ask your vet to check and clean them.

910
Remove loose hair daily

Most cats occasionally vomit up hair balls, especially during the shedding season when they swallow a lot of hair while grooming themselves. The hair balls cause problems if they become impacted in the intestinal tract, however. Symptoms of hair ball impaction include constipation or diarrhea, vomiting hair balls more than once a week, or gagging and unsuccessful attempts to purge a hair ball. To prevent hair balls and resulting constipation, groom your cat every day. Removing loose hair, especially during the spring and the fall when most cats shed heavily, prevents large amounts of hair being swallowed when your cat grooms itself.

Caring for Your Sick Pet

If your cat or dog has a minor injury or a significant illness, you can greatly speed its recovery by providing an optimal healing environment—rest, warmth, healthful food, and tender loving care. However, if you are worried at all, consult your vet.

911
A cozy sleeping place

When your pet is ill, a warm and cozy sleeping place is essential to help it get the rest it needs to recover. Make a soft bed

A cozy place

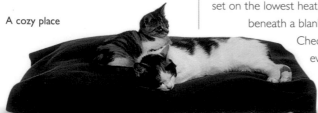

of towels or blankets that can be washed every couple of days. Choose a peaceful, warm, and well-ventilated room, and place the bed away from drafts. During cool weather or if your pet seems cold, warm the bed with a hot-water bottle or a heating pad set on the lowest heat, and place it beneath a blanket or towel. Check your pet every so often to make sure that it is not too hot.

912
A healing environment

A sick pet needs peace and quiet. Give your pet plenty of soothing words and loving attention, but also provide it with the restful quiet it needs for recovery. When you leave the house, turn a radio onto a talk show to keep your pet company. Cats that are sick are prone to depression and need extra attention. Hold it as much as possible, and gently stroke and groom it.

913
Encourage rest

When recovering from an illness or injury, your pet needs to rest as much as possible. Keep it indoors until it is fully recovered, with frequent short periods of supervised time outdoors to relieve itself.

914
Nourishing food

During an illness, your pet may lose its appetite. Nourishing foods are essential for recovering strength and vitality. Try feeding your pet smaller amounts of food several times a day, and give it easy-to-digest foods. For dogs, choose boiled chicken, boiled lamb, white rice, potatoes, and soft cooked eggs; as a special treat, try roast beef, jarred baby food meats, and cottage cheese as long as it is not suffering from digestive upset. For cats, choose boiled chicken and soft scrambled eggs; special treats to encourage it to eat include jarred baby food meats or canned salmon.

915
Mixing pills in food

Getting a pet to swallow a pill is not easy. For dogs, try hiding the pill in a small amount of treat food (such as cottage cheese and peanut butter) or crush a pill and mix it with its regular food—but if the taste is unpleasant, a dog may refuse to eat. For cats, often experts at ferreting out pills hidden in food, mix a crushed pill with a small amount of a strong-tasting treat food, such as mashed sardines.

916
Helping the pills down

If your pet is too sick to eat, you may have to help the pill down its throat. It's best to have your vet show you how to do this to avoid traumatizing your pet. For a dog, talk to it gently, open its mouth, and place the pill at the back of the throat. For a cat, talk to it gently, tilt its head back, open its mouth, and place the pill at the back of the tongue. In each case, hold the mouth shut and massage the throat to help your pet swallow.

917
Giving liquid medicine

For a dog, hold the snout and tilt the head back to about a 45-degree angle. Squirt the liquid into his mouth between the canine teeth with a plastic eyedropper. Gently stroke his throat to encourage him to swallow. For a cat, tilt its head back to the same angle and squirt the liquid into its mouth between the teeth and the cheek, never down the throat.

Cuts & Abrasions

If a cut is small and shallow, you can treat it at home. A deep cut may require stitches, and a cut that will not stop bleeding needs medical attention. An abrasion is a scraped area of skin that may be broken, but not deeply cut. A corneal abrasion causes squinting, eye watering, and possible swelling of the eye. If there is blood in the eye or if the injury is not significantly better within two days, consult your vet. For cuts and abrasions, herbal antiseptics encourage healing and fight infection.

918
First aid for cuts

To stop a cut from bleeding, apply steady pressure directly over the area using a clean folded cloth. Powdered yarrow is a strong astringent and can help stop bleeding; sprinkle the dried powdered herb liberally into the cut. A cut that is more than half an inch (12mm) deep will probably need stitches; take your pet to the vet at once so the wound can heal properly.

919
Healing herbs for cuts

When bleeding has stopped, cleanse a cut under cool running water and rinse with an herbal antiseptic made of equal parts echinacea extract and water. If bleeding starts after cleaning, apply pressure again. Trim hair away from affected area. Apply calendula gel twice daily to encourage healing.

920
Treating an abrasion

Clean the area thoroughly with cool water to remove debris such as embedded dirt or gravel and rinse with an herbal disinfectant made by mixing equal parts echinacea extract and water. Apply calendula ointment twice daily to help the skin heal. If the abrasion shows signs of infection, such as redness, swelling, or discharge, consult your vet.

921
Healing eye wash for corneal abrasions

Abrasions to the cornea of the eye are often caused by a scratch. They are extremely painful for your pet, but usually heal quickly. An herbal eye wash made from calendula blossoms helps soothe the injured eye and speeds healing.

1 cup (250ml) boiling water
1 tablespoon dried calendula flowers
1/8 teaspoon sea salt

Make a strong tea by pouring the water over the calendula flowers and sea salt. Cover, and steep until the tea cools to room temperature. Strain through a clean coffee filter. Saturate a cotton ball with the lukewarm liquid and squeeze several drops into the affected eye four times a day until the abrasion has healed.

Animal Bites & Stings

Most bite wounds, unless severe, can be treated at home with herbal antiseptics such as echinacea. If the bite is deep or jagged, consult your vet. Wasps, yellow jackets, and bees cause painful stings that can become infected if not treated. If your pet has been stung repeatedly or shows signs of allergic reaction such as vomiting, lethargy, or weakness, call your vet at once.

922
Rescue remedy for calming stress

If your pet is stressed or in shock, give it a couple of drops of Rescue Remedy flower essence in a small amount of water and rub a few drops onto its muzzle and paws. Rescue Remedy helps calm emotional distress.

923
Treat a bite wound

Cleanse the wound thoroughly with a gentle natural soap and lukewarm water, and then flush it with a mixture of equal parts of echinacea extract and water. Echinacea is a natural antiseptic and helps kill harmful bacteria.

924
Healing a bite wound homeopathically

Once the wound is clean, apply calendula gel twice daily to encourage healing. Combine this with a dose of ledum, given twice daily. Ledum is a useful homeopathic remedy for any type of puncture wound, including bites. It helps relieve redness, swelling, and pain.

925
Treat a sting

If your pet has been stung by an insect, and if you can see the stinger, remove it by scraping a credit card across the skin. Or pull it out with tweezers, grasping the stinger as close as possible to the skin. Apply a cold pack for up to 15 minutes to relieve the inflammation and swelling. To help draw out toxins and prevent infection, mix up a paste of cosmetic clay and echinacea extract and apply it to the affected area. Let it dry, and reapply twice daily for two days.

926
Relieve a sting

For insect stings, ledum is the homeopathic remedy of choice. It helps ease swelling, redness, and pain. Give one dose, and follow with another after 30 minutes. Repeat every hour until you see improvement.

Homeopathic pills

Skin Burns

Pets can suffer thermal burns from hot liquids or spitting oils in the kitchen, and chemical burns from corrosive substances such as household cleaners, garden chemicals, and automotive products. Treat burns at once to prevent infection but if there is more than a minor burn, consult your vet immediately.

927
Treat a thermal burn

Cooling your pet's skin is the first priority when treating a thermal burn. This will draw out the heat, prevent further damage to the tissues, and relieve pain. Gently apply ice-cold, wet cloths to the burned area for approximately 15 minutes. Follow this by applying calendula gel twice a day to help the skin heal. If you are worried about your pet, contact your vet at once.

928
Treat a chemical burn

Prepare a solution of one teaspoon of baking soda dissolved in two cups (500ml) of lukewarm water. Use this rinse to wash the skin around the chemical burn. Keep your pet from licking the wound; a muzzle or a special cone-shaped collar may be necessary. Consult your vet for advice as soon as possible. To help the skin heal, apply calendula gel to the affected area twice daily.

Abscesses

Cats are more susceptible to abscesses than dogs because bites from other cats cause small puncture wounds that can easily become infected. Abscesses appear as soft, painful swellings, and are filled with pus. If an abscess does not show improvement with home treatment within a couple of days, consult your vet.

Echinacea

929
Treat an abscess

Hot compresses help bring abscesses to a head, draining them naturally. Calendula fights infection and heals.

- 1 cup (250ml) boiling water
- 1 tablespoon dried calendula flowers

Pour boiling water over the calendula. Cover, steep for 15 minutes, and strain. Dip a washcloth in the hot tea (reheat it if necessary) and apply to the affected area for 15 minutes three times a day. The compress should be hot, but should not burn the skin. Rewet the washcloth in the hot tea as needed.

930
Cleaning an abscess

If an abscess bursts, thoroughly clean it with echinacea and goldenseal to combat infection and speed healing.

- 1/2 teaspoon sea salt
- 1 cup (250ml) warm water
- 25 drops echinacea extract
- 25 drops goldenseal extract

Dissolve the salt in the water and mix in the extracts. With a plastic syringe, gently flush the abscess three times a day. Note that goldenseal may stain light-colored fur.

931
Prevent abscesses

Clean all wounds immediately and thoroughly with a mixture of equal parts of echinacea tincture and water. Echinacea is a natural antiseptic and fights the bacteria that cause infection. Clean the area twice daily until the wound heals.

932
Fight infection with echinacea

To rally your pet's immune system to fight an infection, give five drops of echinacea tincture diluted in one teaspoon of water twice a day for up to ten days. Repeat the dosage if necessary after taking a break for three days.

Dandruff

Pet dandruff appears as white or brown flakes in the fur. The coat may be oily with an unpleasant odor. Dietary imbalances, intestinal worms, and nutritional deficiencies are common causes; bathing too often with harsh shampoos can also be a factor. Indoor cats are prone to dandruff because heating, air conditioning, and a lack of fresh air cause skin dryness.

933
Prevent dandruff

Pets have natural oils in their coats that keep both their hair and skin healthy. To prevent your pet's skin from becoming dry and flaky, avoid too many baths. When you do bathe your pet, always use mild natural castile shampoos and dilute them with an equal amount of water. A healthful and varied diet will provide the vitamins and minerals necessary for healthy skin.

934
Flaxseed oil for dry skin

Dry, flaking skin is often a sign of insufficient essential fatty acids, which can be remedied by supplementing the daily diet with cold-pressed flaxseed oil. For dogs, give half a teaspoon of flaxseed oil for each 10lb (4.5kg) of body weight. For cats, add a quarter of a teaspoon of flaxseed oil to your pet's food ration twice a day. Keep the oil refrigerated to prevent rancidity.

935
Herbal skin treatment

Apple cider vinegar restores a healthy acid balance to the skin and calendula helps heal it.

1 cup (250ml) apple cider vinegar
2 tablespoons dried calendula flowers

Heat the vinegar and calendula over a low heat for five minutes; do not allow to boil. Remove from heat, steep until cool, and strain. For dogs, dilute two tablespoons of the herbal vinegar with one cup (250ml) of water. For cats, dilute one teaspoon with a quarter of a cup (60ml) of water. In each case, dip a brush in the solution and brush your pet, rewetting the brush frequently to thoroughly cleanse the fur and skin.

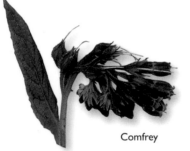

Comfrey

936
Herbal dandruff rinse

An herbal rinse made from thyme and comfrey helps soothe and heal dry, flaking skin.

2 tablespoons dried thyme
2 tablespoons dried comfrey
1 quart (1.25 liters) water

Simmer the herbs and water in a covered pot for five minutes and allow to cool. Strain, and use as a final rinse after bathing your pet.

Fleas & Ticks

Fleas appear as tiny, dark brown, jumping specks in your pet's fur. On dogs, they tend to congregate on the abdomen, around the neck, and along the back. On cats, they are found around the head, ears, neck, rump, and tail. Ticks carry serious diseases such as Lyme disease. They are found more often on dogs than on cats because cats clean themselves so thoroughly.

937
Repel fleas with garlic

Garlic is an excellent natural remedy for repelling fleas. Most dogs like the taste of it. Add half to one clove of finely minced fresh garlic for every 10lb (4.5kg) of body weight to your dog's food each day. As an alternative to fresh garlic, thoroughly mix in the food one to two tablets or capsules of high-potency garlic extract per 10lb (4.5kg) of body weight. Most cats do not like the taste of raw garlic. You may find dried, high-potency garlic extract to be effective. Thoroughly mix in half a capsule of the garlic extract with your cat's food every day. **Caution:** Speak to your vet before feeding garlic to your pet as it may cause health problems in some pets.

938
Supplement the diet with nutritional yeast

Nutritional yeast is a rich source of beneficial B vitamins that can help repel fleas when you include it in your pet's daily diet. For dogs, mix half a teaspoon of nutritional yeast per 10lb (4.5kg) of body weight into their food every day. For a cat, mix half a teaspoon into its food every day.

939
Wash away fleas

If your cat or your dog is infested with fleas, give it a weekly bath to gain control of the parasites. Bathe your pet with a natural, mild castile shampoo diluted with an equal amount of water and rinse its coat with a strong solution of eucalyptus tea. The essential oils in eucalyptus have natural insecticidal properties that help kill the fleas as well as repel them. To make the eucalyptus tea, simmer four tablespoons of the dried eucalyptus leaves in one quart (1.25 liters) of water for five minutes in a covered pot. Cool the brew to room temperature. Strain, and use as the final rinse after shampooing and bathing your pet.

940
Natural flea powder

A powder made from diatomaceous earth and the flea-repellent essential oils of eucalyptus, citronella, and lavender helps control fleas naturally. Diatomaceous earth, a powder made from the microscopic skeletons of tiny marine algae, cuts into fleas and kills them. Buy it from a garden center (the type sold for pools is finely powdered and can injure your pet's lungs).

2 tablespoons eucalyptus essential oil

2 tablespoons citronella essential oil

2 tablespoons lavender essential oil

I cup (225g) diatomaceous earth

Stir the oils into the earth and cover with a cloth. When the powder is dry, mix the oils in with a wire whisk and store in an airtight container. Sprinkle the powder onto your pet as often as needed and rub it into the coat. **Caution:** Do not use on kittens.

Keep your pet free of fleas naturally

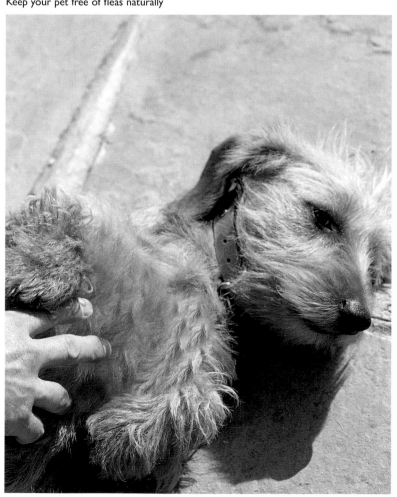

941
Comb out fleas

Daily grooming is an ideal time to de-flea your pet. Flea combs are specially designed with fine teeth to help you remove fleas from your pet's hair as you thoroughly groom it each day. It is essential that you immediately kill the fleas, though, or else they will jump back onto your pet. Prepare a bowl of warm soapy water and dip the comb into the water to drown the fleas as you groom your pet.

942
Flea repellent spray

Make a natural flea spray by mixing eucalyptus, citronella, and lavender essential oils with distilled witch hazel. Spray onto your cat or dog at least once a day. Be sure to keep the spray out of its eyes.

I cup (250ml) distilled witch hazel

1/2 teaspoon citronella essential oil

1/2 teaspoon eucalyptus essential oil

I teaspoon lavender essential oil

Combine the ingredients in a spray bottle and shake well.

943
Soothing rinse for itchy skin

This after-bath herbal rinse helps soothe and heal the itchy rash caused by flea allergies.

2 tablespoons dried calendula

2 tablespoons dried comfrey

2 tablespoons dried chamomile

I quart (1.25 liters) water

Simmer the dried herbs and water in a covered pot for about five minutes. Remove from the heat and let steep until cool. Strain, and pour over your pet as a final rinse after bathing.

944
Eradicate fleas from your home

To successfully rid your pet of fleas, you must at the same time eradicate fleas in your home. To kill fleas and their eggs, wash your pet's bedding at least once a week in hot water with a mild natural laundry detergent and dry in a hot dryer. Wash the floors and thoroughly vacuum everything, including carpeting, furniture, and drapes. Remove and dispose of the bag in your vacuum cleaner after cleaning to prevent reinfestation.

945
Rid carpeting of fleas with borax

Fleas are tenacious and can survive in carpeting for months. If you find them jumping onto you or your pet, try treating your carpeting with borax, a naturally occuring mineral that can help eliminate the pesky parasites. Sprinkle a thin layer of borax onto carpeting and rugs. Leave overnight, and vacuum thoroughly in the morning. Dispose of the vacuum cleaner bag immediately to prevent reinfestation of fleas.

946
Treating flea allergies

Some pets are allergic to flea bites, and suffer symptoms such as severe scratching and significant hair loss. A key to preventing flea allergies is to feed your pet an optimal diet; a healthy immune system makes your pet more resilient. Be sure to include garlic and nutritional yeast (see *Nos. 937, 938*) in your pet's diet to help repel fleas. Flaxseed oil is rich in essential fatty acids that protect hair and skin. For dogs, add half a teaspoon of flaxseed oil for every 10lb (4.5kg) of body weight to their daily food ration. For cats, add a quarter of a teaspoon of flaxseed oil.

947
Removing a tick safely

If you find a tick in your pet's skin, gently grasp the tick as close as possible to the skin with a pair of blunt tweezers, and pull it out with smooth, steady pressure. Twisting or yanking the tick only increases the possibility of leaving part of it embedded in the skin. Wrap the tick in a tissue and immediately flush it down the toilet.

948
Treat a tick bite

When removing a tick, it is not uncommon for part of the tick's head to remain in the skin, which can cause inflammation or local infection. Clean the area with a cotton ball soaked in equal parts of echinacea extract and water. Using a cotton swab, dab on a drop of tea tree essential oil, a powerful antiseptic that will help prevent infection.

Ear Mites

Ear mites are tiny, highly contagious parasites. They burrow into the ear canal and lay eggs, causing irritation, inflammation, and itching. Symptoms include ear scratching, head shaking, and a dark wax in the ear canal. Ridding a pet of ear mites requires patience and persistence and may require your vet's help.

949
Cleaning your pet's ears

First clean excess wax and debris out of the ears. Warm a metal teaspoon of almond oil in a small pot over low heat or candle flame. Test the oil on the back of your hand to make sure it is a comfortable temperature. Use an eye dropper to put the oil into the ear canal and gently wedge a cotton ball into the ear. After several hours, use a rubber syringe or a plastic eyedropper to flush out the loosened wax with a solution of equal parts of lukewarm water and white vinegar. Gently remove the wax with cotton swabs. Repeat the treatment for three days in a row, and then as often as needed.

950
Garlic oil ear drops

Garlic oil helps rid the ear of mites and wards off reinfestation. To make the oil, mince one bulb of fresh garlic and place in a small heavy pot. Add olive oil to an inch (25mm) above the surface of the garlic. Cover, and warm gently over a low heat for about an hour. Strain the oil through cheesecloth and store refrigerated in a covered glass jar. Warm the oil in a metal teaspoon over a candle flame. Use the back of your hand to ensure the oil is not too hot. After cleaning the ear, put several drops into the ear with an eye dropper and plug with a cotton ball. Repeat twice daily. If your pet is prone to ear mites, use the drops twice a week as a preventive.

Ringworm

Ringworm is a fungal infection of the skin. In dogs, it has a characteristic circular, raised shape, and often occurs on the head. In cats, the fungus creates small, circular, scabby areas and hair loss, most often on the face, ears, neck, and tail. Ringworm is contagious, and can spread to other dogs, cats, and even to humans.

951
Strengthen immunity

A healthy pet with a strong immune system is naturally resistant to fungal infections. Feed your pet a high-quality diet free from sugars and chemicals. Supplement its diet with a quarter of a teaspoon of flaxseed oil once a day. To bolster immunity and improve the condition of the skin and hair, add vitamin E daily: for dogs, add 50 units per 10lb (4.5kg) of body weight; for cats, add 100 units.

952
Herbal antifungal bath

Trim the hair around the affected area. Add three drops of tea tree oil to a teaspoon of mild natural castile shampoo or pet shampoo and bathe your pet weekly. If you are bathing a big dog, double the amounts. After bathing use this rinse.

2 tablespoons dried thyme
2 tablespoons dried eucalyptus
2 tablespoons dried lavender
1 quart (1.25 liters) water

Simmer the ingredients in a covered pot for five minutes. Remove from the heat and steep until cool. Strain, and use the herbal tea as a final rinse.

953
Antifungal treatment

Apple cider vinegar restores the healthy acidity of the skin, making it more resistant to the growth of fungi. Lavender essential oil is antimicrobial and soothes itching as well as inflammation. Tea tree essential oil is a potent natural antifungal.

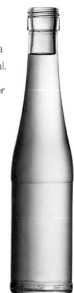

½ cup (125ml) apple cider vinegar
½ teaspoon lavender essential oil
½ teaspoon tea tree essential oil

Mix the ingredients and shake well. Apply to the affected areas twice daily with a cotton ball.

Apple cider vinegar

Conjunctivitis

Conjunctivitis, or pinkeye, is most often caused by debris, such as dust or grit. Symptoms include redness, a discharge, and a crusty accumulation on the eyelid. It can also be caused by an allergy, bacterial infection, or an upper respiratory infection. If home care brings no improvement in 24 hours, call your vet.

954
Treat conjunctivitis

This eyewash soothes irritation and helps heal the eye.

1 cup (250ml) boiling filtered water
1 teaspoon dried calendula
1 teaspoon dried chamomile

Pour the water over the herbs, cover, and steep for 15 minutes. Strain through a coffee filter. Soak a cotton ball in the lukewarm solution and squeeze liquid into the affected eye several times a day until the eye has healed. If there is no improvement within 24 hours, consult your vet.

955
Tips for preventing conjunctivitis

Bring your cat or dog inside when the weather is extremely windy or the air is very dusty. Try to prevent your pet from entering into a dusty environment. If you have a dog, do not let it hang its head out of the window when it rides with you in the car; flying particles of dust and grit can irritate the eyes and cause conjunctivitis. If you have a cat with long hair, keep it clipped short around the eyes to prevent irritation of the membranes of the eye.

Allergies

Allergies cause symptoms such as skin irritation, hair loss, hives, sneezing, runny nose and eyes, diarrhea, and vomiting. Allergies can be triggered by specific foods, pollens, molds, insects, chemicals, and environmental pollutants. Pinpointing allergies takes time and patience so ask your vet for help. Most important is to improve your pet's general health, which helps the body come back into balance.

956
Dietary factors in allergies

Try eliminating certain foods from your pet's diet for a month. For dogs, the most common food allergens are soy, yeast, wheat, corn, and beef. Switch to a nonallergenic diet of rice, lamb, chicken, vegetables, yogurt, and olive oil. For cats, switch to a nonallergenic diet of chicken, vegetables, and cooked whole grains (but don't include wheat). After one month, test other healthful foods one at a time by adding a small amount back into your pet's diet every day for one week. If you notice any allergy symptoms returning, eliminate that food permanently from your pet's diet.

957
Strengthen digestion

Improving digestive function can often help alleviate allergies. One way to keep your pet's digestive system functioning optimally is to add a small amount of the beneficial bacteria *Lactobacillus acidophilus* to its daily food ration. For a dog, give one tablespoon of live yogurt per 10lb (4.5kg) of body weight. For a cat, add a quarter of a capsule of powdered acidophilus to her food. Powdered digestive enzymes that have been formulated especially for your pet will also provide extra support.

958
Create a healthful environment

Molds, dust, household chemicals, cleaning products, and insecticides can all cause allergic reactions. Avoid the use of chemicals in and around your home; natural household cleansers and garden products are safer for you and your pet. Wash your pet's bedding weekly in a mild natural laundry detergent and rinse thoroughly. Chemicals such as dyes and fragrances in conventional laundry products can irritate your pet's skin and respiratory system.

Hypothermia

Hypothermia, or a dangerously low body temperature, can occur when a pet has suffered overexposure to cold water or cold weather. Symptoms of hypothermia include shivering, lethargy, and a body temperature below 99°F (37.2°C). If hypothermia is not treated immediately, the pet may die. Pets most susceptible are small or short-haired breeds of dog and cats that are wet and left outdoors.

959
Treat hypothermia

If you think your pet is suffering from hypothermia, immediately wrap it in a blanket or a sweater, and move it into a warm room. If your pet is wet, vigorously dry its coat with a towel; this will also help stimulate its circulation. Make up a warm bed with hot-water bottles or a heating pad wrapped in towels and cover your pet with a blanket. If it continues to show symptoms of hypothermia, call your vet at once.

960
Stress remedy

Rescue Remedy is a subtle yet effective emergency treatment for relieving stress and anxiety. It is a homeopathic remedy that is composed of five flower essences. Rescue Remedy helps alleviate shock and calm emotional distress at times of crisis. Give your pet a couple of drops of Rescue Remedy in a small amount of water and gently rub a few drops onto its muzzle and paws.

Parasites

Various parasites, such as roundworms, hookworms, and tapeworms, can cause serious health problems if left untreated. A healthy immune system is the best defense. Have your pet checked twice a year for parasites. If your pet shows signs of an infestation, such as the appearance of worms in the feces, as well as diarrhea, vomiting, or lethargy, consult your vet for advice.

961
Prevent parasites

Many parasites are picked up through contaminated soil, garbage, or contact with infected feces. Keep your yard clean and free of animal wastes where infestations can breed. To prevent tapeworm, control fleas. Dog owners should use garbage cans with tight-fitting lids and discourage their pet from roaming unsupervised. Cat owners should keep their pets' litterbox clean, and discourage them from eating rodents or birds.

962
Feed your pet garlic

Garlic is an antimicrobial that helps kill parasites in the intestinal tract. For dogs, feed them daily half a clove of raw garlic for each 10lb (4.5kg) of body weight. To treat an infestation of parasites: two cloves of minced garlic for each 10lb (4.5kg) of body weight. for several days. Mix the garlic with food. For cats, mix half a teaspoon of powdered garlic extract with their daily food. **Caution:** Speak to your vet before feeding garlic to your pet.

Digestive Upsets

Digestive upsets, such as stomach problems, flatulence, diarrhea, or constipation, usually result from a dietary imbalance or when your pet eats spoiled food or a nonfood substance. Diarrhea can also be a symptom of more serious conditions. Consult your vet if you suspect that your pet has ingested a poisonous substance, or if symptoms worsen or persist for more than 24 hours.

963
Treat an upset stomach

Fast your pet for 24 hours to give its stomach time to recuperate. Give it plenty of water and reintroduce solid foods by feeding small amounts of boiled chicken and plain white rice.

964
Soothing chamomile tea

To help ease stomach upset, give your pet chamomile tea. Chamomile contains soothing antispasmodic compounds and can relieve stomach and intestinal cramping. Make a tea by pouring one cup (250ml) of boiling water over two teaspoons of dried chamomile. Cover, and steep for ten minutes. Strain, and cool to room temperature. Using a large plastic dropper, give an adult dog two teaspoons three times a day, and a puppy one teaspoon twice a day. For cats, give one teaspoon three times a day.

965
A flatulence-free diet

Experimenting with dietary changes is often the key to eliminating flatulence. Notorious gas-producing foods include milk, legumes, and vegetables from the cabbage family such as broccoli. For dogs, avoid foods made with soy products or cornmeal, and provide two meals a day to avoid overloading the digestive tract. For cats, provide a high-quality daily diet with plenty of raw, high-fiber foods such as grated carrot.

Dietary changes may eliminate gas

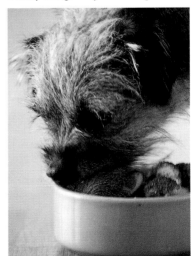

966
Gas-relieving herbs

Fennel seed tea has antispasmodic and gas-relieving properties and helps ease flatulence problems.

1 cup (250ml) water
1 teaspoon crushed fennel seeds

Make a tea by simmering the seeds and the water in a covered pot for five minutes. Cool to lukewarm and strain. For dogs, feed one teaspoon per 10lb (4.5kg) of body weight twice daily as needed. For cats, feed one teaspoon twice daily as needed.

967
A healthy intestine

Include *Lactobacillus acidophilus* in your pet's daily diet to help establish a healthy internal environment and to prevent excess gas. For dogs, provide one to two tablespoons of live yogurt per 10lb (4.5kg) of body weight every day. For cats, add a quarter of a capsule of powdered acidophilus to their food twice a day.

968
Prevent constipation

A varied, high-fiber diet usually prevents constipation. Raw meat has a laxative effect and foods rich in fiber (whole grains such as oatmeal, bulgur, and brown rice, as well as fresh vegetables and fruits such as carrots and apples) act as intestinal cleansers. To keep digestion working efficiently, give your pet plenty of fresh water and encourage it to take regular exercise or be engaged in active play.

969
Add additional fiber to your pet's diet

Some pets may need extra fiber to prevent constipation. Psyllium husks are an excellent, tasteless source of fiber. For dogs, add a quarter of a teaspoon of powdered psyllium husks per 10lb (4.5kg) of body weight to your dog's food and mix it in well. For cats, mix an eighth of a teaspoon of powdered psyllium husks and an eighth of a cup (30ml) of water with your cat's food. In each case, provide your pet with plenty of water.

Garlic

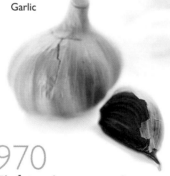

970
Fight microorganisms with garlic

Garlic is a natural antimicrobial and is effective against many of the microorganisms that can cause diarrhea in your pet. For dogs, add half a clove of minced fresh garlic for each 10lb (4.5kg) of body weight to your dog's food each day. This will help keep the intestinal tract healthy, free from pathogenic microorganisms, and prevent diarrhea. For cats, add half a 500mg capsule of concentrated garlic to their food each day. **Caution:** Speak to your vet before feeding garlic to your pet as it may cause health problems in some pets.

971
Fasting to help relieve diarrhea

Fasting is one of the quickest, most effective treatments for diarrhea. Withhold all food from your pet for 24 hours, but provide plenty of fresh water and plain chicken broth. Gradually add back easily digestible foods such as white rice and boiled chicken. **Caution:** Only try fasting with otherwise healthy adult pets.

972
Soothe irritation with goldenseal

Goldenseal extract is astringent and helps soothe the intestinal tract lining. It also helps to fight microbes that may be causing the diarrhea. For dogs, dilute goldenseal extract (a sixteenth of a teaspoon per 10lb (4.5kg) of body weight) in warm water. For cats, dilute five drops of goldenseal extract in one teaspoon of warm water. In each case, give three times a day until the diarrhea stops.

973
Replenish healthy bacteria after diarrhea

Following a bout of diarrhea, give your pet *Lactobacillus acidophilus* to help replenish the friendly flora that normally inhabit the intestinal tract. For dogs, add an eighth of a capsule of powdered acidophilus for each 10lb (4.5kg) of body weight to their food each day for a week. For cats, add an eighth of a teaspoon to their daily food ration for one week.

Urinary Tract Infections

These infections occur when bacteria travel up the urethra and into the bladder. Cats also suffer from feline urologic syndrome. Symptoms of the ailments include frequent but scanty urination and possible blood in the urine. If your pet passes blood each time it tries to urinate or if symptoms do not improve within 24 hours, call your vet at once.

974
Prevent bladder infections

The best way to prevent your pet from developing a bladder infection is to make sure it drinks plenty of fresh water. Encourage it to drink after exercising or active playing. This keeps the bladder flushed out and prevents bacteria from gaining a foothold. It also minimizes the risk of mineral crystals forming in the bladder. Cranberry juice makes the walls of the bladder slippery and also stops bacteria from accumulating. For dogs that are prone to bladder infections, mix an eighth of a cup (30ml) of unsweetened cranberry juice per 10lb (4.5kg) of body weight with their food ration every day. Alternatively, you can give your pet half a 400–500mg capsule of powdered cranberry concentrate per 10lb (4.5kg) of body weight every day. For cats, avoid a dry foods diet, which contributes to the formation of mineral stones. Instead, provide a high-quality diet with plenty of raw foods. If cystitis is a recurring problem, permanently restrict organ meats and fish, which can create irritating mineral crystals.

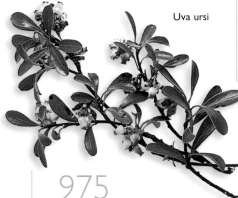

Uva ursi

975
Fight infections with herbal antiseptics

A combination of uva ursi, echinacea, and goldenseal makes a potent antiseptic formula for fighting urinary tract infections.

1fl oz (30ml) uva ursi extract
½fl oz (15ml) goldenseal extract
½fl oz (15ml) echinacea extract

Combine the ingredients in a dark glass bottle and shake well. For dogs, give an eighth of a teaspoon of the mixture per 10lb (4.5kg) of body weight in their food twice every day. For cats, give five drops of the mixture diluted in one teaspoon of water three times daily. In each case, continue giving the herbs for several days after the symptoms abate to be sure all the harmful microorganisms have been eradicated.

976
Vitamin C to prevent infections

Supplementing your pet's diet with vitamin C in the form of ascorbic acid can help prevent and heal bladder infections. Ascorbic acid makes urine acidic, and creates an environment that is inhospitable to bacteria and discourages the formation of mineral stones. For dogs, add a sixteenth of a teaspoon per 10lb (4.5kg) of body weight of powdered ascorbic acid to your dog's daily food ration. If your dog is suffering from a bladder infection, give it a sixteenth of a teaspoon of ascorbic acid per 10lb (4.5kg) of body weight— dilute it in water or chicken broth twice daily. For cats, add a sixteenth of a teaspoon of powdered ascorbic acid to their food twice daily. At the first symptom of urinary distress, increase the dosage to four times daily.

977
Give acidophilus after antibiotics

If your pet has been given antibiotics to treat a bladder infection, feed her *Lactobacillus acidophilus* supplements to help replenish the beneficial bacteria in the gastrointestinal tract. For dogs, mix in a quarter of a capsule of powdered acidophilus per 10lb (4.5kg) of body weight to their food once every day for two weeks. For cats, mix in half a teaspoon of liquid acidophilus or a quarter of a capsule of powdered acidophilus to their food twice daily for two weeks.

Obesity

Obesity is common in pets, especially as they get older, and is primarily caused by lack of activity and overfeeding. Excess weight can cause a variety of health problems such as joint disorders, cardiovascular and kidney disease, and lethargy as well as shortening your pet's life.

978
Exercise your pet daily

An overweight pet may need to be encouraged to exercise. For dogs, try to walk at least 45 minutes daily, easing it in gradually to avoid overexertion and muscle soreness. For cats, try to play with it at least 30 minutes daily, engaging in activities such as chasing a ping-pong ball or scarf or playing with a favorite toy.

979
Adjust your pet's food intake

Regulating the amount of food your pet eats will help bring its weight down and into a healthy range. Do not starve your pet, but reduce the amount of food it is eating by approximately one third until it has achieved its optimal weight.

980
Healthy food choices for weight loss

Adjust your pet's diet to enable it to lose weight and, to ensure that it is getting all the nutrients it needs to stay healthy, include a high-potency vitamin and mineral supplement with its daily food ration. For dogs,

include plenty of high-fiber, low-fat foods to help it feel satisfied with less food. Rely on lean chicken, fish, turkey, cottage cheese, and eggs for protein. Add plenty of cooked and grated raw vegetables such as carrots, leafy greens, zucchini, and broccoli. For cats, if you provide a high-quality diet with plenty of raw foods they may never become overweight. Do not allow your cat to snack throughout the day. Instead, feed it twice a day and remove food after 30 minutes.

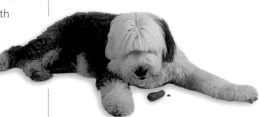

A healthy diet equals a healthy pet

Muscle Strains & Sprains

Sudden limping is often the sign of a muscle injury, particularly if the affected muscle is swollen and tender to the touch. Overexertion, playing too hard, or engaging in unaccustomed activities can cause a muscle strain or sprain. Muscle fibers are actually torn during an injury and need time to heal.

981
Apply ice to a strain

Place a cold gel pack on your pet's injured muscle for up to 15 minutes, several times a day. Secure it with an elastic bandage, but not too tightly. Your pet should rest for the first day or two. If the pain or swelling persists for more than 48 hours, consult your vet at once.

982
Herbal healing

Turmeric is an anti-inflammatory that encourages the healing of muscle and joint injuries. For dogs, mix an eighth of a teaspoon of powdered turmeric per 10lb (4.5kg) of body weight into their food every day. For cats, mix a sixteenth of a teaspoon of powdered turmeric into their food twice a day. In each case, continue with the turmeric until the pain and swelling have subsided.

983
Arnica pain relief

To ease the pain of a muscle strain or sprain, give your pet arnica pills several times each day. Arnica is a homeopathic remedy that relieves pain, reduces swelling, and speeds the healing of muscle injuries.

Arthritis

Arthritis is an inflammation of the joints, causing pain, stiffness, joint swelling, and limping. Older pets or large breeds of dog are most susceptible to arthritis, but this painful condition also affects pets who have nutritional deficiencies or who have suffered physical trauma from accidents. In general, arthritis is less common in cats than in dogs and symptoms are less severe.

984
Nutritional support

A health-supportive diet is essential for helping prevent and relieve arthritis. Follow the dietary guidelines in this chapter and give your pet flaxseed oil. The fatty acids in the oil help lubricate joints and prevent inflammation. Keep the oil fresh in a refrigerator. For dogs, add half a teaspoon per 10lb (4.5kg) of body weight to their daily food. For cats, add half a teaspoon each day.

985
Detox with barley grass

A gentle cleansing program can help relieve arthritis. Add a daily dose of powdered, freeze-dried barley grass to your pet's food. This is a rich source of chlorophyll, which helps detoxify the body, and antioxidants, which help prevent cell damage. For dogs, add an eighth of a teaspoon of barley grass per 10lb (4.5kg) of body weight. For cats, add an eighth of a teaspoon of barley grass daily.

Arthritic pets need comfortable beds

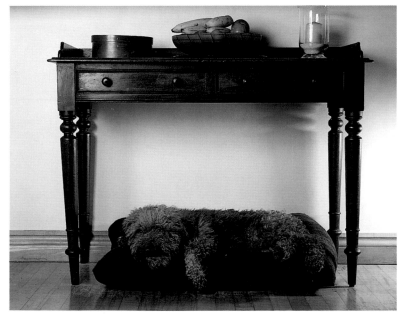

986
Glucosamine sulfate for healing

Glucosamine sulfate is a substance that is naturally found in the joints. It can help repair joints and ease the pain and inflammation associated with arthritis. Glucosamine sulfate is safe and can be given indefinitely as a supplement; it may take a month or longer to see results. For dogs, give a daily dose of 250mg of glucosamine sulfate per 10lb (4.5kg) of body weight. For cats, give 200mg of the supplement daily.

987
Exercise to relieve stiffness

Exercise helps keep your pet's muscles strong and joints flexible; a gentle walk lubricates joints and prevents them from stiffening. For a dog, take it for at least a 30-minute walk every day but let it set the pace. For a cat, engage it in gentle play for 15 minutes twice a day.

988
A comfortable bed

A soft, supportive, and warm bed helps relieve the pain and stiffness of arthritic joints. Keep the bed in a warm, dry room to stop symptoms from worsening. For dogs, a thick foam pad provides enough padding to keep joints off hard surfaces; a warm blanket makes a comfortable bed. For cats, provide a soft blanket and a comfortable pillow, and keep it away from drafts.

Upper Respiratory Viruses

These viruses are more common in cats than dogs and are known as cat flu. Symptoms include congestion, fever, appetite loss, lethargy, sneezing, and runny nose and eyes. The healthier the immune system, the less likely your pet is to come down with a cold. Treat symptoms at once to prevent bronchitis.

989
Diet for recovery

Do not be concerned if your ailing pet refuses food for a day or two. Offer lukewarm chicken broth, and keep plenty of fresh water available to prevent dehydration. You can also offer easy to digest foods such as boiled chicken, soft scrambled eggs, and jarred baby food meats. Add half a teaspoon of concentrated garlic powder to its food to bolster its immune system and 100 units of vitamin E daily.

990
Relieve cold symptoms

Clean crusty secretions from your pet's eyes and nose with a soft cloth dipped in warm water. Provide a warm and cozy sleeping place, and use a vaporizer in the room to keep the air moist and make breathing easier. To ease congestion, add a few drops of eucalyptus essential oil to the vaporizer.

991
Herbal decongestant

To boost your pet's immune function, give five drops of echinacea tincture diluted in one teaspoon of warm water three times a day for one week. To help loosen bronchial congestion, give mullein tea. Pour one cup (250ml) of boiling water over one teaspoon of dried mullein leaf, cover, and steep for 15 minutes. Strain, and give one teaspoon three times a day.

992
Clear a stuffy nose

If your pet has difficulty breathing through its nose, use a solution of mild saline drops to open up the nasal passages and shrink swollen membranes. Dissolve an eighth of a teaspoon of sea salt in half a cup (125ml) of boiling water. Cool to lukewarm. Gently tilt your pet's head back so that the nostrils are facing up, and place three drops of the saline solution into one nostril. Allow a few seconds for the drops to run down into the throat, and then repeat on the opposite nostril.

Kennel Cough

This respiratory infection of dogs causes a harsh, persistent cough that usually lasts for about two weeks. The dog otherwise seems normal. Care must be taken to avoid secondary infections such as bronchitis and pneumonia. If your dog is coughing and has a fever, is lethargic, or lacks appetite, call your vet at once.

993
Peppermint tea to ease coughing

A tea made from peppermint and honey can help calm your dog when he is coughing.

- 1 cup (250ml) boiling water
- 1 teaspoon of dried peppermint
- 1 tablespoon of honey

Make the tea by pouring the boiling water over the peppermint. Cover and steep for 10 minutes. Strain, and add the honey. The dose depends on the size of your dog. In general, give one teaspoon to a small dog and one tablespoon to a large dog every couple of hours.

994
Aromatherapy to relieve coughing

Peppermint and eucalyptus essential oils have antispasmodic properties and can help relieve your pet's coughing. Place a couple of drops of each essential oil into an aromatherapy diffuser and keep it near your dog's sleeping area. Make sure the diffuser is out of the dog's reach. Replenish the essential oils every couple of hours until the coughing subsides.

995
Herbal cough relief

An herbal liquid cough suppressant made with white horehound helps loosen the mucus in the respiratory tract and relieve your pet's coughing. The dose depends on the size of your dog. In general, give half a teaspoon to a small dog and one teaspoon to a large dog every four hours as needed.

996
Fight the infection with garlic

Garlic is an antimicrobial and helps combat infection. Give your dog half a teaspoon of liquid garlic extract or half a clove of minced raw garlic for every 10lb (4.5kg) of body weight. **Caution:** Speak to your vet before feeding garlic to your dog as it may cause health problems in some dogs.

997
Moisten the air

Keeping the air moist helps ease a dog's kennel cough. Place a vaporizer near your dog's bed and keep it running all day and night.

Traveling with Your Pet

Pets are light travelers, but a few essentials will make any journey easier: a leash for venturing out of the vehicle; a no-spill water dish; a container of fresh water; and a bag of treats. Cats are most comfortable and safest in a pet carrier that has plenty of ventilation and soft bedding.

998
Calm a restless traveler

Rescue Remedy, a stress-relieving blend of flower essences, is good for an anxious pet. It usually takes effect within about 15 minutes. Repeat the dosage every 30 minutes if you need. For a dog, put two drops into a small amount of water and offer it before traveling, or simply open its mouth and squirt in the drops. You can also massage a few drops onto its paws and around its muzzle. For a cat, massage a few drops onto its paws and around its cheeks.

999
Valerian for calming anxiety

If your pet becomes especially anxious when traveling, give it valerian capsules 30 minutes before your departure. Give approximately half a 300–500mg capsule for each 10lb (4.5kg) of body weight. Valerian is a safe, natural sedative with no harmful side effects for your pet.

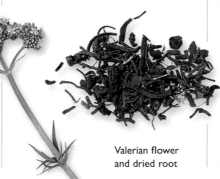

Valerian flower and dried root

1000
Prevent motion sickness in your dog

Some dogs are prone to motion sickness, which can make even the shortest car trip miserable. A good measure to prevent your dog from suffering motion sickness is Nux vomica, a homeopathic remedy. Give it as drops or pills approximately 30 minutes prior to your departure and at least 15 minutes before a meal. You can also give Rescue Remedy to help ease the stress associated with motion sickness. Rub a couple of drops of the remedy on your dog's muzzle or give a couple of drops in a small amount of water.

1001
Prevent heatstroke

Leaving your pet in a car on a hot day can be deadly. It only takes a few minutes for a car to heat to dangerous temperatures, and your pet can quickly succumb to dehydration and heatstroke. If you must leave your pet in a car, make sure you park in a shady spot and leave the windows partly open for fresh air. For a dog, make sure there is enough water in a bowl. For a cat, make sure it is secure in its carrier and with water available.

Plant Names

The recipes in this book rely on plants of different kinds. Their common names are given in the text, but if you want to confirm you have the right species, see below.

Aloe vera *(Aloe vera)*
Anise *(Pimpinella anisum)*
Anise hyssop *(Agastache foeniculum)*
Arnica *(Arnica montana)*
Astragalus *(Astragalus membranaceus)*

Basil *(Ocimum basilicum)*
Bay leaves *(Laurus nobilis)*
Bergamot *(Monarda didyma)* *(Citrus bergamia as bergamot essential oil)*
Bilberry *(Vaccinium myrtillus)*
Black cohosh *(Cimicifuga racemosa)*
Black currant *(Ribes nigrum)*
Borage *(Borago officinalis)*
Burdock *(Arctium lappa)*

Calendula *(Calendula officinalis)*
Carrot seed *(Daucus carota)*
Cascara sagrada *(Rhamnus purshiana)*
Catmint *(Nepeta spp.)*
Catnip *(Nepeta cataria)*
Cayenne pepper *(Capsicum annuum)*
Cedar *(Cedrus spp.)*
Cedarwood *(Cedrus atlantica)*
Chamomile *(Matricaria recutita)*
Chaste tree berries *(Vitex agnus castus)*
Chives *(Allium schoenoprasum)*
Cinnamon *(Cinnamomum cassia)*
Citronella *(Cymbopogon nardus)*
Clary sage *(Salvia sclarea)*
Cloves *(Syzygium aromaticum)*
Comfrey *(Symphytum officinale)*
Cornflower *(Centaurea cyanus)*
Cramp bark *(Viburnum opulus)*
Cypress *(Cupressus sempervirens)*

Dandelion *(Taraxacum officinale)*
Dill *(Anethum graveolens)*

Echinacea *(Echinacea spp.)*
Elderberry *(Sambucus nigra)*
Eucalyptus *(Eucalyptus globulus)*
Evening primrose *(Oenothera biennis)*
Eyebright *(Euphrasia officinalis)*

Fennel *(Foeniculum vulgare)*
Feverfew *(Tanacetum parthenium)*
Forget-me-nots *(Myosotis spp.)*
Foxglove *(Digitalis purpurea)*

Frankincense *(Boswellia carteri)*
French marigolds *(Tagetes patula)*

Garlic *(Allium sativum)*
Garlic chives *(Allium tuberosum)*
Gentian *(Gentiana lutea)*
Geranium *(Pelargonium graveolens)*
Ginger *(Zingiber officinale)*
Ginkgo *(Ginkgo biloba)*
Goldenseal *(Hydrastis canadensis)*
Golden marguerite *(Anthemis tinctoria)*
Grapefruit *(Citrus x paradisi)*
Green tea *(Camellia sinensis)*
Gymnema *(Gymnema sylvestre)*

Hawthorn *(Crataegus oxyacantha)*
Hibiscus *(Hibiscus spp.)*
Hops *(Humulus lupulus)*
Horse chestnut *(Aesculus hippocastanum)*

Jasmine *(Jasminum officinale)*
Juniper *(Juniperus communis)*

Kava *(Piper methysticum)*

Lamb's quarter *(Chenopodium album)*
Lavender *(Lavandula angustifolia)*
Ledum *(Ledum palustre)*
Lemon *(Citrus limon)*
Lemon balm *(Melissa officinalis)*
Licorice root *(Glycyrrhiza glabra)*
Lime *(Citrus aurantifolia)*
Linden *(Tilia x vulgaris)*
Lupin *(Lupinus spp.)*

Marjoram *(Origanum majorana)*
Marshmallow *(Althaea officinalis)*
Milk thistle *(Silybum marianum)*
Mint *(Mentha spp.)*
Mullein *(Verbascum thapsus)*
Myrrh tree *(Commiphora molmol)*

Neem *(Azadirachta indica)*
Neroli *(Citrus aurantium)*

Orange *(Citrus aurantium)*

Palmarosa *(Cymbopogon martinii)*
Parsley *(Petroselinium crispum)*

Passionflower *(Passiflora incarnata)*
Patchouli *(Pogostemon cablin)*
Peppermint *(Mentha piperita)*
Petitgrain *(Citrus aurantium var. amara)*
Pine *(Pinus spp.)*
Purslane *(Portulaca oleracea)*

Raspberry leaf *(Rubus ideaus)*
Red clover *(Trifolium pratense)*
Rosemary *(Rosmarinus officinalis)*
Rose *(Rosa spp.)*
Rue *(Ruta graveolens)*

Sage *(Salvia officinalis)*
Sandalwood *(Santalum album)*
Sarsaparilla *(Smilax officinalis)*
Saw palmetto *(Serenoa repens)*
Siberian ginseng *(Eleutherococcus senticosus)*
Skullcap *(Scutellaria lateriflora)*
Spearmint *(Mentha spicata)*
Spruce *(Tsuga canadensis)*
St. John's wort *(Hypericum perforatum)*
Stinging nettle *(Urtica dioica)*
Sweet alyssum *(Lobularia maritima)*
Sweet orange *(Citrus sinensis)*

Tansy *(Tanacetum vulgare)*
Tea tree *(Melaleuca alternifolia)*
Thyme *(Thymus vulgaris)*
Turmeric *(Curcuma longa)*

Uva ursi *(Arctostaphylos uva-ursi)*
Valerian *(Valeriana officinalis)*
Vetiver *(Vetiveria zizanoides)*

White horehound *(Marrubium vulgare)*
White willow bark *(Salix alba)*
Wild black cherry bark *(Prunus serotina)*
Witch hazel *(Hamamelis virginiana)*
Wormwood *(Artemisia absinthium)*

Yarrow *(Achillea millefolium)*
Ylang ylang *(Cananga odorata)*

Index

Page numbers in *italics* refer to the Natural Pet Care section

Acknowledgments

· ·

PUBLISHERS' ACKNOWLEDGMENTS
The publishers wish to thank Dave King for new photography, Sue Bosanko for the index and Carla Masson for proofreading.

Photo Credits
All images © DK except 5: Photonica; 22: Rex Interstock Ltd/Organic Picture Library; 66: James Merrell; 151: Bruce Coleman Ltd/P.Kaya; 160–1 Photonica; 171: RSPCA/Angela Hampton.

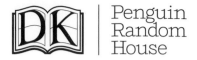

DK UK
Project Editor Kate Meeker
Senior Art Editor Glenda Fisher
Editorial Assistant Amy Slack
Jacket Designer Harriet Yeomans
Producer, Preproduction Catherine Williams
Senior Preproducer Tony Phipps
Senior Producer Stephanie McConnell
Creative Technical Support Sonia Charbonnier
Managing Editor Stephanie Farrow
Managing Art Editor Christine Keilty

DK INDIA
Preproduction Manager Sunil Sharma
DTP Designer Anurag Trivedi

DK US
US Managing Editor Lori Cates Hand
US Publisher Mike Sanders

First American Edition, 2003
This edition published in the United States in 2016 by
DK Publishing, 345 Hudson Street, New York, New York 10014

Copyright © 2003, 2016 Dorling Kindersley Limited
Text copyright © 2003 The Philip Lief Group, Inc. and Weider Publications, Inc.
DK, a Division of Penguin Random House LLC
16 17 18 19 20 10 9 8 7 6 5 4 3 2 1
001–296963–Oct/2016

A catalog record for this book is available from the Library of Congress.
ISBN 978-1-4654-5878-0

DK books are available at special discounts when purchased in bulk for sales
promotions, premiums, fund-raising, or educational use. For details, contact:
DK Publishing Special Markets, 345 Hudson Street, New York, New York 10014
SpecialSales@dk.com

Printed and bound in China

All images © Dorling Kindersley Limited
For further information see: www.dkimages.com

A WORLD OF IDEAS:
SEE ALL THERE IS TO KNOW

www.dk.com

"Burp!" said Kate.
"Is everything all right?" asked Mother.
"It is now," Arthur answered.

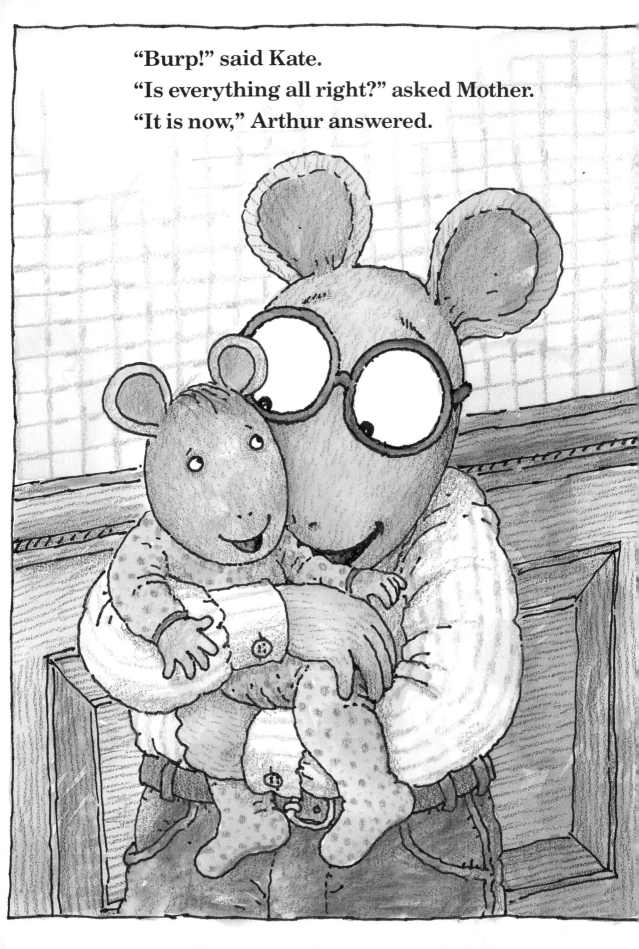

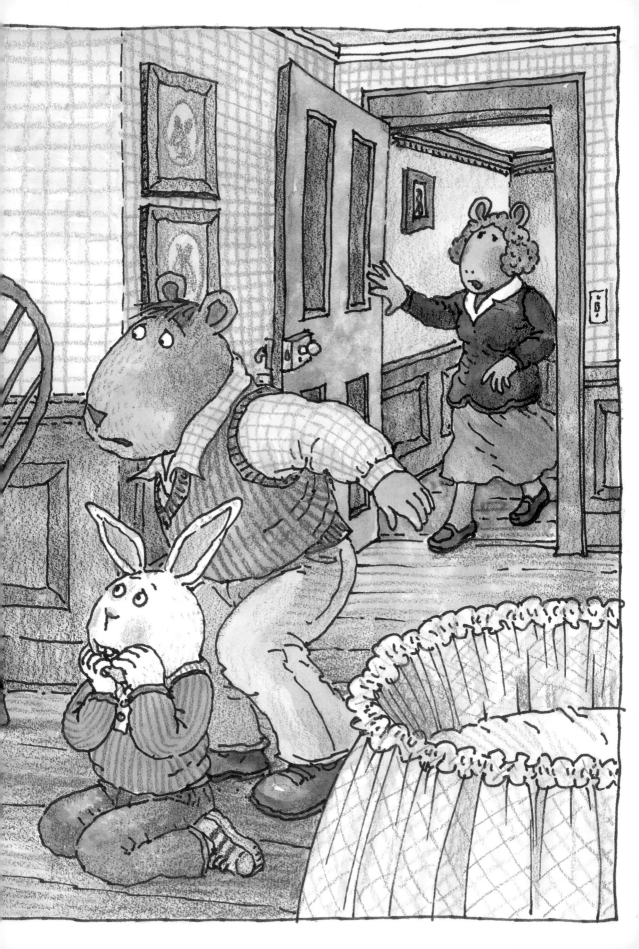

"Arthur, quick! Do something!" D.W. said.
"She's your baby, too."
"All of a sudden she's *my* baby," said Arthur.
"Why is she crying?" asked D.W.
"She's trying to tell you something," said Arthur.
"What?" asked D.W.
"Listen carefully," said Arthur.

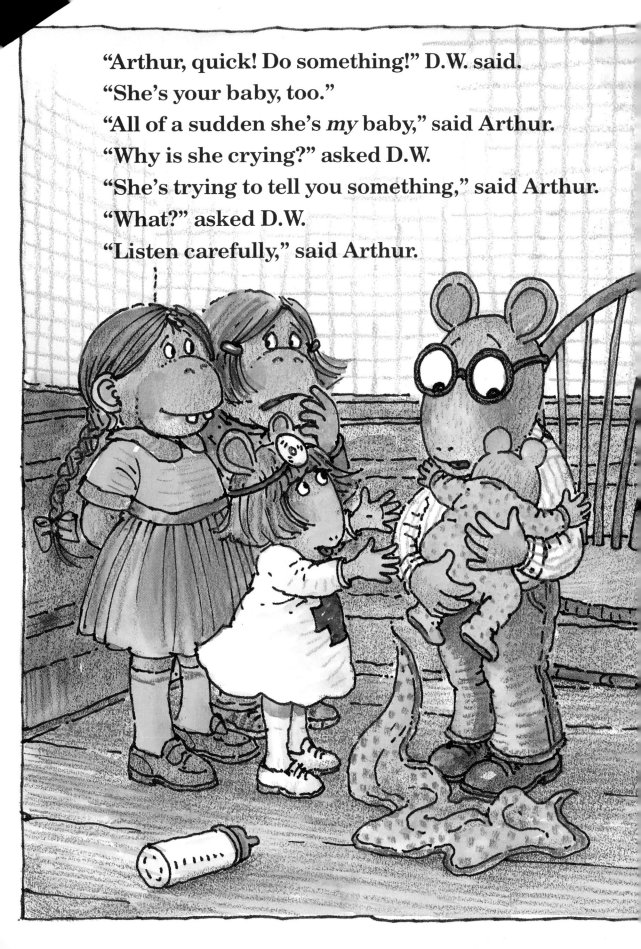

D.W. gave Kate a kiss.
Kate cried louder.

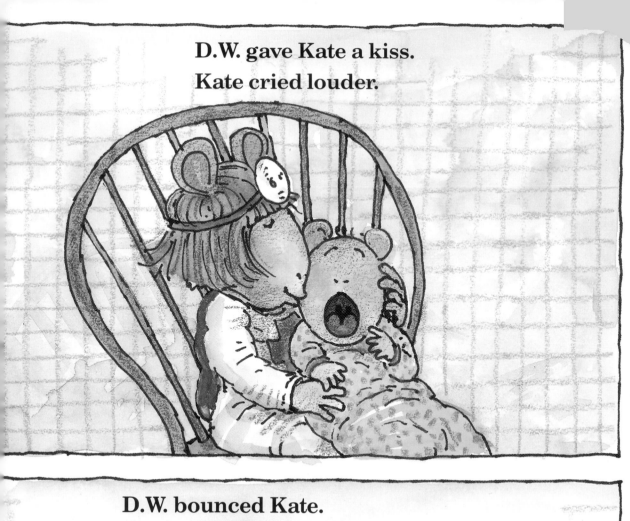

D.W. bounced Kate.
Kate screamed.

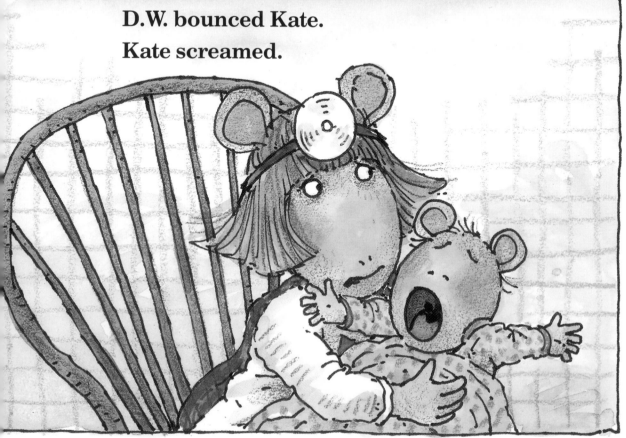

Kate drank her bottle in a flash.

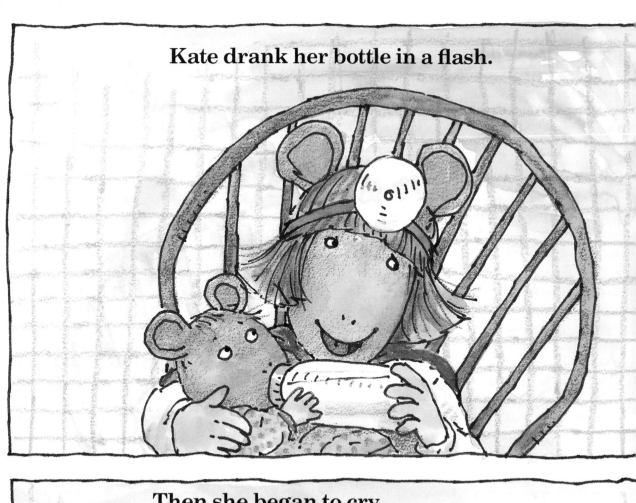

Then she began to cry.
"Everyone remain calm," said D.W.

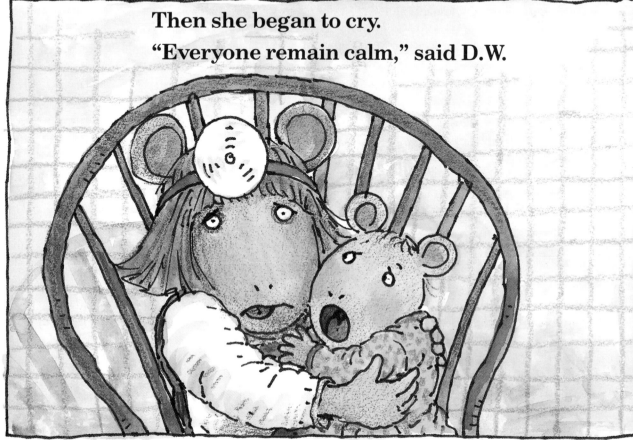

"Look!" said Francine. "She opened her eyes."
"Stand back," said D.W. "She wants her bottle."

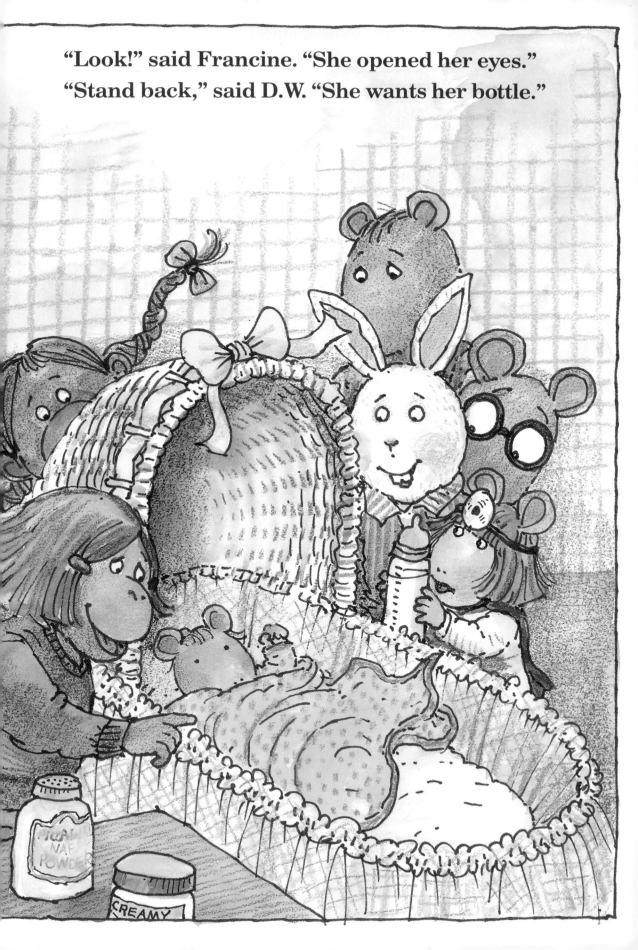

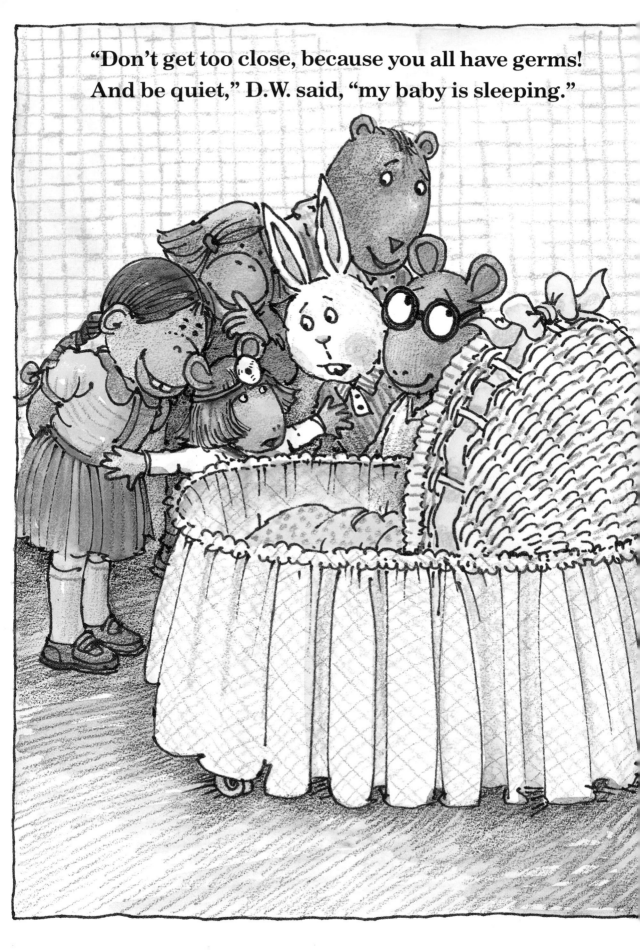

"Don't get too close, because you all have germs!
And be quiet," D.W. said, "my baby is sleeping."

When the doorbell rang, D.W. answered the door.
"Arthur can't play," she said. "He has to babysit.
But you can come in and see my baby."

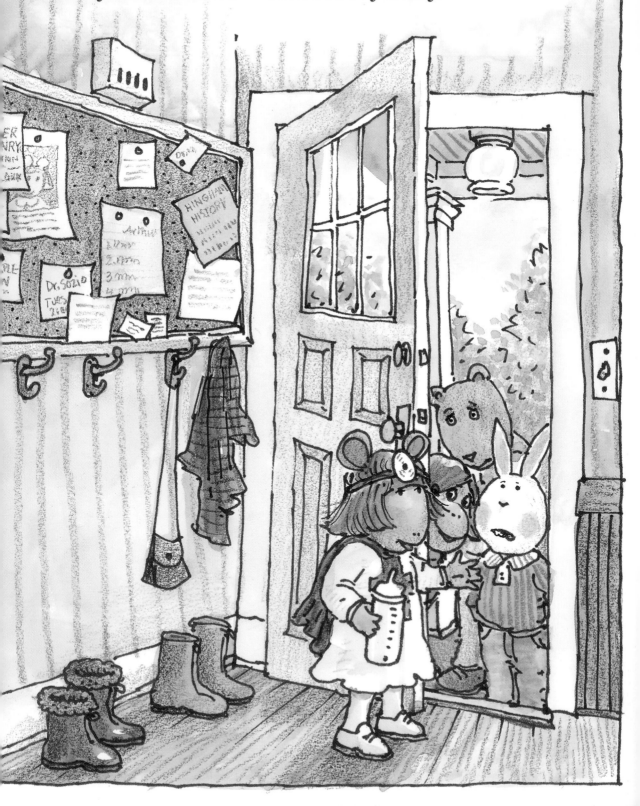

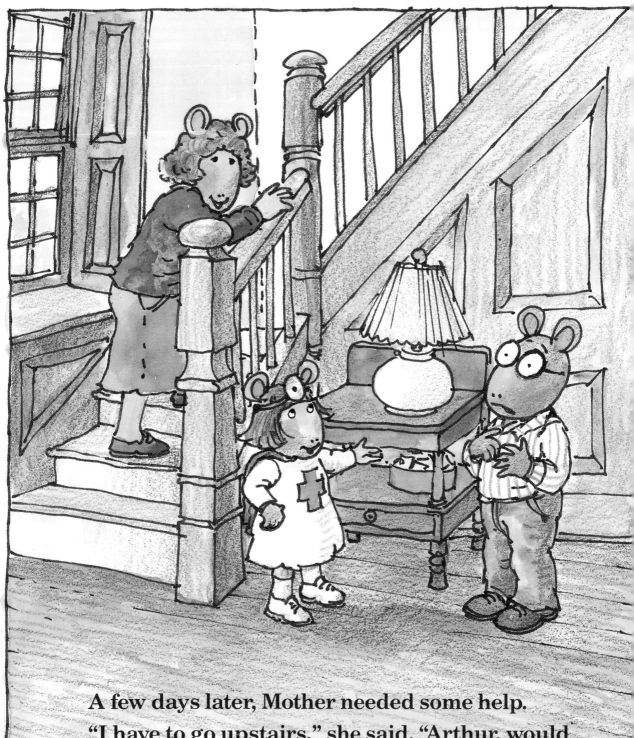

A few days later, Mother needed some help.
"I have to go upstairs," she said. "Arthur, would
you watch Kate?"
"*Me*?" asked Arthur. "What do I do?"
"Don't worry," said D.W. "I'll take care
of everything."

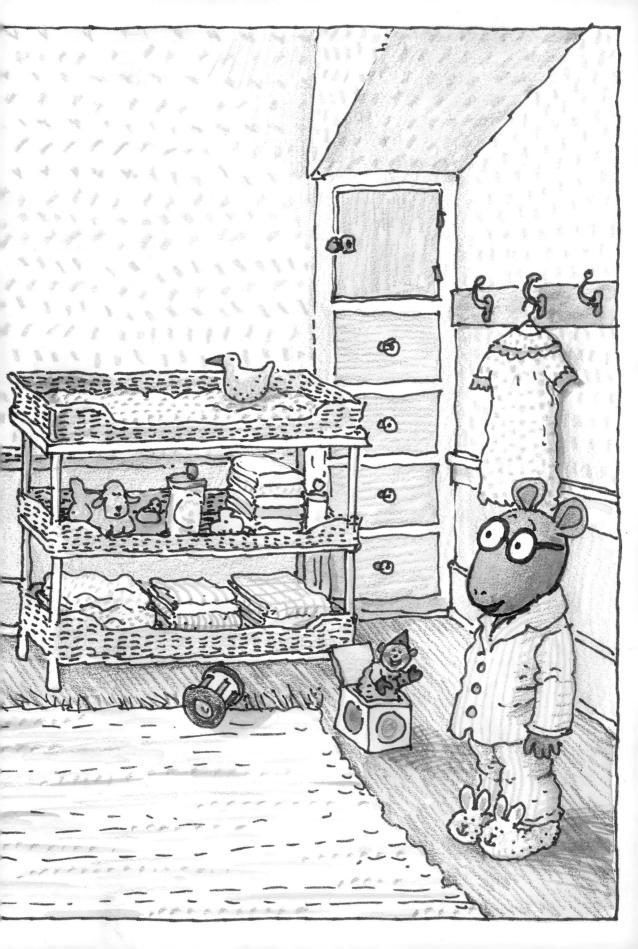

"Arthur, don't you want to try holding Kate?"
Mother asked.
"Can I have another turn first?" asked D.W.
"It's Arthur's turn," Mother said.
"I'd rather look," said Arthur.
"It's just as well," said D.W.
"Arthur doesn't know beans
about babies."

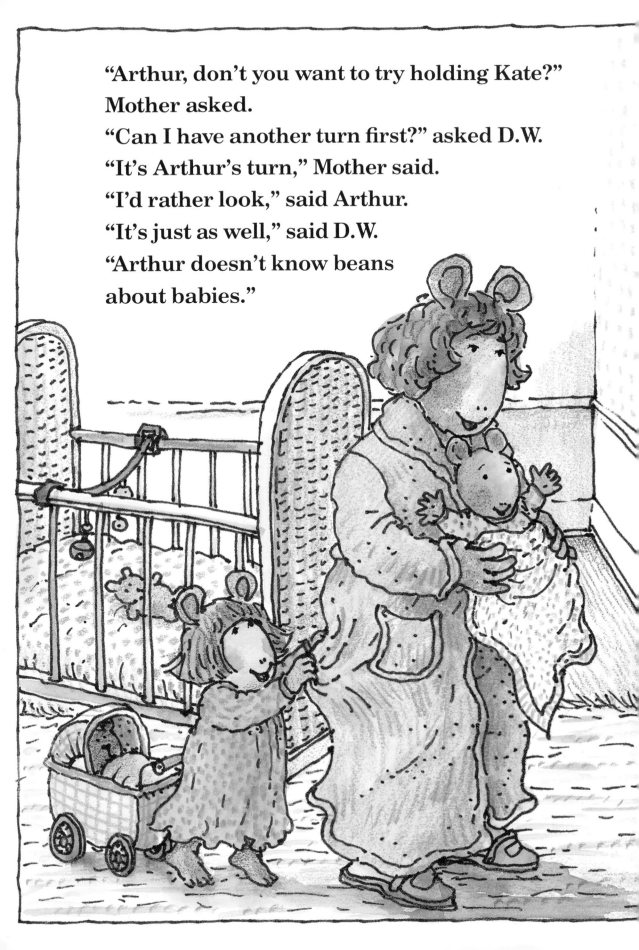

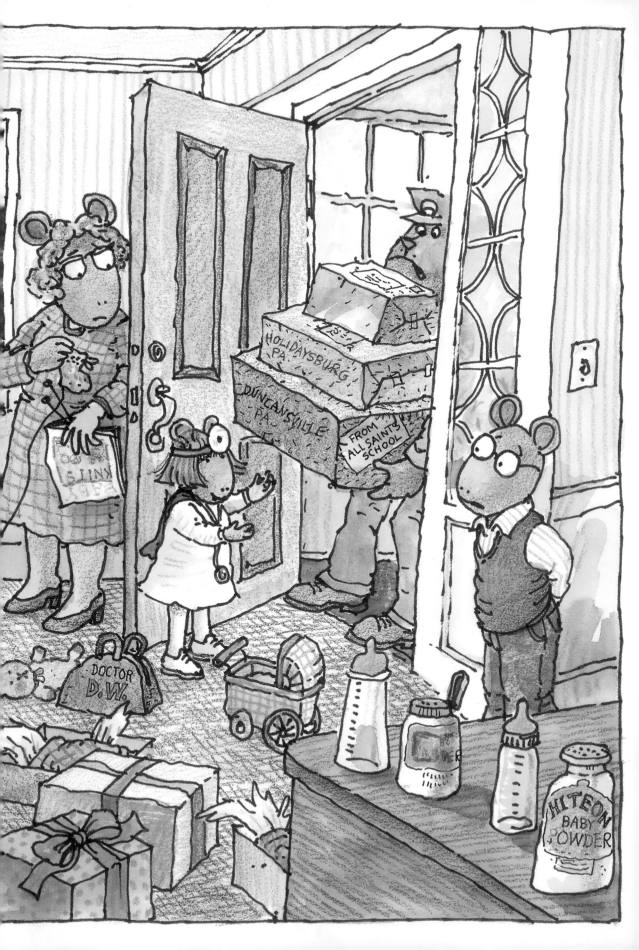

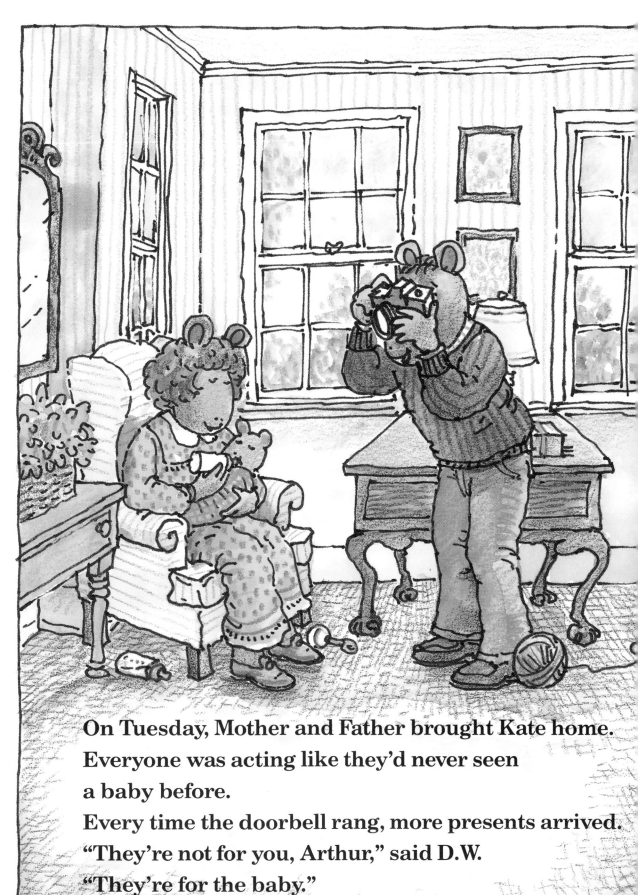

On Tuesday, Mother and Father brought Kate home.
Everyone was acting like they'd never seen
a baby before.
Every time the doorbell rang, more presents arrived.
"They're not for you, Arthur," said D.W.
"They're for the baby."

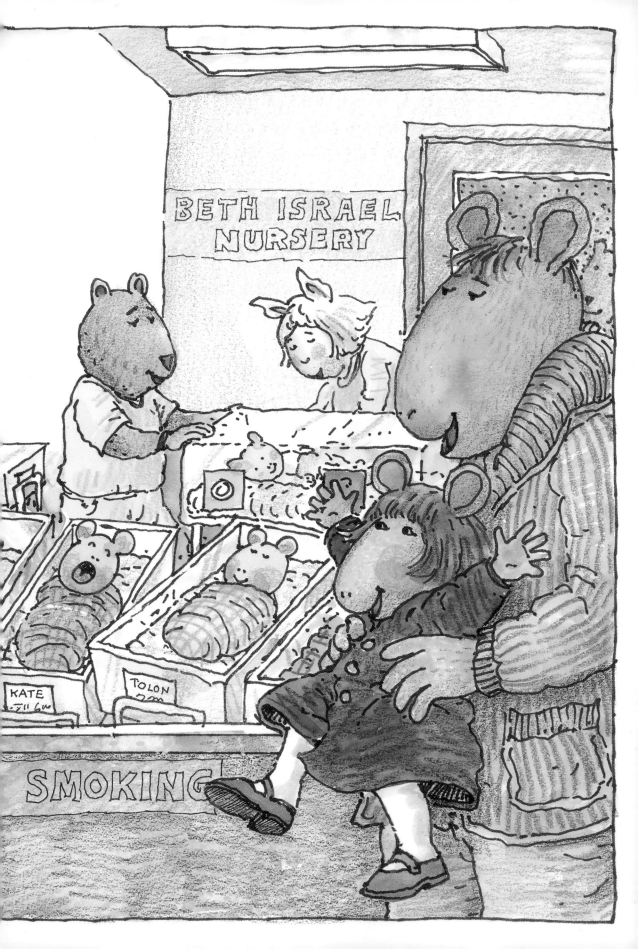

The next day, they went to the hospital to see the new baby.

"We named her Kate," said Father.

"I think she has your nose, Arthur."

"I think she has D.W.'s mouth," said Arthur.

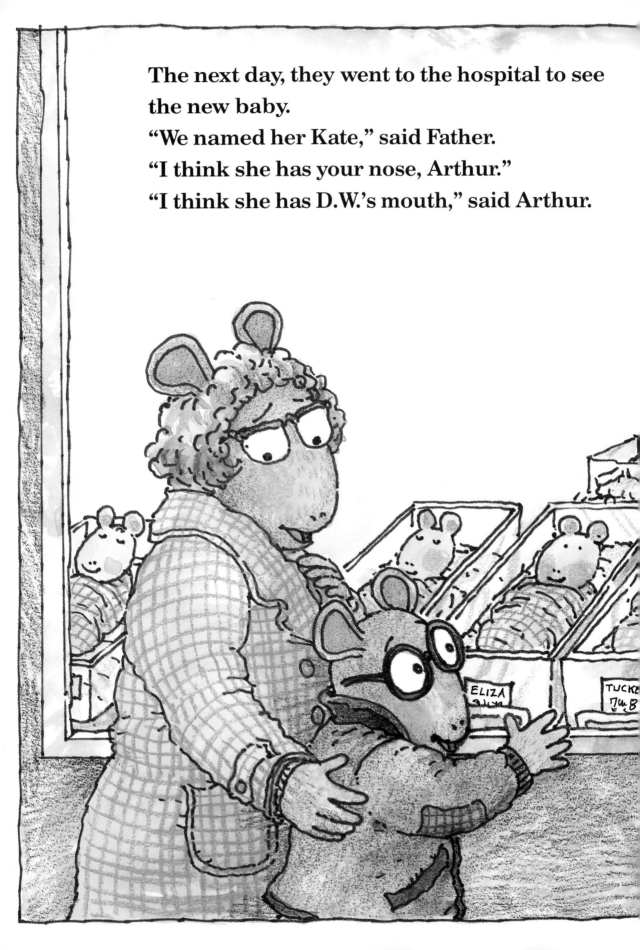

Sunday morning, Arthur and D.W. found
Grandma Thora fixing breakfast.
"You have a new sister!" she said.
"Yippee! Yippee! Yippee!" said D.W. "She'll be
just like me!"
"That's what I'm afraid of," said Arthur.

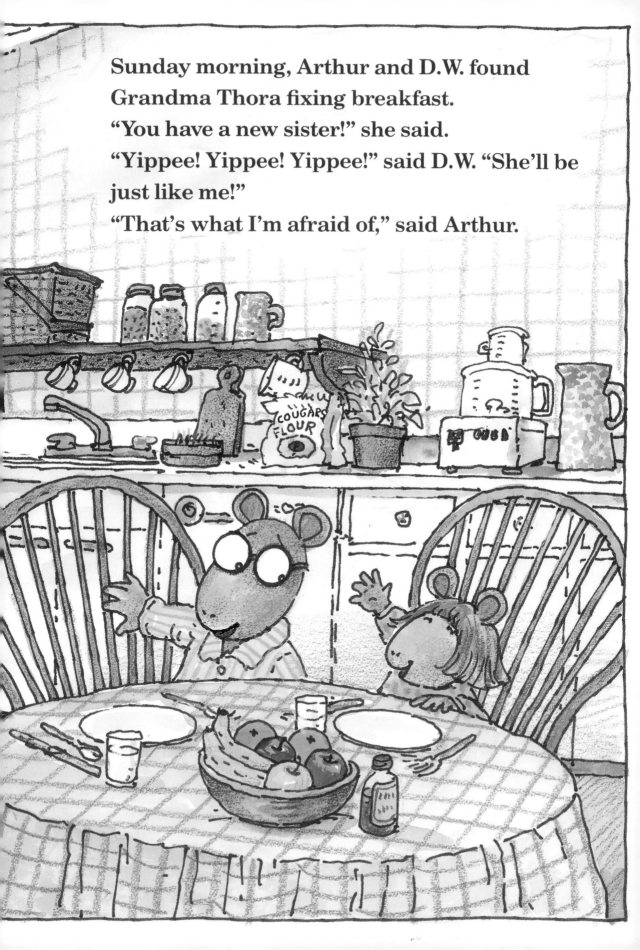

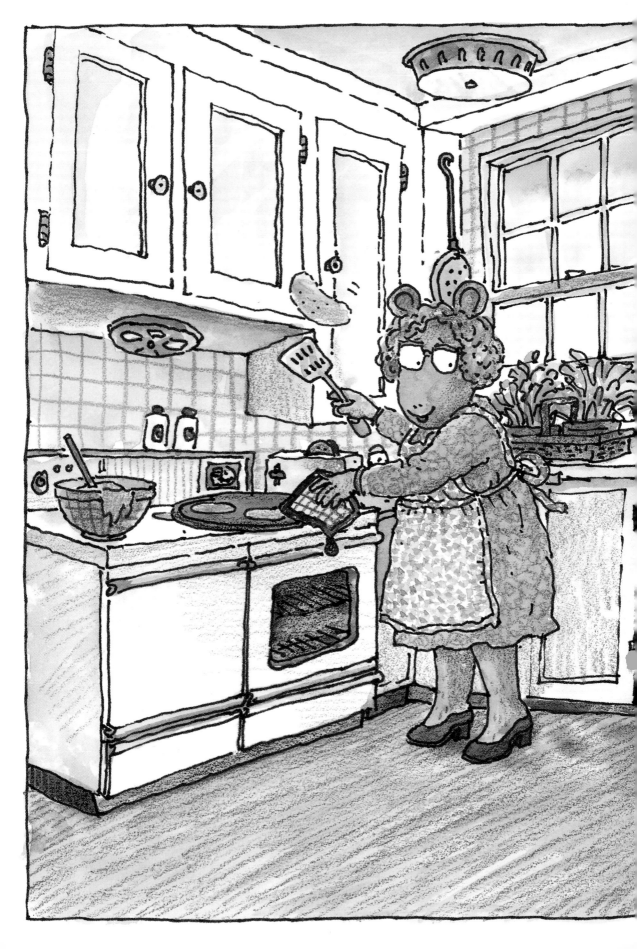

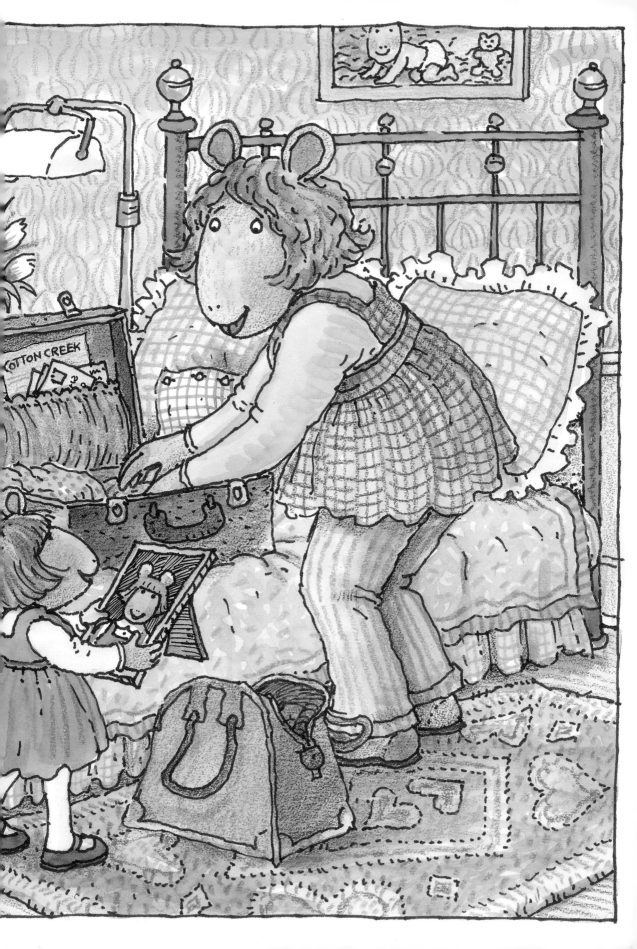

That Saturday morning, Mother took out her
suitcase.

"Where are you going?" asked Arthur.

"The baby could come any day now," said Mother.

"I need to be ready for the hospital."

"Here," said D.W. "Something for you to look
at while you're there."

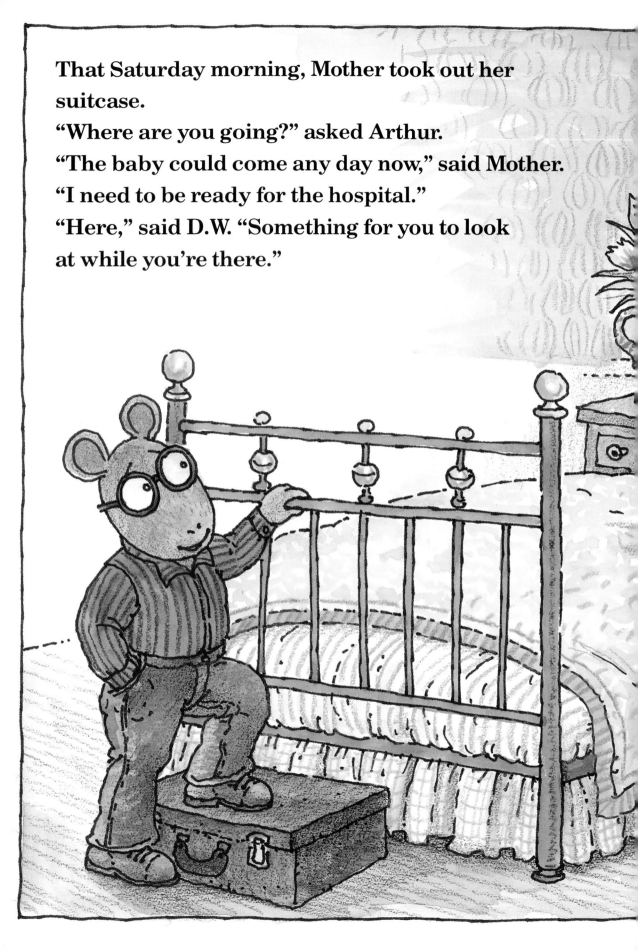

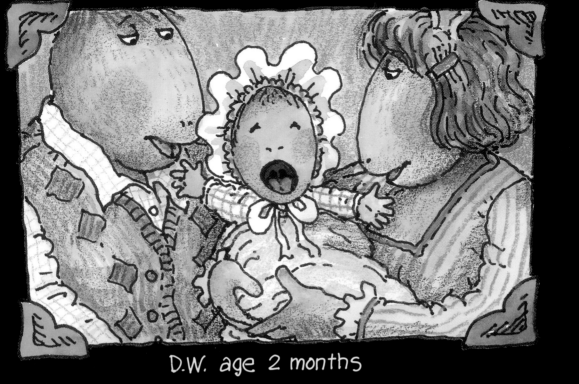

D.W. age 2 months

"Look," said D.W. "This is me with Mommy and Daddy. Don't I look adorable?"

D.W. age 5 months

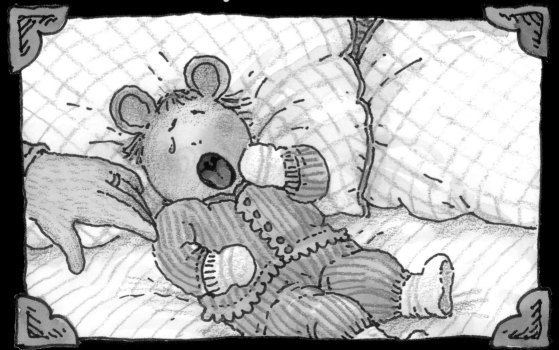

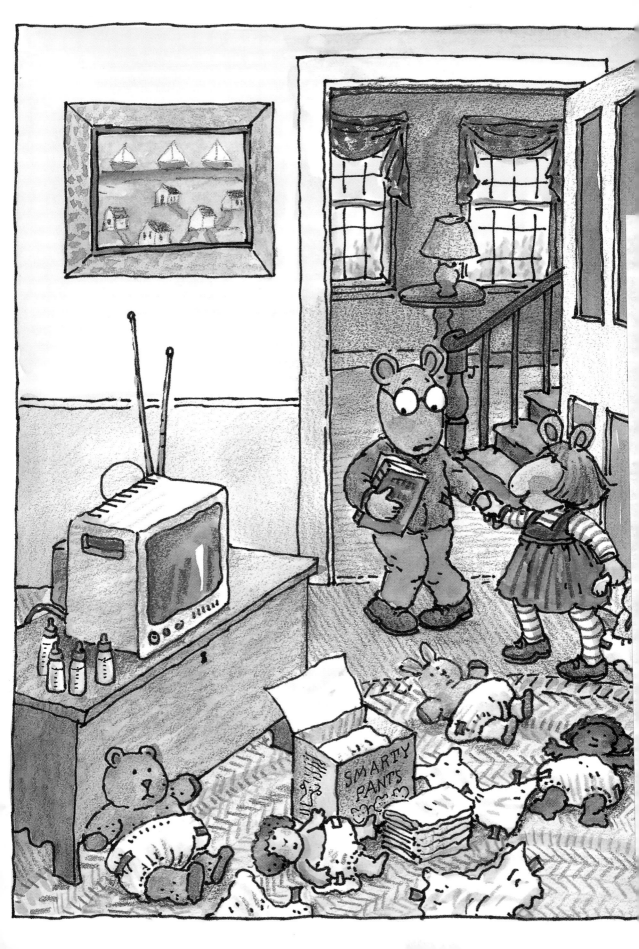

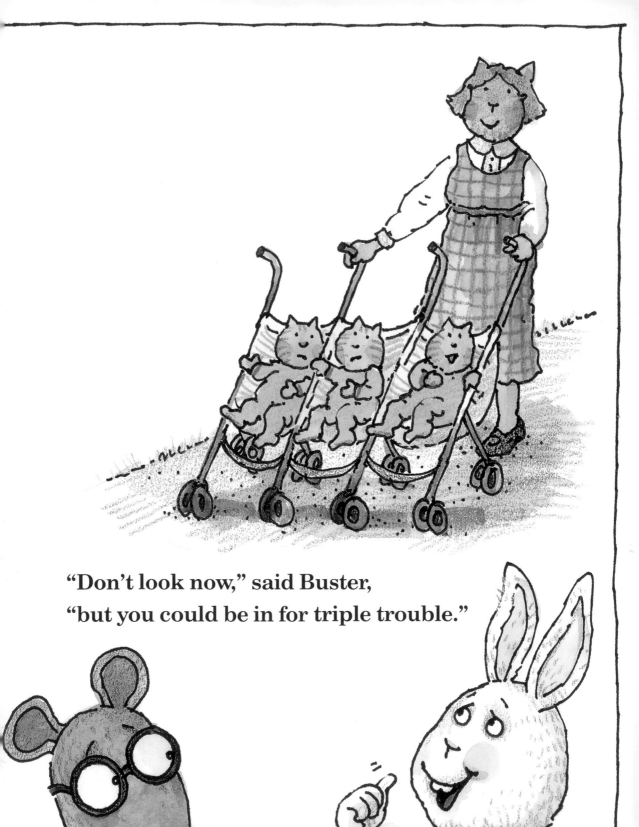

"Don't look now," said Buster,
"but you could be in for triple trouble."

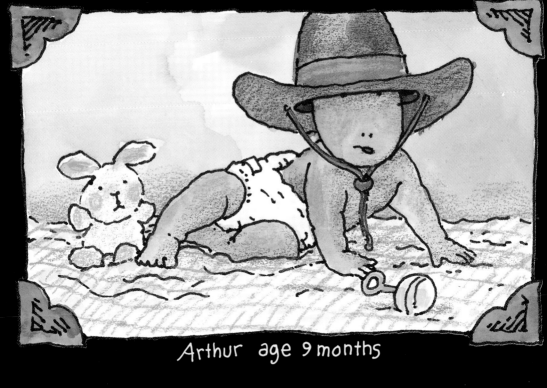

Arthur age 9 months

"Is that really me?" asked Arthur.
"Yes," said Mother. "You were such a cute baby."

Arthur age 1 year

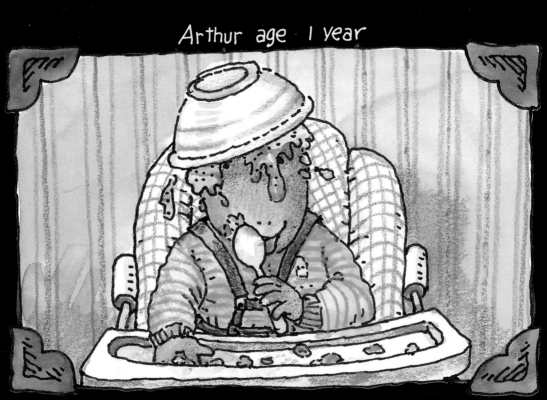

One day after school, D.W. grabbed
Arthur's arm.
"I will teach you how to diaper a baby," she said.
"Don't worry about diapers," said Mother.
"Come sit next to me. I want to show you
something."

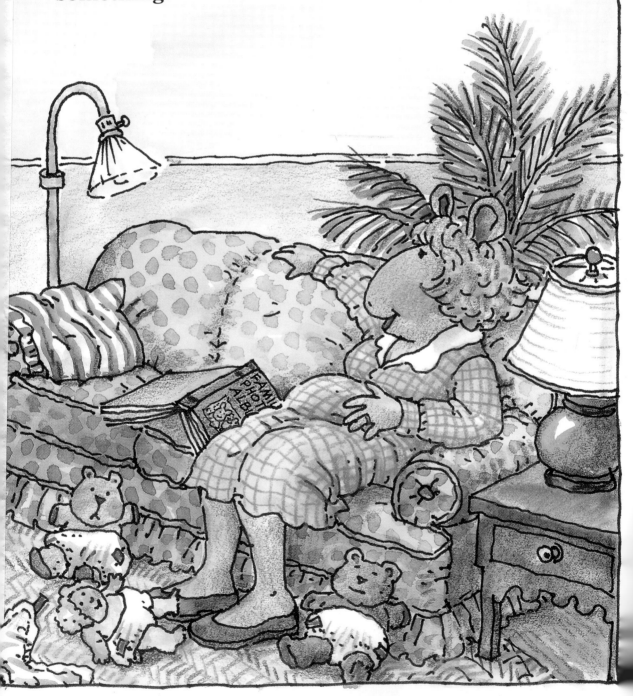

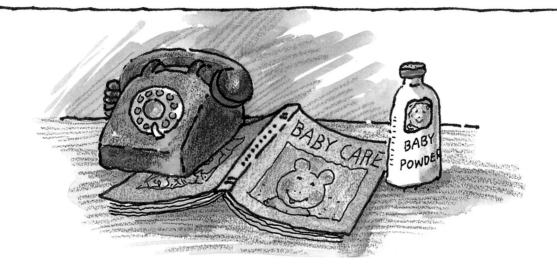

For the next few months, everywhere
Arthur looked there were babies — more
and more babies.

"I think babies are taking over the world!"
said Arthur.

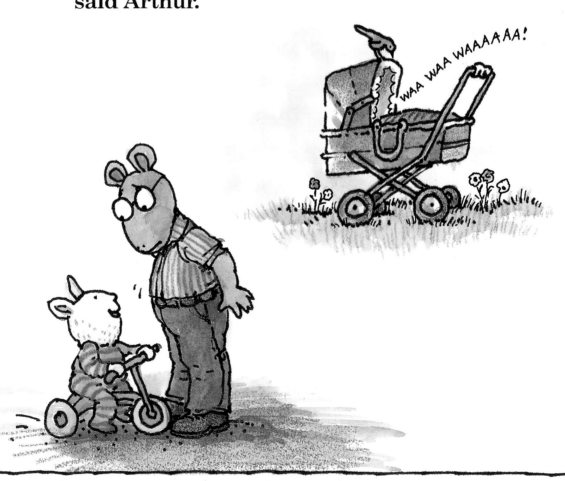

WAA WAA WAAAAAA!

"You'll have to change all those dirty diapers!"
said Muffy.

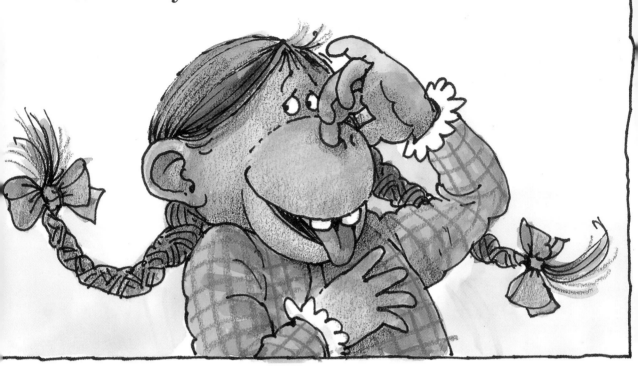

"And you'll probably start talking baby talk,"
said Francine. "Doo doo ga ga boo boo."

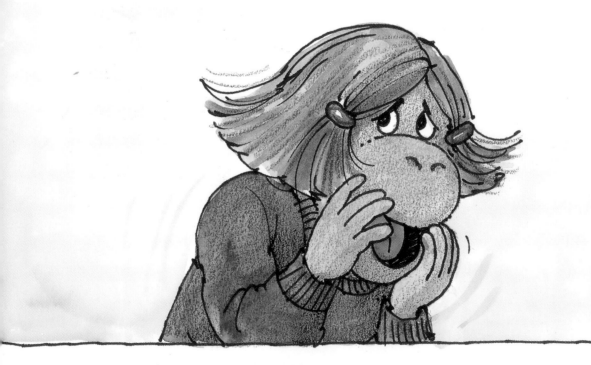

Arthur's friends had lots of advice.
"Better get some earplugs," said Binky Barnes,
"or you'll never sleep."

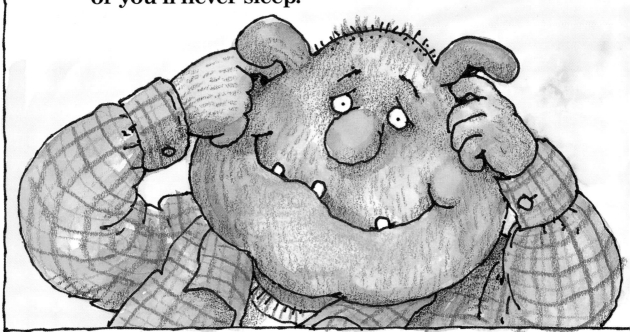

"Forget about playing after school," said Buster.
"You'll have to babysit."

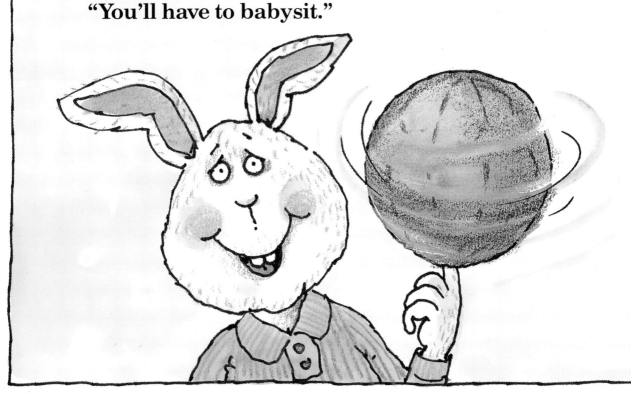

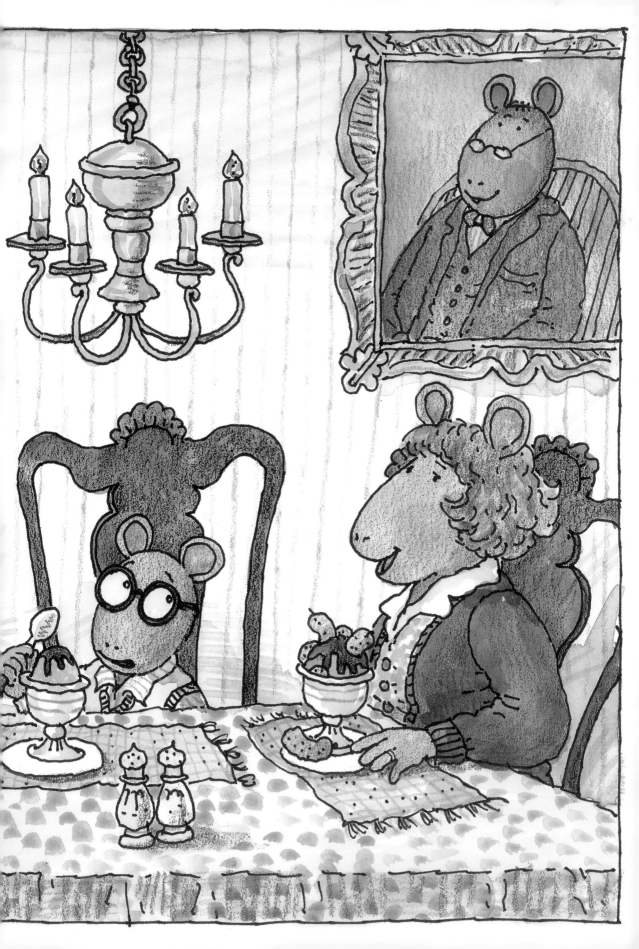

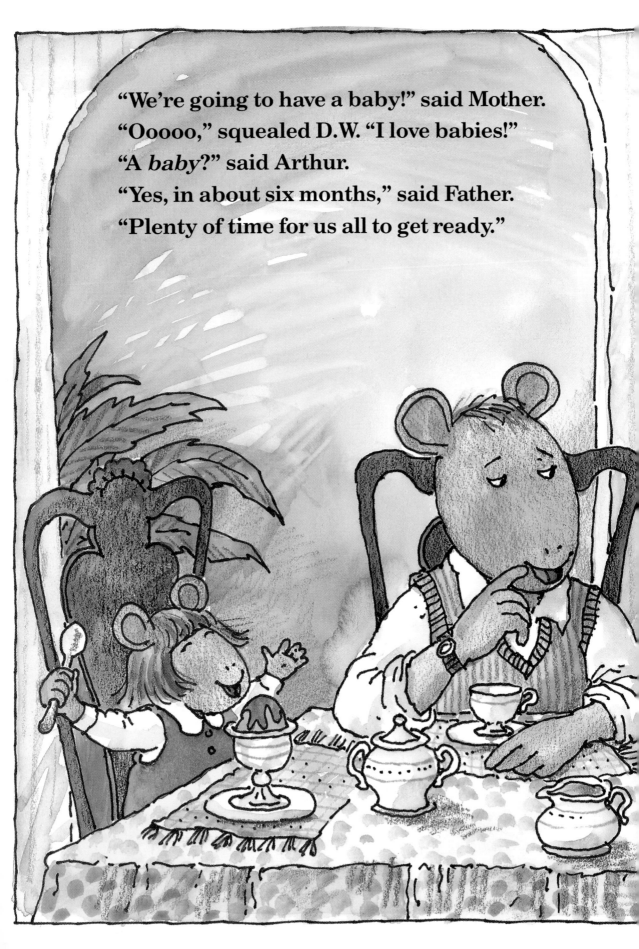

"We're going to have a baby!" said Mother.

"Ooooo," squealed D.W. "I love babies!"

"A *baby*?" said Arthur.

"Yes, in about six months," said Father.

"Plenty of time for us all to get ready."

"We have a surprise for you," said Mother
and Father.
"Is it a bicycle?" asked Arthur.

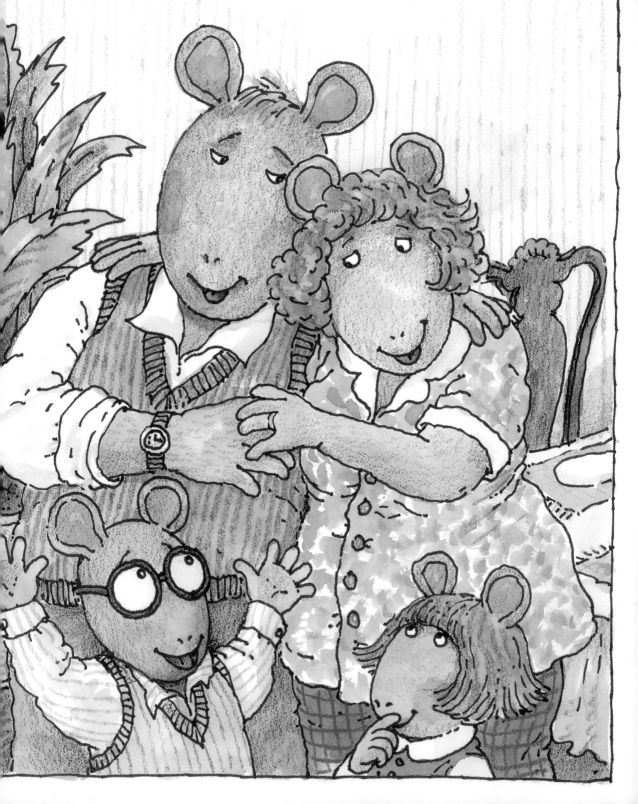

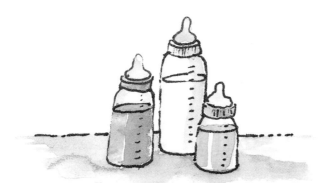

◇FOR TOLON, TUCKER AND ELIZA◇
my three babies

Little, Brown and Company

Time Warner Book Group
1271 Avenue of the Americas, New York, NY 10020
Visit our Web site at www.lb-kids.com

Library of Congress Cataloging-in-Publication Data

Brown, Marc Tolon.
  Arthur's baby.

  Summary: Arthur isn't sure he is happy about the
new baby in the family but when his sister asks for his
help in handling the baby, Arthur feels much better.
  [1. Babies—Fiction. 2. Brothers and sisters—
Fiction] I. Title.
PZ7.B81618Aok 1987   [E]   87-3988
HC:ISBN 0-316-11123-6
PB: ISBN 0-316-11007-8

        HC: 20 19 18 17 16 15 14
          PB: 20 19 18
              SC

Manufactured in China

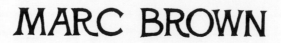

MARC BROWN

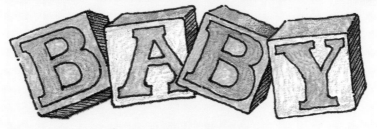

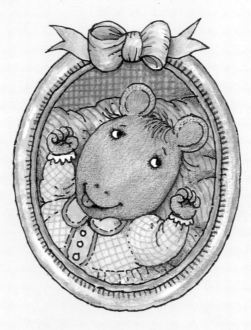

LITTLE, BROWN AND COMPANY

New York ❧ Boston

P9-CJC-396